"This program is going to change the face of the emergency services in our country."

"O2X has motivated me to become the best I can be."

"O2X has developed a program that addresses the total wellness of our members. They have truly earned our trust and acceptance. The [department] will go into the future with the concepts of O2X as a guiding force in maintaining good physical and emotional health for our members and their families."

"After O2X I have a better understanding of how vital it is to take care of my overall health as a firefighter. We put more stress on our bodies than the average human being. If we neglect to take care of ourselves, we could face significant health problems down the road. I would certainly recommend the program to a coworker. There are many simple changes we can make to live a healthier lifestyle."

"Thrive has had a lasting impact on me personally. While all of us are aware of nutrition and exercise the elements of the Thrive component are probably what is most lacking and misunderstood in our community. As first responders we are exposed to trauma, injury, and loss of life. The thrive philosophy is the guide to bouncing back from the physical and mental toll we pay to do this job. This is a complete package that will give you the knowledge of how your mind and body are connected."

"I gave O2X a shot, put in the sweat effort, stayed disciplined and dedicated with their nutrition programs, and eventually the results made me a believer for life. I'm in the best shape of my life because I bought into their exercise, nutrition, and mindset philosophies."

"The tactical athlete philosophy has worked as a bridge from military service to fire service and has transformed our culture."

"This program is an asset for first responders' health and wellness. An investment in wellness provides for a healthy career, minimizing injuries and mitigating stress."

"You guys are going to save the lives of firefighters. You won't ever know their names or when you saved them. And they will never know that you saved them. This is life saving/changing training for many of our guys."

"We feel that O2X is not only giving us an edge on our competition but is also making us better leaders and citizens. We look forward to continuing to work and grow with them."

"The O2X program taught me so much more about myself and lifestyle changes that I need to make to create a well balanced way of life that not only makes me a more effective firefighter and paramedic but a better, healthier and happier person and family man."

Human Performance for Tactical Athletes

Human Performance for Tactical Athletes

O2X Human Performance

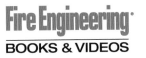

BOOKS & VIDEOS

Disclaimer

The recommendations, advice, descriptions, and methods in this book are presented solely for educational purposes. The author and publisher assume no liability whatsoever for any loss or damage that results from the use of any of the material in this book. Use of the material in this book is solely at the risk of the user.

800.752.9764
+1.918.831.9421
info@fireengineeringbooks.com
www.FireEngineeringBooks.com

Senior Vice President: Eric Schlett
Operations Manager: Holly Fournier
Sales Manager: Joshua Neal
Managing Editor: Mark Haugh
Production Manager: Tony Quinn
Developmental Editor: Chris Barton

Cover Designer: Dylan Kaufman
Book Designer: Robert Kern

Library of Congress Cataloging-in-Publication Data

Names: O2X Human Performance, author.
Title: Human performance for tactical athletes / O2X Human Performance.
Description: Tulsa, Oklahoma : Fire Engineering Books & Videos, [2019] | Includes bibliographical references and index.
Identifiers: LCCN 2018059941 | ISBN 9781593704766
Subjects: LCSH: Physical education and training. | United States. Navy. SEALs--Physical training. | Nutrition.
Classification: LCC GV481 .O23 2019 | DDC 613.7--dc23

Printed in the United States of America

4 5 6   23 22 21 20 19

DEDICATION

This book is written for tactical athletes: the firefighters, law enforcement officers, EMS, and military personnel who dedicate their lives to making our cities, our towns, and our nation better, safer places to live.

What is Human Performance for Tactical Athletes?

As a tactical athlete, you face heightened levels of mental and physical stress daily in order to do your job and keep your community safe. You have also chosen a career that is inherently dangerous and where mistakes can have serious consequences. Our goal is to provide comprehensive, science-backed training and education in all pillars of human performance—nutrition, conditioning, stress management, sleep, and resilience—so you can finish your career as strong as you started. By focusing equal attention on each pillar of our EAT SWEAT THRIVE curriculum, you will be able to make small, incremental changes that lead to major lifestyle improvements and optimal performance.

CONTENTS

FOREWORD

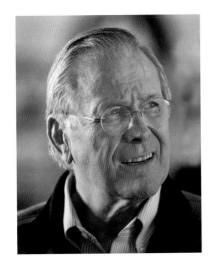

"Send me." That is the request of a remarkable group of volunteers who have raised their hands and sworn an oath. Soldiers, sailors, airmen and marines, firefighters, law enforcement officers and emergency medical service providers—each stands ready to answer the call. Not conscripted, but driven by a desire to help others.

What is asked of these folks is dedication, long hours, time away from family, deployments and physically demanding assignments. They each respond willingly, without hesitation, and perform their duties as professionals, often at great personal risk.

You go to war with the army you have, not the army you might wish to have. The O2X Human Performance team and the contributors to this guide understand this, many having served in the U.S. military and worked with some of our country's most elite units. No matter the battlefield, the time for preparation has passed when the action begins.

This comprehensive manual offers guidance for enduring success. The O2X team is making an important and valuable contribution in creating this guidebook for those who serve and protect us.

—Donald H. Rumsfeld
13th and 21st U.S. Secretary of Defense

AUTHORS' NOTE

O2X Human Performance was born from more than 50 years of combined experience in special operations. In the SEAL teams, we benefited from a tremendous wealth of human performance (HP) resources to support our units and maximizing performance was an essential part of our lives. Upon separating from service, our passion for elite performance, service, and helping others drove us to build O2X. Through the company's development, it became clear that the issues plaguing the Special Operations community were also prevalent in other tactical communities like the fire service, law enforcement, and conventional military as well as various elite organizations and we were uniquely positioned to do something about it. We looked hard at the programs we had in the military, both the successful elements and the gaps, and used that as the roadmap for O2X Human Performance. Before getting too far into *what* we do, here is the brief story on *why* we are writing this book.

The company's first outward manifestation of helping people maximize their performance was a series of base-to-peak mountain running races. These races—Summit Challenges—took place in rugged mountain towns across North America and attracted people who wanted to tackle an unknown challenge, beyond their comfort zone.

The Summit Challenges were unlike anything else. The physical aspect of running up a mountain was only one element of the two-day event. The heart of the Summit Challenges was Basecamp, a gathering place for athletes that included healthy food, a bonfire, mountainside camping, and a fireside chat the night before the race start. The fireside speakers acknowledged the mental side of performance and were select people who had chased maximum performance in their personal pursuits including athletes, veterans, and scientists who shared experiences of overcoming obstacles; you will hear a few of their stories later in this book. These lessons on the pillars of human performance were effective and powerful. Elite specialists discussing their areas of expertise to an audience that stood to benefit directly from it—we were on to something. From here the O2X program began to take shape and our holistic curriculum was born.

We knew that tactical athletes also wanted and needed comprehensive human performance training. Based on our military DNA, our desire to help others, and our collective passion for pushing boundaries both physically *and* mentally, the connection between O2X and tactical athletes was (and remains) a natural fit.

During our ongoing evolution, we made other important progressions. We decided to focus exclusively on HP education, geared specifically for tactical athletes and elite organizations. The need was obvious, the demand was high, the connection felt right, and the reception was overwhelmingly positive. We were working to increase sustainability, durability, and performance in groups that needed it most. During this time, we bucketed the five pillars—conditioning, nutrition, sleep, stress management, and resilience—into an EAT SWEAT THRIVE framework. This book is the guide to that unique, cutting-edge curriculum, designed as a resource to improve the health and lives of our nation's heroes.

Firefighters, law enforcement officers, EMTs, and other tactical athletes are experiencing a national health crisis: elevated cancer rates and mental health issues, high incidence of cardiac events, and painful orthopedic injuries specific to their professions. On top of all that, first responders must be mentally and physically prepared daily, *for decades*, to deal with the most challenging jobs in the country. These tactical athletes are required to perform physically, face consistent life-or-death decisions, deal with extreme trauma, and do it all in dangerous environments. When tactical athletes leave work, they must relate with family and friends who may not have a full appreciation for the daily demands of the job. Finally, in addition to planning for retirement, tactical athletes must also focus on getting there in one piece and being able to thrive in it. Their duties, their career trajectories, and their lives are uniquely dangerous. They need and deserve a resource to address these adverse conditions.

This book was the next natural step for O2X. The objective: to write a practical, comprehensive, world class book on human performance—tailored for tactical athletes—that reflects our passion, complements our training, and serves as an ongoing reference. It's our goal that it teaches the fundamentals and key principles of a complete Human Performance program, in a practical way so you can finish your career as strong as you started.

—*O2X founders: Paul McCullough,*
Adam La Reau, Gabriel Gomez,
Craig Coffey

ACKNOWLEDGMENTS

Tactical athletes work in teams. Whether serving in the military, fire service, or law enforcement all members rely on the support of one another to be successful. Different strengths, weaknesses, and specialties blend into a cohesive group capable of nearly anything. This book is the result of a similar effort, built with the collaboration and hard work of the entire O2X Human Performance team.

At our core, O2X is a training and education company with the goal of providing tactical athletes the tools they need to finish their careers as strong as they started. To do this we rely on an elite group of the nation's top specialists in the fields of conditioning, nutrition, sleep science, stress management, and mental resilience. These folks have dedicated hours and days of their precious free time to the development and delivery of O2X programs nationwide and this book is an extension of that mission.

Dr. Maria Urso, O2X nutrition specialist, former Army Major, scientist, and elite marathon runner, served as our go-to expert on this project; acting as a one stop reviewer, fact checker, and author of more than a few significant sections. Dr. Christine Sanchez and Dr. Tracy Heller expertly crafted and edited the Mental Performance sections. Mike Sanders, Dr. Antigone Vesci, Adrian Wright-Fitzgerald, Dr. Shumi Rawlins, Dr. Rachel Markwald, Dylan Polin, and Annie Okerlin each put pen to paper and shared their combined centuries of experience to fill this text with EAT, SWEAT, and THRIVE content. Maria Trozzi reviewed sections within her area of expertise with great precision, as did Valerie Cogswell and Dr. Cheryl Zonkowski. Arno Ilgner, Geoff Krill, Matt Cady, Andy Haffle, and Paralympic Gold medalist Dan Cnossen each brightened the text with their personal anecdotes.

We have also benefited from a tremendous resource of expert advisors who have helped shape not only this text, but the O2X curriculum and indeed company as a whole. Dr. Michael Hamrock, Dr. Dustin Allen, Dr. Laura Moretti, Dr. Mike Donato, Dave McQuade, Dr. Paul Sargent, Shaun Huls, Rob Skinner, Zach Weatherford, and Mike Hooper. Thank you each for your dedication and guidance.

Team O2X is an impressive one. A group of motivated and passionate people from diverse and interesting backgrounds, each playing a vital role in bringing these pages to life. Dylan Kaufman and Ali Levy spearheaded this project, bringing it from concept to reality. Along with our team members past and present: Brice Long guided this book across the goal line; Eamonn Burke, Josh Stuart-Shor, John Hall, Spencer Schnell, Lewyn Poage, and Scott Rosenthal.

Chief Bobby Halton introduced us to the rockstar group from PennWell, including Mark Haugh and Andy Kantola, who shepherded us through the final stages along with their team of editors, fact checkers, and designers.

Family and friends, you each deserve recognition for your patience and dedication to O2X. Without you we wouldn't be here to publish this book.

Finally, to all tactical athletes, for whom this book is written, thank you for your service and sacrifice. The thousands we trained over the years have shaped us to who we are today. We learned from you and molded our program to meet the demands and dynamic environments you face. It's our hope that this serves as a resource, but also a testament to your hard work, dedication, and the tremendous effort required to be successful in your chosen career.

—O2X founders

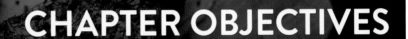

CHAPTER OBJECTIVES

This chapter provides a comprehensive, practical overview of diet and nutrition, with the perspective of maximizing physical and mental performance for tactical athletes. You will learn a number of key takeaways, including:

- Why stabilizing your blood sugar levels is paramount
- Why maintaining proper hydration will keep you healthier
- How the quality, quantity, and timing of your food intake affects your performance
- How to calibrate your food intake
- How to make healthier choices
- How to approach a grocery store

WELCOME TO EAT

Welcome to EAT, the chapter designed to provide information on how small, incremental changes in *what* you eat and *how* you eat can help to improve your health, performance, and overall well-being. We are excited to share input from several nutrition educators who work directly with O2X helping to merge the science of nutrition with the practice of performance.

My approach as an O2X specialist is to help our athletes incorporate quality eating that is sustainable and substantiated, both factors that are important to me for personal reasons. As a former member of the military, a self-proclaimed athlete, frequent traveler, and a scientist, I understand how critical it is to choose foods wisely to optimize everything from performance to mental health, to sleep. I have used my own trials and tribulations with nutrition, as well as my background as a scientist, to develop an approach to healthy eating that is shared in this chapter.

Before you dive in, I need to give you a bit more background on my passion for nutrition education. First is the concept of sustainable eating. While there are thousands of "diets" that have been introduced and tried by millions over the years, science has shown us that a comparison of those diets reveals one thing: real food always comes out on top. It has also revealed that it is difficult to maintain restrictive eating for long periods of time, why many people who lose weight end up regaining it. There is nothing more critical than adopting a nutrition plan that you can follow for life. A sustainable nutrition plan is one that works at home, on the road, at parties, and when having dinner with friends.

The second concept is that of substantiated information. When it comes to claims about nutrition, health, and the body, I have always done my due diligence in reading the literature to understand the difference between hype and fact. There is a dizzying array of claims around purported superfoods and special diets, but very few of the claims are substantiated with actual data. I cannot stress the importance of asking "why" or "how" when you are faced with nutritional information that seems suspect. Remember, your goal is to incorporate natural foods that taste good, provide as many macronutrients as possible, and stabilize your blood sugar. Commit those rules (and staying hydrated!) to memory and you are destined to realize performance gains from faster recovery post-workout to improved focus.

Finally, somehow over the past few decades we have become a culture that focuses on what is *not* in foods, versus what *is* in foods. Food is necessary for life, so why have we become so exclusionary? It is my hope that this chapter helps you to incorporate nutrient-dense foods based on what they do have, rather than the things they don't have (e.g., fat, sugar, gluten, dairy). Best of luck on your continued journey with O2X.

Bon appetEAT!

—*Maria L. Urso, PhD; O2X HP Expert; Major, US Army (Ret.); All-Army Marathon Team; Fellow, American College of Sports Medicine*

INTRODUCTION

Nutrition is the fuel that powers human performance. Proper nutrition will help you optimize your daily mental and physical potential by keeping you alert, and prepared. In contrast, poor nutrition will slash your physical readiness and mental acuity, and undermine your conditioning efforts and overall well-being. As a tactical athlete, proper habits will keep you safer, stronger, and more resilient so you can finish your career as strong as you started. That is the overarching goal of the O2X curriculum and this book.

The foundational elements of a successful nutrition plan are: (1) stabilizing your blood sugar levels; (2) maintaining proper hydration; and (3) controlling the quality, quantity, and timing of your food intake. In this chapter, we will explain these foundational elements, teach a little metabolic and nutritional science so you understand why the fundamentals matter, and give you practical suggestions on how to manage your nutrition so you can maximize your performance. After we cover these topics, we will teach you practical information on fueling for exercise, supplements, caffeine, vitamins, and how to navigate the grocery store well. But first, let's step back and look at a key concept in the O2X science-backed approach: diet.

Diet
A diet, as a general term, describes the kinds of foods that a person most commonly eats.

When we hear the word **diet**, we have been conditioned to think of specific gimmicks or plans, usually aimed at weight loss. O2X's nutrition curriculum does not advocate for extreme calorie restriction or following a strict inflexible plan. Instead, we want you to understand the basics, learn some practical science, and adopt healthy long-term habits. Remember, give a man a fish and he eats for a day, teach a man to fish and . . . he eats for a lifetime. Well, that's what we want to do here: teach you how to fish.

We begin this book with nutrition because it is critically important to not only your human performance as a tactical athlete, but also your overall health and well-being. Proper nutrition habits decrease your risk of disease, provide greater energy for daily activities, help you get the most benefit from workouts, reduce your risk of on-the-job injury, improve your mood, and help you sleep better. Whether you are a first responder awoken from a sound sleep to respond to a life-threatening call, an Olympic athlete at the starting line, or climbing over a wall into an enemy compound at night, everyone needs to be properly fueled to optimize, and maximize, their performance.

BLOOD SUGAR STABILIZATION

Glucose
A simple sugar and an important energy source. Glucose circulates through the blood and is a key source of fuel for the human body.

Putting it simply, our muscles run on sugar (aka glucose, carbs), and our blood carries that sugar to our muscles for fuel. For a number of important reasons, we will explain how stabilizing the levels of **glucose** in our blood through proper nutritional habits will optimize your overall performance and be fundamental to a successful nutrition plan. In contrast, we will explain why widely swinging blood sugar levels cause unneeded fat storage, counterproductive muscle depletion, and unhealthy food cravings. Unstable blood sugar levels sap your energy, reduce your cognitive ability, and impact your ability to sleep and recover.[1] Before we dig into *how* to regulate your blood sugar levels, let's explore the science of *why* it is so important.

Optimal Blood Sugar Stabilization

Our blood sugar level—technically, milligrams of glucose per deciliter of blood, or mg/dl— fluctuates according to what we eat and how much energy we burn. As illustrated in the graph (fig. 1–1), somewhere between 80 and 120 mg/dl is the healthy range in which your body optimally metabolizes simple sugars and fat for energy.

In this healthy mid-range, because you have enough glucose to fuel your activity, your body does not need to metabolize lean muscle mass for energy, thereby preserving it.[2] And, because your body is not overfueled, you will not store excess sugars as fat. In short, you will feel stable, healthy, energized, and efficient.

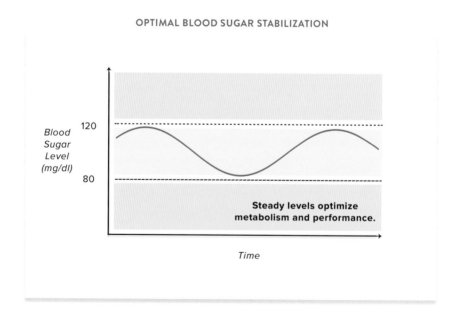

Figure 1–1. Optimal blood sugar stabilization

Low Blood Sugar Levels

The range of glucose below 80 mg/dl can have negative effects for a few notable reasons. First, because our body lacks an efficient, ready energy source, we begin to feel weak and groggy. This can be dangerous because it can slow reaction time, dull mental acuity, and may make us faint and irritable. It is also counterproductive **metabolically** because in the absence of glucose, our bodies begin to burn the next readily available energy source—lean muscle. Not only does this eat into our strength, it also robs us of the most efficient calorie burning mass in our body. Finally, it causes us to crave sugar and binge on unhealthy snacks. Along with adding unnecessary calories to our intake, it causes our blood sugar levels to spike past the healthy range and into +120 mg/dl territory. This craving and binging cycle is an adaptive response that can be traced back to evolution and survival: "I'm starving! Find food! Eat . . . Survive!"

Metabolism
The build-up and breakdown of substances. Metabolism describes the body's process of converting food into fuel.

High Blood Sugar Levels

Beyond energy spikes, high blood sugar levels can be unhealthy and impact our overall performance. First, we can be impaired with a "sugar high" that causes jitters and racing thoughts. Metabolically, long term, the consequences can be even worse. When your body detects that your blood sugar levels are too high, it releases **insulin** from your **pancreas**, which grabs the extra sugar and stores it for future use, when nourishment is hard to find. Again, this is a natural adaptive response that for thousands of years improved our survival. The bad news is that the excess glucose is stored in the form of fat, specifically triglycerides, in your body.[3]

Insulin
A fuel-regulating hormone secreted from the pancreas, typically in response to a stimulus like glucose after a meal.

Pancreas
An organ that makes insulin and enzymes for digestion.

Blood Sugar Roller Coaster

Looking at figure 1–2, imagine the roller coaster your blood sugar levels may follow: if your glucose/blood sugar levels are low, it will lead to food cravings and consuming too many calories or carbohydrates, or both. Basically, your caveman instinct kicks in, and you crave easily digestible sugar and carbs, and you binge. This causes your glucose levels to spike well above the healthy levels, and your body reacts by releasing insulin to remove the glucose from your blood. As expected, the insulin causes a drastic absorption of glucose into cells of the brain, muscles, and liver, eventually leading to triglyceride (fat) storage in the body. The fast absorption leads blood sugar levels to drop again even though a large "carb/sugar" heavy meal was recently consumed.[4] This simple real-world roller coaster example not only replaces healthy lean muscle with fat, but it also leaves you right back at the starting point—with a low blood sugar level—to start the cycle all over again. This is why, scientifically and metabolically, stabilizing your blood sugar levels is so critical to your overall performance and success.

What common poor habits can lead us to this unproductive, downward spiral? First, restrictive diets—eliminating carbs, fats, or a combination of the two—can lead your blood sugar to drop quickly and cause cravings. Skipping a meal sounds productive on the surface, but can also cause a significant drop in glucose levels, resulting in a binge cycle.

Staying up late can lead to binging, not just because your inhibitions are lowered, but also because you are used to fasting overnight yet your body is still using fuel, so your blood sugar levels will naturally drop. Therefore, if you are awake at midnight instead of asleep, you will get cravings and adopt unhealthy habits. Finally, another major cause of this roller coaster is exercising on an empty stomach or training without proper fuel in your tank. Not only will your body lack the energy to perform the exercises, but you will be burning muscle for fuel and finish with a major craving for sugar. The downward spiral starts again. While optimizing your blood sugar levels through nutrition may take some trial and error, it will ultimately provide you with the most noticeable benefits in the short term, and may help to prevent disease later in life.

We have covered unhealthy habits that can impact blood sugar levels, but there are sustainable habits that will help consistently maintain stable blood sugar levels. These healthy habits require a fundamental understanding of nutrition science, which O2X breaks into the categories quality, quantity, and timing (i.e., what am I eating, how much am I eating, and how frequently am I eating). We will start by looking at nutrition science and hydration, and then jump into the practical elements of O2X's methodology.

KEY TAKEAWAYS

Blood Sugar Stabilization

- Stabilizing blood sugar levels is fundamental to maximizing performance
- Too much glucose causes spikes, fat storage
- Too little glucose saps energy, consumes lean muscle
- The sugar/glucose binge and crash cycle is unhealthy
- Stability results from balanced, nutrient dense meals and snacks at regular intervals

BASIC SCIENCE OF NUTRITION

Body Composition

To understand how nutrition fuels the engine we call the human body, let's look first at what that unique engine is made up of as it relates to performance and burning fuel. Weight wise, each one of us made up of roughly 50% water, 25% fat, and the remaining 25% a combination of protein, minerals, carbs, and other essential substances. Figure 1–3 highlights the minor average differences between the sexes, and provides a helpful way to visualize our bodies' composition.

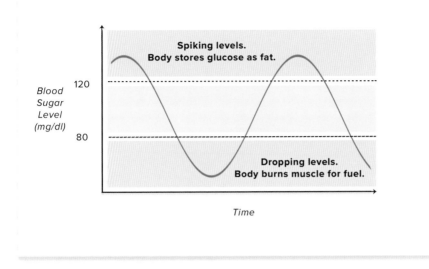

Figure 1–2. Poor blood sugar stabilization

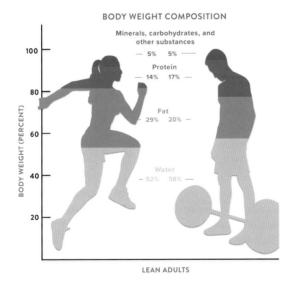

Figure 1–3. Body weight composition

Two takeaways from figure 1–3: first, it is easy to see why hydration is an essential component of proper nutrition and performance. Second, because protein (i.e., muscle) is the only chart element in your body that *consumes* fuel, we can see how important it is to calibrate the quality, quantity, and timing of our food/fuel intake.

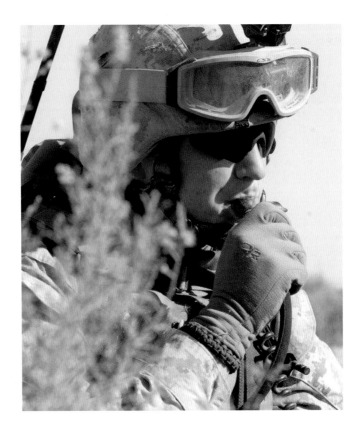

Hydration

Because roughly 50% of our body weight is water, **hydration** is critical to maintaining, and maximizing, our performance as tactical athletes. Water lubricates our joints, acts as a shock absorber when we move, transports essential nutrients through our bodies, and helps us maintain our proper body temperatures.[5]

A minor drop in hydration—even 2%—can decrease our cognitive and physical performance.[6] Specifically, mild dehydration decreases our ability to concentrate, reduces our reaction times, and impacts our visual motor tracking. And *extreme* dehydration can cause dangerously low blood pressure, headaches, nausea, fever, and a rapid heartbeat. Figure 1–4 compares how various levels of dehydration and intoxication affect reaction times.[7]

A simple rule of thumb for maintaining proper hydration: we should aim to consume roughly 2.5 liters of water daily, with adjustments up and down, depending on your body weight, activity level, temperature, and environment. Figure 1–5 is a helpful chart converting 2.5 liters to other measurements.

DEHYDRATION CAUSES EFFECTS SIMILAR
TO INTOXICATION BY ALCOHOL
Reaction Time
1 2 3 4 5
Dehydration
(% Body Weight)
SOLUTION: Drink 16 oz. of water as soon as you wake up

Figure 1–4. Effects of dehydration on reaction time

RECOMMENDED DAILY WATER INTAKE

LITERS	8oz CUPS	32 OZ WATER BOTTLE	GALLONS
2.5	*10*	*3*	*0.66*

Figure 1–5. Recommended daily water intake

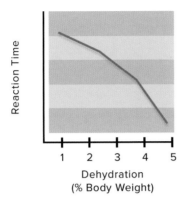

Other practical considerations: consistently hydrating each day makes us more resistant to dehydration and performance deficits on the days that we exercise intensely, or in the heat. Not only does consistency buffer your body against tough conditions, it also reduces the likelihood of bloating and hyponatremia (too much water), the latter condition happening when we drink too much water all at once to catch up.

Spreading your suggested intake evenly throughout the day is beneficial, and a practical way to accomplish this is having a glass of water with every snack and meal. Carrying a water bottle to work and in the car is another helpful habit. If this is a big change for you, start slowly. Gradually increase your water intake each week until you reach 2.5 liters per day so you are not adding too much water too quickly at one time.

On exercise days, particularly in the heat, it helps to drink 10–20 ounces of water 1–2 hours *before* exercising, another 10–20 ounces immediately *after* exercising, and 8 ounces per hour for another 2–3 hours thereafter. Of course, these are rough guidelines and amounts will vary depending on how much you sweat and your body weight.

As a general rule, the best way to assess hydration is through the "pee test." Your urine when you first wake up each morning should be the color of pale lemonade or closer to clear (see fig. 1–6 for a reference). If it is darker than that (amber or dark yellow), you are dehydrated. If it is clear, you have consumed too much water (or not enough nutrients). Warning: if you have been exercising intensely, you have all-over body aches, and your urine begins to look like cola (dark, almost brown), seek medical attention immediately.

Pay attention to the way your diet affects hydration as well—if your diet is low in salt and other electrolytes (or if you do not have enough sugar in your bloodstream because you skipped a meal), your body will release water that it needs. You may also try drinks that are supplemented with electrolytes, or taking electrolyte tablets.

Whether you are operating in extreme conditions and variable temperatures, or on the job for extended periods of time, hydration is critical. As a tactical athlete, focusing on consistent hydration daily will help ensure that you have the physical energy and cognitive focus to respond to a call at any moment.

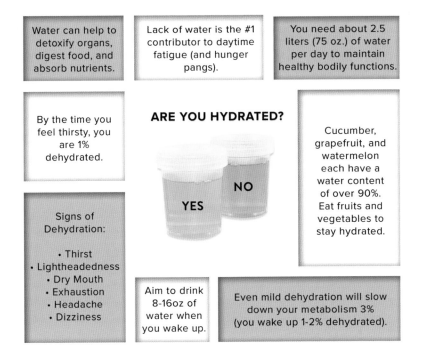

WATER AND DEHYDRATION

Water can help to detoxify organs, digest food, and absorb nutrients.

Lack of water is the #1 contributor to daytime fatigue (and hunger pangs).

You need about 2.5 liters (75 oz.) of water per day to maintain healthy bodily functions.

By the time you feel thirsty, you are 1% dehydrated.

ARE YOU HYDRATED?

NO

YES

Cucumber, grapefruit, and watermelon each have a water content of over 90%. Eat fruits and vegetables to stay hydrated.

Signs of Dehydration:

- Thirst
- Lightheadedness
- Dry Mouth
- Exhaustion
- Headache
- Dizziness

Aim to drink 8-16oz of water when you wake up.

Even mild dehydration will slow down your metabolism 3% (you wake up 1-2% dehydrated).

Figure 1–6. Water and dehydration[8]

KEY TAKEAWAYS

Hydration

⬦ Proper hydration is an essential component of maximizing performance

⬦ 2.5 liters (or ten 8 oz cups) daily is a good rule of thumb

⬦ Rehydrate first thing in the morning—we lose at least 1 liter overnight

⬦ 50% of our body weight is water, which lubricates joints, absorbs impacts

⬦ Water transports nutrients throughout our bodies

⬦ A 2% drop in hydration significantly impacts cognitive and physical performance

REFINE YOUR ROUTINE—MARIA URSO

I challenge anyone to spend 15 minutes online scrolling through social media without encountering some sort of health or fitness-related "sell." It is nearly impossible to keep up with the number of supplements, exercise regiments, wellness trends, and 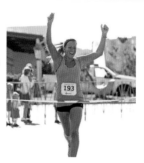 food pyramids that cross our paths throughout our daily routine. As a scientist with a background in physiology and nutrition, I made it my business to stay abreast of what new trends were based on science and what new trends were based on snake oil. However, in the midst of all of this, I lost track of the fundamental pillars of health and human performance.

Before any new supplement, food pyramid, or exercise regimen is introduced, it is critical that a foundation of proper nutrition, sleep, and hydration is intact. I ran into trouble about 4 years back when a change in my daily routine nearly derailed my fitness and performance. I was always a distance runner and consistently ran 8–10 miles per day during the week, followed by a long run on the weekends of 13–20 miles, depending on the event that I was training for. I had a well-rounded diet that was high in protein, I slept 6–7.5 hours per night, and I drank 7–9 cups (57–72 ounces) of water each day. I recovered from my workouts well and I rarely had a performance decrement that was related to poor nutrition or hydration. Additionally, I never took water on my long runs and trusted that I was hydrated enough to get me through the 1.5–2.5 hour workout.

About 4 years ago, I was conducting a research study that had me up early and performing surgeries in a very warm room (88°F) for 6–8 hours per day. About that time, I started to have extreme stomach pains and it seemed as if any food that I ate was irritating my stomach. At the same time, while I was able to complete my long runs on the weekends (I was training for my 8th Boston Marathon), I would have to spend the 3 hours following my long run in the fetal position on my bed. I could not eat or drink anything, and it felt as if I was too depleted to raise my head off the pillow. My stomach would get terribly upset, I would have excruciating headaches, and while I tended to recover a few hours later, I had a difficult time sleeping at night and would experience intense, sudden calf cramps that would stop me in my tracks.

After a battery of tests on my stomach, the doctor concluded that I was simply hypohydrated (more commonly known as dehydrated). This seemed nearly impossible, as my symptoms were so severe; the proposed solution of drinking more water seemed too easy. However, on closer thought, I realized that the change in my routine changed not only how much water I was drinking, but the frequency of my meals and the amount that I was sweating on a regular basis, all of which would likely contribute to a hypohydrated state. My first change was to never leave the house without my own water bottle that had 50 ounces of water in it. My second change was to add small snack breaks during the extended surgeries, as I knew that my body would not retain water if my blood sugars and my electrolytes (e.g., sodium) were too low—especially since I was going 6–8 hours between meals. My final change was to start "water loading" before big runs, in a similar manner to the way people used to "carbo-load" several decades ago. In the days leading up to a long run or event, I would consciously increase my water intake so that I was urinating every 2–3 hours. I began to monitor the color of my urine to avoid hyponatremia (hyperhydration), and found that within the span of a month, my running performance was back on track. I was also able to eat most foods without any intestinal irritation, and I no longer had trouble with calf cramps and headaches after a long run.

Fast-forward a few years and instead of prolonged surgeries, I am spending a lot of time in airports and on long haul flights. After one of my first long flights on a particularly busy trip, I noticed that my body started to "revolt" with performance decrements that lingered for 24 to 48 hours after my long flight. I recalibrated my pillars while en route to my destination, and as a result have been able to train as well on the road as I train at home.

To this day, I am amazed by the extreme discomfort that I endured following those runs and how a simple change in my daily routine contributed to the drastic change in my performance and recovery. As with any setback, it was critical that I assess the situation and changes that I had made in my lifestyle and looking into ways that I could compensate to bring my body back to equilibrium. With proper training, no workout should sideline you in the hours afterwards; if this is happening, be sure to assess your pillars and your own lifestyle. If left unchecked, you risk illness and injury that may derail your training program for weeks or months.

—Dr. Maria Urso, O2X Nutrition Specialist, former Army Major, scientist, and elite marathon runner

Calories

Now, let's turn to the concept of food as fuel. **Calories** are the unit of measurement that quantifies how much energy/fuel any given food provides us. While the scientific definition is important, a more practical and useful way to think about how many calories are contained in our foods is detailed in figure 1–7.

Calorie
The amount of energy needed to increase the temperature of 1 kilogram of water by 1 degree Celsius.

WHAT DOES 150 CALORIES LOOK LIKE?

A 200 pound man and a 150 pound woman
burn approximately 150 calories per mile of running.
Here is what 150 calories looks like in common food and drink:

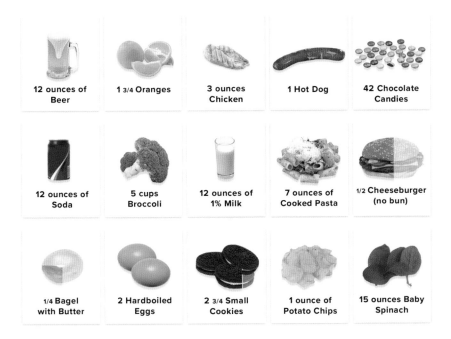

12 ounces of Beer	1 3/4 Oranges	3 ounces Chicken	1 Hot Dog	42 Chocolate Candies
12 ounces of Soda	5 cups Broccoli	12 ounces of 1% Milk	7 ounces of Cooked Pasta	1/2 Cheeseburger (no bun)
1/4 Bagel with Butter	2 Hardboiled Eggs	2 3/4 Small Cookies	1 ounce of Potato Chips	15 ounces Baby Spinach

Figure 1–7. What does 150 calories look like?

When looking at the diagram, consider the fact that a 200 lb man and a 150 lb woman each burn approximately 150 calories per mile of running. For example, 10 miles of running would burn 420 pieces of chocolate candy, 10 hot dogs without the buns, or 50 cups of broccoli. We are not recommending this approach at all—just pointing out how food energy works and can be measured. Also: watch out for calories that may sneak up on you, such as the ones in sugary drinks (fig. 1–8).

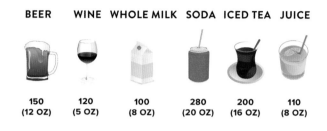

CALORIES IN SUGARY DRINKS (1 Standard Serving Size)

BEER	WINE	WHOLE MILK	SODA	ICED TEA	JUICE
150 (12 OZ)	120 (5 OZ)	100 (8 OZ)	280 (20 OZ)	200 (16 OZ)	110 (8 OZ)

Figure 1–8. Calories in sugary drinks

Along with sugary drinks, alcohol can be a source of unnecessary calories. Alcohol contains 7 calories per gram, and does not provide a metabolically useful form of energy. Additionally, alcohol can cause dehydration, prevent muscle growth and recovery, increase fat storage, and disrupt sleep cycles and memory. Rather than providing fuel like the calories found in macronutrients, alcohol interferes with fat burning by diverting your metabolism from breaking down fats consumed in food.[9]

Caloric Intake The number of calories the body needs to maintain balance and have the energy necessary to function well.

Understanding calories and how they impact your metabolism is key to creating a diet that will help optimize your performance. To estimate the right amount of food for you, begin by determining your "ideal **caloric intake** window", which represents the optimal range of calories you should be consuming each day based on your body weight, exercise level, and weight goals. As you see in the key takeaways, and in an example calculation later in this chapter, the recommended amounts are anywhere from 11 to 18 calories per pound of body weight, per day, depending on activity levels and goals. Not all calories are created equal; the next sections will highlight the three different macronutrients our bodies use as fuel.

KEY TAKEAWAYS

Calories

◇ Calories are a measurement of fuel (like miles per gallon)

◇ "Caloric Intake Window" is our healthy range

◇ Daily intake guidelines per pound of body weight:

» 11–13 calories/lb for weight loss, inactive people

» 14–16 calories/lb for maintenance, moderate activity

» 16–18 calories/lb for weight gain, very active people

Nutrients

With an understanding of calories and caloric intake, we can discuss the food we eat, which serves two equally important nutritional purposes. First and foremost, food provides fuel: some of the nutrients from our food intake provide energy. These energy sources are called **macronutrients**. Specifically, our body uses macronutrients as energy for behind-the-scenes functions such as pumping blood, repairing muscles, building tissues, and maintaining our immune systems. Macronutrients also provide fuel for our conscious activities, such as walking, running, thinking, moving around—basically living our lives. It stands to reason that without enough calories from macronutrients, our bodies and minds would not properly function.

On the other hand, certain other nutrients from food intake provide us *no* energy, but they do enable essential biological functions to help our bodies perform better. These are called **micronutrients**. Figure 1–9 highlights how our bodies utilize both macro- and micronutrients. If we were cars, the macronutrients would be the gas, and micronutrients would be the oil. And, just like a car, because they rely on one another, proper amounts of these two elements are equally important to our health and survival.

Macronutrients
Foods that are required in the human diet. These include protein, fats, and carbohydrates, which provide energy in the form of calories.

Micronutrients
Vitamins and minerals that are required in small amounts in the human diet. Consuming the proper amounts of micronutrients helps maintain health and avoid disease.

MACRONUTRIENTS

Imagine a dinner of steak, hot off the grill, with an ear of buttered corn. Though it may not sound like a meal for someone watching their caloric intake, you are looking at a meal containing all three macronutrients: protein (steak), carbohydrates (corn and steak), and fats (butter, corn, and steak). These three macronutrient categories provide 100% of the energy/calories we need to survive. More on this later, but as you read about protein, carbohydrates, and fats, please keep in mind *every* meal should ideally contain all three macronutrients.

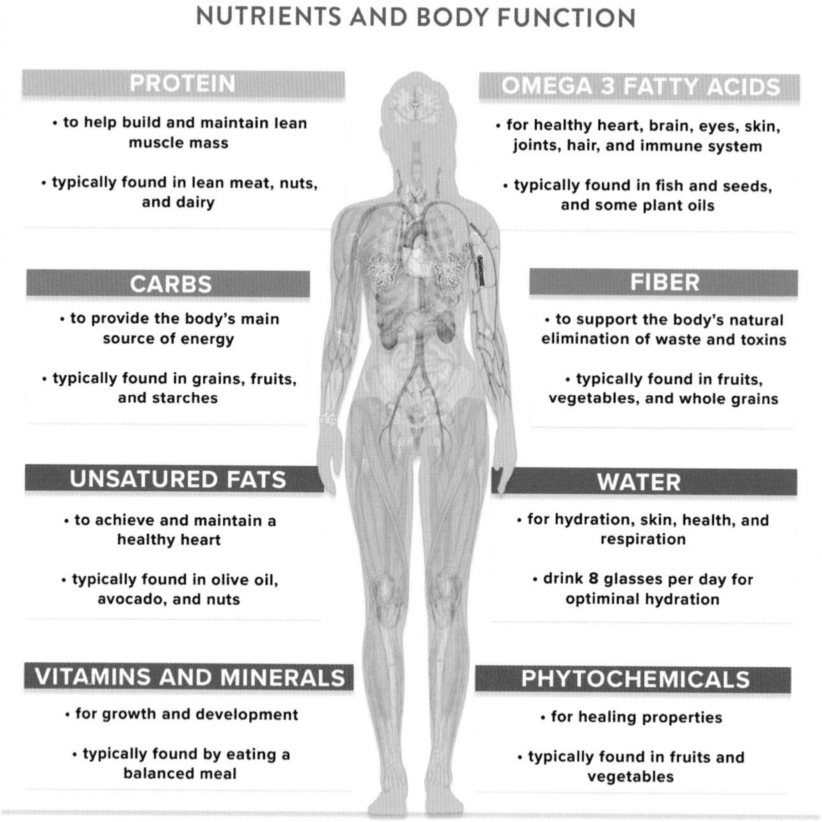

NUTRIENTS AND BODY FUNCTION

PROTEIN
- to help build and maintain lean muscle mass
- typically found in lean meat, nuts, and dairy

CARBS
- to provide the body's main source of energy
- typically found in grains, fruits, and starches

UNSATURED FATS
- to achieve and maintain a healthy heart
- typically found in olive oil, avocado, and nuts

VITAMINS AND MINERALS
- for growth and development
- typically found by eating a balanced meal

OMEGA 3 FATTY ACIDS
- for healthy heart, brain, eyes, skin, joints, hair, and immune system
- typically found in fish and seeds, and some plant oils

FIBER
- to support the body's natural elimination of waste and toxins
- typically found in fruits, vegetables, and whole grains

WATER
- for hydration, skin, health, and respiration
- drink 8 glasses per day for optiminal hydration

PHYTOCHEMICALS
- for healing properties
- typically found in fruits and vegetables

Figure 1–9. Nutrients and body function

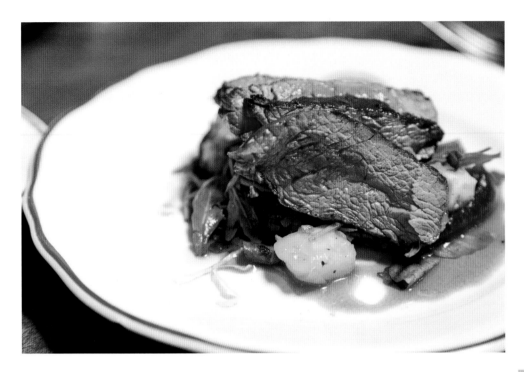

Protein

We cannot overstate the primary role **protein** plays in healthy nutrition and maximum performance. Its most important role is building lean muscle mass. On top of this, proteins replace and repair damaged cells, build enzymes that speed up chemical reactions, and make antibodies, a vital component of your immune system that fends off infections and illnesses. In fact, there are approximately 100,000 different proteins in the human body including muscles, enzymes, hormone receptors, skin, neurotransmitters, organs, glands, hair, and nails.[10] More mind-boggling is the fact we have over one trillion cells in our bodies, and *each* cell makes and uses proteins all day long.

This is why protein is the macronutrient around which every meal should be planned. As a starting point, consider that protein should provide approximately 10%–35% of your total calories each day, depending on your overall health, activity level, and age. The questions then become: are proteins different, on which ones should I focus, and how can I tell the difference? A little more nutritional science will help answer those questions.

Proteins are made up of chains of either **essential** or **nonessential amino acids**. *Essential* amino acids are labeled "essential" because our bodies do not produce them, and they can only be obtained through the food we eat. Therefore, it is *essential* we eat them. One example is Tryptophan, found in turkey. Other essential amino acids include Isoleucine, Leucine, and Lysine.[11] *The body produces nonessential amino acids naturally* and thus it is not necessary we ingest them from food. For this reason, we do not need

Protein
A macronutrient composed of a chain of amino acids linked together. It is essential for cell functioning.

Essential amino acids
Amino acids that the body does not produce and can only be obtained through food.

Nonessential amino acids
Amino acids that the body produces naturally and do not need to be consumed in food.

to cover nonessential amino acids in this book. Instead, we will focus on how to get the *essential* amino acids needed to optimize our performance.

The essential amino acids can be found in *complete* proteins. Complete proteins come from animals like chickens, cows, and fish. Soybeans are the only source of complete protein that does not come from animals. Finally, complete proteins contain essential amino acids in the right proportions for your bodily requirements. The chart in figure 1–10 provides a helpful list of various foods and whether they contain complete, or incomplete, proteins.

TYPES OF PROTEIN

COMPLETE PROTEIN
Contain all the essential amino acids

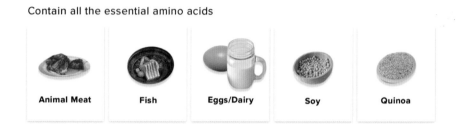

INCOMPLETE PROTEIN
Contain some, but not all, of the essential amino acids

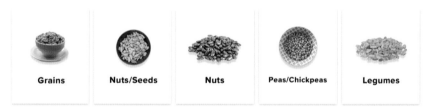

Figure 1–10. Types of protein

As you can likely guess, *incomplete* proteins do not contain *all* the necessary essential amino acids, but they do contain some. Incomplete proteins come from plants, like beans, grains, rice, legumes, and nuts. Vegans, for example, often combine two or more complementary, incomplete proteins to provide all essential amino acids they need. However we choose to get there, our focus should always be obtaining complete proteins (even if that means combining two incomplete proteins). Now that we know complete proteins are the important focus, let's look at some practical considerations.

First, you should include protein, ideally complete, at every meal because it helps slow the post-meal rise in blood sugar levels. Second, if you can eat the proper amount of protein with every meal—a good rough estimate is approximately 20 grams—it will help satiate you longer, which is another way of saying it will slow hunger. Finally, snacks with complete proteins are also an excellent idea: milk, cheese, meats, and eggs help keep your healthy eating on track, and convenience items like protein bars and supplement drinks with enough protein (watch the sugar content) help when you need something on the go.

KEY TAKEAWAYS

Protein

- ◇ 1 gram of protein = 4 calories
- ◇ Healthy target range: 15%–35% of daily calories
- ◇ Roughly 20 grams per meal, depending on goals, activity
- ◇ Focus on complete proteins with essential amino acids
- ◇ Build each meal around protein as start point
- ◇ Consistent protein intake helps stabilize blood sugar levels
- ◇ Proteins build and repair muscle and other essential functions

Carbohydrates

As we discussed with the craving and binging cycle, **carbohydrates** are the primary source of overall energy for our bodies—both quick energy boosts (think: sugar), and the more sustained energy stores we need. Aside from the obvious ones (candy, bread, and chocolate, for example), carbohydrates also come in many enjoyable and healthy forms that provide sustained energy, energy that allows us to live, work out, move, and think.[12]

Carbohydrates A compound of carbon, hydrogen, and oxygen. Carbohydrates are an immediate source of energy present in most foods, but mainly found in natural sugars and starches

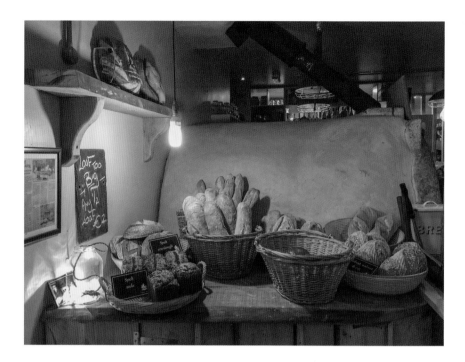

Carbohydrates get a bad reputation because many people picture "convenience" foods such as white bread, pretzels, processed pastas, candy, and other sugary snacks as being extremely high in carbohydrates and low in most other valuable nutrients. They are correct about the convenience foods. However, that does not mean all carbohydrates should be avoided. High-quality carbohydrates that contribute to overall health and wellness, including fruits, vegetables, and **whole grains**, should be eaten often. Bottom line: carbohydrates play a fundamental role in fueling and optimizing our performance and, as you recall from our steak, corn, and butter example, *every* meal should ideally contain all three macronutrients, including carbohydrates.

Like we did with protein, let's review rough guidelines for consuming carbohydrates. First, carbohydrates should comprise roughly 45%–65% of your total caloric intake each day, depending again on your overall health, activity level, and age. And, to help reduce the growing **type II diabetes** problem in the United States, the World Health Organization (WHO) recommends no more than 10% of your total caloric intake should come from added sugars. For most people, this is about 25 grams per day (this does not include sugar from dairy, fruits, and vegetables).[13] Another helpful, *general* rule is to try to fill half of every meal plate up with carbohydrates such as fruits and vegetables.

This last sentence raises the questions: how are various carbohydrates different from one another, on which ones should you focus, and how can you tell the difference? The following is a little nutritional science to help you understand the "why," so that "what" and "how" become second nature.

The first thing to know is carbohydrates come in two forms: simple and complex (fig. 1–11). Simple carbohydrates are made up of either one or two sugar molecules (monosaccharides and disaccharides, respectively). Your body burns through simple carbohydrates (table sugar, honey, and soda, for example) very quickly, providing immediate bursts of energy.

Complex carbohydrates, on the other hand, are made up of many sugar molecules chemically bound together (polysaccharides). These complex carbohydrates are digested slowly, thereby providing long-lasting, stable energy for your body. Oatmeal, whole grain bread, and high fiber cereal are excellent examples of complex carbohydrates.

TYPES OF CARBOHYDRATES

COMPLEX CARBOHYDRATES
Digested slowly, providing long-lasting, stable energy for your body

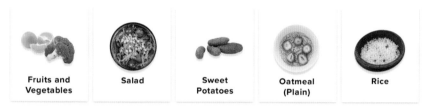

| Fruits and Vegetables | Salad | Sweet Potatoes | Oatmeal (Plain) | Rice |

SIMPLE CARBOHYDRATES
Digested very quickly, providing immediate bursts of energy

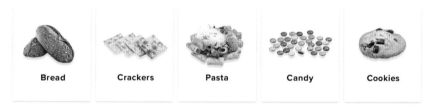

| Bread | Crackers | Pasta | Candy | Cookies |

Figure 1–11. Types of carbohydrates

For a carbohydrate to be useful energy for our bodies, it must be a mono- or disaccharide. Simple carbohydrates (table sugar, honey, etc.) are already in this form when we eat them, and thus can be used as energy *immediately*. Complex carbohydrates, on the other hand, need to be metabolized (i.e., broken down into mono- or disaccharide form) before the body can use them. All complex carbohydrates can be broken down into glucose (fig. 1–12).

BREAKING DOWN CARBOHYDRATES

Carbs are broken down into glucose, then converted to ATP, which provides your body with the energy it needs.

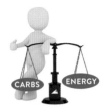

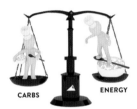

When your level of carb intake is balanced with your energy needs, you will maximize your performance.

When your level of carb intake is heavier than your energy needs, the excess carbs will be converted to fat and you will feel sluggish with an increased risk of long-term complications.

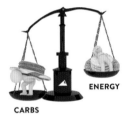

Figure 1–12. Breaking down carbohydrates

Let's combine what we know about carbohydrates with our earlier discussion on stabilizing blood sugar levels. Specifically, if we eat too many fast-burning, simple sugars in one sitting, the surge of available glucose causes our blood sugar levels to spike, and our bodies react by releasing insulin. In turn, this insulin converts and stores the abundance of sugar as fat. If the body is consistently forced to produce insulin in response to large meals made of simple carbohydrates, the pancreas becomes overworked and "sluggish," eventually contributing to illnesses like type II diabetes.[14]

In contrast, if we eat complex carbohydrates, our bodies need more time to break them down into a usable state (glucose), thereby creating a slow-release of glucose into our bloodstream. As a practical example, let's look at the positive ripple effects of 10 grams of simple carbohydrates with 10 grams of complex carbohydrates. First, we experience steadier, more consistent energy levels that sustain us over longer periods of time. Secondly, we stay off of the *blood sugar roller coaster* (fig. 1–13) and do not experience the highs and lows of sugar cravings.[15] Finally, we minimize the fat storage associated with spikes, and we avoid having to metabolize our healthy **lean muscle** as energy. Bottom line: if we minimize our intake of simple carbohydrates, and instead focus on eating complex carbohydrates, we will help maximize our performance in the short and long term.

Lean Muscle
The amount of muscle present in the body independent of the amount of fat, bones, and other tissues.

BLOOD SUGAR REGULATION

The flatter the curve, the better you'll feel!

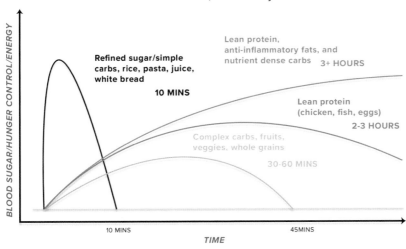

Figure 1–13. Blood sugar stabilization

Because nutritional information and labels do not always differentiate between complex and simple carbohydrates, prioritizing fruits, vegetables, and whole grains is a good way to ensure you are consuming the right carbohydrates. Depending on where you are on the couch-potato-to-ultra-marathoner activity spectrum, you will need to eat fewer (less active) or more (more active) carbohydrates. We will get into specific math of plate construction later in this chapter. Finally, as we keep hammering home, *every* meal should contain all three macronutrients, including carbohydrates. This habit will provide needed energy and prevent low blood sugar and cravings.[16]

Fats

Are fats delicious? Yes. Are they always bad for you? No. Contrary to popular thought, fats are not always bad for you. Go back to our bedrock: *every* healthy meal should contain all three macronutrients, including fats. At a conscious level, fats provide great flavor and the "full" feeling that keeps you from oversnacking between meals. On a metabolic and physiological level, fats provide us a secondary form of heat and an energy source used during rest or low-intensity exercise. Fats are also needed to build the sheaths covering our nerves, assist in blood clotting and inflammation, and build exterior membranes around every cell in our bodies.[17] Regarding nutrition, fats also aid in the absorption of some vitamins and minerals. So, if fats are helpful, then how much of them do we need?

After accounting for our daily protein and carbohydrate intake detailed above, fats should roughly comprise the remaining 25%–35% of our total caloric intake each day. Again, this is a general rule of thumb and should be calibrated according to our individual health status, activity level, and age. Good news: we should be eating fats as part of a healthy diet. Therefore, we need to know: are various fats different from one another, on which ones should we focus, and how can we tell the difference? Let's again dig into a little nutritional science (fig. 1–14).

First and foremost, there are both unhealthy and healthy fats. Let's begin with the unhealthy variety. *Hydrogenated* fats (aka trans fats) are the most unhealthy and are generally regarded as having no known health benefits. They increase our risk of heart disease, type II Diabetes, stroke, and other negative outcomes. They also increase the amounts of cholesterol in our bodies. These unhealthy fats show up on nutritional labels as "hydrogenated fats," "partially hydrogenated oil," and "trans fat." Dealing with this one is easy: avoid them completely.[18] (As of the writing of this book, these harmful fats are being phased out of the food supply).

In the middle of the pack are *saturated* fats. These fats show up naturally in animal products and some plant-based products: for example you will find saturated fats in red meat, whole milk dairy products, coconut oil, and a lot of commercially baked goods. Saturated fats also show up in some artificially hydrogenated vegetable products. There is a reasonable ongoing debate on the negative impacts of saturated fats (they can raise our risk of heart disease if eaten in excess), but they do provide us with the essential fatty acids needed to support optimal nutrition. For this reason, use of hydrogenated vegetable products and animal-based saturated fats should be used sparingly. As a guideline, many nutritionists recommend limiting saturated fats to under 10% of our daily caloric intake.

Next, we get to the healthier fats, and they fall into two broad categories: mono- and polyunsaturated. Monounsaturated fats can be found in olive oil, peanut oil, canola oil, avocados, and most nuts. Some studies reveal that despite a high-fat diet, some populations with monounsaturated fats (olive oil) as their primary fat source have enjoyed relatively low rates of heart disease. The relative comparison was other populations who ate primarily animal fats (i.e., saturated fats) and experienced higher rates of heart disease. Accordingly, where possible, we should seek to replace trans and saturated fats with monounsaturated fats (and polyunsaturated fats, more on that in a moment) as often as possible.[19]

UNDERSTANDING FATS

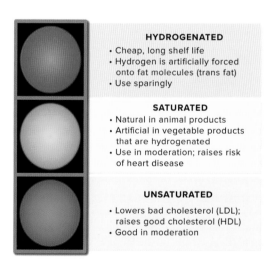

Figure 1–14. Understanding fats

Finally, we get to the more beneficial healthy fats (fig. 1–15), polyunsaturated fats, also known as *essential* fats (most specifically, two essential fatty acids are relevant in this class of fats—linoleic and alpha-linoleic—not the entire class). *Essential* means they are required by our bodies to properly function, but our bodies cannot make them: therefore getting them from food is *essential*.[20] Most of the positive roles of fats (clotting, building cell membranes and nerve sheathing, lowering harmful LDL cholesterol, etc.) are attributed to polyunsaturated fats. One more distinction before we're done with macronutrients: there are two main types of polyunsaturated fats—omega-3 fatty acids and omega-6 fatty acids.

Some excellent sources of omega-3 fatty acids are eggs, leafy vegetables, walnuts, chicken, salmon, mackerel, flaxseeds, canola oil and certain soybean oils. Omega-3s are considered "anti-inflammatory" and supportive of cell turnover and nerve repair. Adequate consumption of omega-3 fatty acids has been shown to reduce the incidence of heart disease and alleviate the symptoms of arthritis.[21] Omega-6 fatty acids can be found in vegetable oils such as safflower, soybean, walnut, and corn oils. One final note on omega-3 and omega-6 fatty acids: an ideal intake ratio is 1:4 (omega 3:omega 6). Since many Western diets consist of high amounts of breads and cereals, it is common for people to overconsume omega-6 fatty acids and not get enough omega-3s—the typical Western diet is closer to 1:10.[22] We should counteract this trend, and rebalance toward the more appropriate ratio, by trying to incorporate foods rich in omega-3s at every meal.

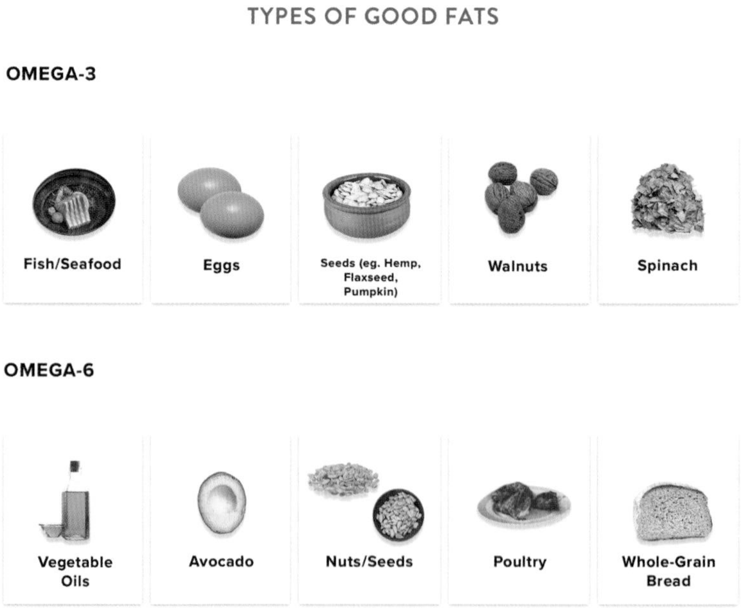

TYPES OF GOOD FATS

OMEGA-3

| Fish/Seafood | Eggs | Seeds (eg. Hemp, Flaxseed, Pumpkin) | Walnuts | Spinach |

OMEGA-6

| Vegetable Oils | Avocado | Nuts/Seeds | Poultry | Whole-Grain Bread |

Figure 1–15. Types of good fats

The bottom line with fats: limit them to 1/4 to 1/3 of your plate at meals (roughly 25%–35% of your daily caloric intake), focus mostly on unsaturated fats that can be found, among other places, in salmon, nuts, mackerel, and vegetable oils, and limit your intake of saturated fats (red meat, whole milk products, for example) to no more than 1/10 of your meal plate (or 10% of your daily caloric intake). If you follow these guidelines and incorporate them into every meal you reasonably can, then you will be on the path to maximizing your performance.

KEY TAKEAWAYS

Fats

⋄ 1 gram of fats = 9 calories

⋄ Healthy target range: 25%–35% of daily calories

⋄ Roughly 45–60 grams per day, depending on goals, activity

⋄ Focus on unsaturated fats with essential fatty acids

⋄ Good sources include fish, poultry, eggs, seeds, vegetable oils

⋄ Consistent intake keeps us "full" and helps stabilize blood sugar levels

CHOLESTEROL

Cholesterol
A waxy, fat-like substance used to make hormones, cell membranes, and vitamin D. It helps aid digestion of foods. The body makes all the cholesterol it needs. However, cholesterol is also found in some foods.

Before we shift from fats to micronutrients, let's take a look at an important nutritional consideration related to fats: **cholesterol**. There are two types: "bad" cholesterol (LDL, or low-density lipoproteins), and "good" cholesterol (HDL, or high-density lipoproteins). Don't construe the labels "good" and "bad" too literally: the body needs both LDL and HDL to function properly. LDL is considered "bad" cholesterol because its deposits are sticky and lodge themselves into your tissues. LDLs also "deliver" cholesterol that builds up over time, contributing to clogged arteries. You can see why elevated levels can increase our risk of heart disease. HDLs, on the other hand, tend to be too large to become lodged in tissues and blood vessels.[23] Instead, they act as "sweepers" in the circulation, ridding the body of deposits or debris on the artery and vein walls.

From a practical standpoint, you should know cholesterol is only found in animal fats, not vegetable fats. The recommended daily allowance of cholesterol is 300 mg, and, interestingly, because we need cholesterol to provide structure and support to cells, our bodies make about 1,200 mg of cholesterol per day. This is why it is difficult to lower cholesterol through diet alone. Exercise, and consuming unsaturated fats, will help to lower our total cholesterol levels and improve our HDL levels.

Dietary fiber is another factor in managing cholesterol. A high **fiber** diet has many important benefits, including normalizing bowel movements, managing cholesterol levels, stabilizing blood sugar levels, and keeping us feeling "full," thereby helping to maintain a healthy body composition. Healthy sources of dietary fiber include whole grain products, nuts, seeds, veggies, and fruits. A good rule of thumb when you are planning a balanced nutrition plan is to focus on whole grains and dietary fibers as often as possible.

While macronutrients lay the foundation for your diet and offer you the caloric fuel you need to get the job done day-in and day-out, micronutrients are also essential for your body to function. The next section will provide greater insight into how micronutrients help turn food into fuel.

MICRONUTRIENTS

Micronutrients, unlike their macro siblings, do not have calories and do not provide energy to our body. But, if you recall the "macronutrients-are-gas, and micronutrients-are-oil" analogy, you will remember that micronutrients are essential for your body to function properly. Vitamins, minerals, and water are common micronutrients.

What do micronutrients do? Vitamins, both the water-soluble and oil-soluble variety, assist in metabolism of the macronutrients listed above, they facilitate nerve signal transmission, and are involved in other bodily chemical reactions.[24]

As for minerals, they are the catalysts for many biological reactions within the body, including the digestion and utilization of nutrients in foods, the production of hormones and tissues, and, like vitamins, signal transmission through the nervous system.

Finally, water is considered a micronutrient because it provides no energy (i.e., it has no caloric value), but is essential to life. Water transports nutrients in your body, serves as a shock absorber and lubricant, and helps regulate your body temperature. Water makes up roughly 50% of your body weight, so even small deviations in hydration status can affect how you function and perform. Water is an extremely important topic, and was already covered in depth in the Hydration section of this chapter.

Ideally, you would receive all of the vitamins and minerals you need through a healthy, well-balanced nutrition plan. If for some reason you are not eating a well-balanced diet, or are under the care of a healthcare provider, you may benefit from a multi-vitamin and mineral supplement, which you will learn more about later in the chapter. Next we will jump into the importance of using quality, quantity, and timing as practical guidelines for your nutrition planning.

KEY MINERALS AND THEIR ROLES

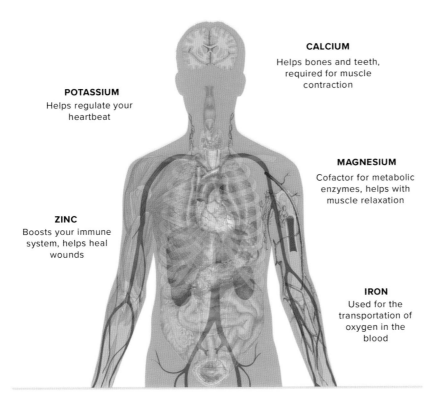

Figure 1–16. Key minerals and their roles

QUALITY, QUANTITY, AND TIMING

While what you eat is important, it is not the whole story. You also have to pay attention to how much and how often you eat. Now that we have a basic understanding of nutrition science, let's take a closer look at the specifics of the quality of calories we consume, the quantity we consume, and the timing of when we consume them. These three factors are separate, but extremely dependent on one another. To give you the tools to succeed, we will provide some helpful guidelines in each category, a practical dose of science and math, straightforward tailoring methods to meet your goals, and finally concrete ways to implement best practices in your career and lifestyle as a tactical athlete.

CALORIC INTAKE PLANNING

STEP 1: *Determine your activity level and weight goals*

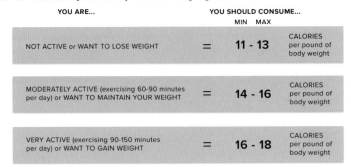

STEP 2: *Calculate your caloric window (your ideal range of calories per day)*

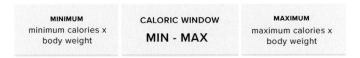

STEP 3: *Select your plate construction, and then calculate calories per macronutrient*

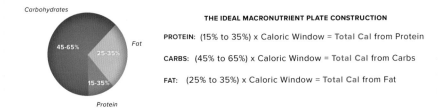

FINAL STEP: *Convert calories to grams per day*

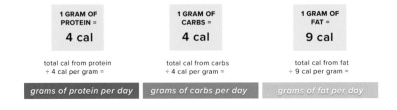

Figure 1–17. Caloric intake planning

CALORIC INTAKE PLANNING (EXAMPLE)

STEP 1: *Determine your activity level and weight goals*

For this example, let's assume you are a 200 lb man who wants to lose weight

YOU ARE...		YOU SHOULD CONSUME...	
		MIN MAX	
NOT ACTIVE or WANT TO LOSE WEIGHT	=	**11 - 13**	CALORIES per pound of body weight

STEP 2: *Calculate your caloric window (your ideal range of calories per day)*

MINIMUM	CALORIC WINDOW	MAXIMUM
11 calories x 200 lbs = 2,200 calories	**2,200 - 2,600**	13 calories x 200 lbs = 2,600 calories

STEP 3: *Select your plate construction, and then calculate calories per macronutrient*

For this example, let's assume your ideal caloric intake is 2,500 calories per day and your ideal plate construction is 25% protein, 50% carbs, 25% fat

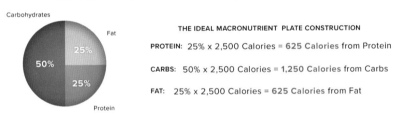

THE IDEAL MACRONUTRIENT PLATE CONSTRUCTION

PROTEIN: 25% x 2,500 Calories = **625 Calories** from Protein

CARBS: 50% x 2,500 Calories = **1,250 Calories** from Carbs

FAT: 25% x 2,500 Calories = **625 Calories** from Fat

FINAL STEP: *Convert calories to grams per day*

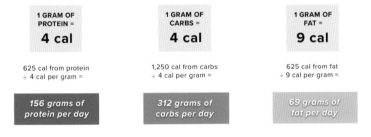

1 GRAM OF PROTEIN = **4 cal**	1 GRAM OF CARBS = **4 cal**	1 GRAM OF FAT = **9 cal**
625 cal from protein ÷ 4 cal per gram =	1,250 cal from carbs ÷ 4 cal per gram =	625 cal from fat ÷ 9 cal per gram =
156 grams of protein per day	**312 grams of carbs per day**	**69 grams of fat per day**

Quality

> Would you put cheap gas into a Ferrari? Choosing high-quality protein, fats, and carbohydrates ensures that your body is running optimally. Your energy is better, your body looks and feels stronger, and you get the added bonus of improving your health overall, which can add years to your life.
>
> —*Laura Moretti MS, RD, CSSD, LDN, and O2X*
> *Nutrition Specialist*

The overall rule when considering *quality* is focusing on eating balanced, nutrient dense, and unprocessed foods as often as possible (we do not suggest or expect anyone should completely rule out "cheat" meals or snacks—it is not sustainable, and does not acknowledge the fun and human side of performance). For each fuel category, this means focusing on complete proteins, complex carbohydrates, and healthy fats. Understanding the science of quality's importance in nutritious eating helps healthier options become more appealing and easier to choose during an everyday meal.

The first guideline in *quality* is a reiteration of what we emphasized when discussing macronutrients: aim for meals and snacks to have a balance of protein, carbohydrates and fat. Protein signals the release of a hormone called glucagon; carbohydrates signal the release of a hormone called insulin; and when eaten together, they counterbalance each other to keep blood sugar levels stable. Finally, a little fat in each meal slows the rate of digestion and keeps you satisfied until your next meal. This is why if you *just* eat a bowl of cereal (95% carbohydrates), or just a piece of fruit or crackers (100% carbohydrates), your blood sugar spikes and you are starving and craving more carbohydrates within a few hours, or even minutes. In contrast, a *balance* of protein, carbohydrates, and fats should help stabilize our blood sugar levels, and provide sustained energy.

Next, let's look at the concept of nutrient dense foods. People often label foods as "good" and "bad"—but those labels are inaccurate and not helpful. Instead, we should begin to think about foods on a spectrum between being nutrient dense and having limited nutritional value.

For proteins, *complete* proteins are nutrient dense choices, and when choosing proteins we should always be conscious of their fat content. Meat, poultry, fish, eggs, and so on—the items listed in the earlier Complete Proteins diagram on page 18—are excellent examples and should be included as the centerpiece of each meal, and a significant part of your daily diet.

For carbohydrates, *fibrous complex* carbohydrates such as fibrous fruits with skins intact, minimally processed starches/whole grains, and most vegetables, are nutrient dense. Berries are also nutrient dense, have a high dietary fiber content, and are a natural anti-inflammatory due to their anthocyanins, flavonoids, and resveratrol. A practical rule of thumb to obtain adequate amounts of nutrient dense foods is filling half of each meal plate with fruits (with the skin intact) and/or vegetables. Also, when eating carbohydrates like bread and pasta, look for minimally processed, whole grain options rather than simple, processed carbohydrates. There are delicious multi-grain, unprocessed bread options, and the whole grain pasta options have gotten much, much better in recent years. Evidence supports that adults who eat more whole grains, particularly those higher in dietary fiber, have a lower body weight compared to adults who eat fewer whole grains.[25]

For fats consider the following: if your protein and carbohydrates do not already contain fat, add a small amount of unsaturated (non-animal), heart-healthy fat to your meals. In contrast, avoid saturated animal fats (butter, lard, fat found in ice cream), and trans/hydrogenated fats found in many processed food products, as much as possible.

One other consideration similar to nutrient density is caloric density (fig. 1–18). For example, 3.3 tablespoons of oil has the same calories as *8 cups* of mixed vegetables. Think of how full you'd feel on 8 cups of veggies, and how you may not even notice 3 tablespoons of oil mixed into it. Eating healthy, calorie dense foods helps you feel full, longer.

The quality of foods you eat provides the foundation for proper nutrition, and the next area of focus will be how much you need to eat in order to stay fueled. In our discussion of quantity, we will help you break down the amounts of calories and nutrients you need to maximize your performance.

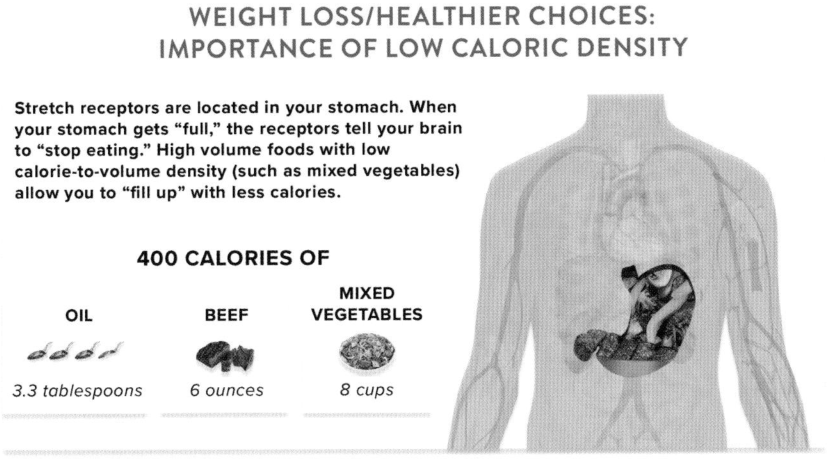

WEIGHT LOSS/HEALTHIER CHOICES: IMPORTANCE OF LOW CALORIC DENSITY

Stretch receptors are located in your stomach. When your stomach gets "full," the receptors tell your brain to "stop eating." High volume foods with low calorie-to-volume density (such as mixed vegetables) allow you to "fill up" with less calories.

400 CALORIES OF

OIL	BEEF	MIXED VEGETABLES
3.3 tablespoons	6 ounces	8 cups

Figure 1–18. Weight loss/healthier choices: importance of low caloric density

KEY TAKEAWAYS

Quality

- Every meal, and ideally every snack, should contain protein, carbs, and fats
  - **Proteins:** focus on complete proteins with essential amino acids
  - **Carbohydrates:** focus on complex carbohydrates and avoid added sugar content
  - **Fats:** focus on unsaturated fats from, e.g., plants, fish, seeds, and poultry
- Overall, focus on nutrient dense, and high fiber, foods

Quantity

The overall rule when considering quantity is consuming just enough healthy, balanced meals and snacks to feel *satisfied*, but not full. We will focus on providing guidelines to help you calibrate food intake based on exertion levels (just as a car needs more gas for a two-hour drive than it does for a trip down the street, we require more, or less, fuel depending our activity levels). By learning some basic calculations that allow us to manage portion size and macronutrient balance (fig. 1–19) we should know how to meet the demands of our daily activity levels, and personal performance goals.

MACRONUTRIENT : CALORIES

CARBOHYDRATES	1g = 4 calories
PROTEIN	1g = 4 calories
FATS	1g = 9 calories

Figure 1–19. Macronutrient calories

Managing the correct quantity of your food will depend on four factors: your current weight, desired weight, current activity levels, and your body composition goals. You can find caloric intake calculations and an example of how to calculate your caloric intake needs a few pages back in this chapter. Don't forget: no matter how these four factors impact our quantity calculations, the guidelines of quality and timing always apply.

Some practical concepts can help you control quantity:

1. We tend to underestimate the calories in meals considered "healthy"—by half.
2. Using smaller plates will help maintain healthy portion sizes.
3. Serve your food at the counter and bring only the portioned meals to the table.
4. Be mindful of serving sizes.

To find the right quantity of food for you, begin by determining your ideal caloric intake window, which represents to the ideal range of calories you should be consuming each day based on your body weight, exercise level, and weight goals.

These calculation guidelines will help you find a nutritional balance that optimizes your performance. Obviously, the needs of an active training or operations day look very different from a day spent on the couch watching television. Here is what can change on a day to day basis: your overall intake (i.e., you can shift from the low to high end of your caloric intake window) and your plate construction (i.e., your allocation between proteins, carbs, and fats). Finally, if you are training for a race or trying to lose weight, you will have to make additional modifications. We will cover fueling for exercise later in the chapter.

KEY TAKEAWAYS

Quantity

⋄ Ideal "caloric intake window" depends on goals, weight, and activity level

⋄ Daily intake guidelines per pound of body weight:

  » 11–13 calories/lb for weight loss, inactive people

  » 14–16 calories/lb for maintenance, moderate activity

  » 16–18 calories/lb for weight gain, very active people

⋄ It takes 20 minutes for your brain to learn your stomach is full

⋄ So eat slowly and deliberately until satisfied, not stuffed

⋄ Using smaller plates is a helpful portion control technique

⋄ Planning meals ahead of time reduces impulse snacks and meals

A HUNGRY WOLF—DAN CNOSSEN

One important side effect of nutrition is how it translates into body weight. Even if we eat healthy, if we overeat we will gain weight. If the calories in exceed the calories burned, weight will be gained, and the types of foods our calories come from can also play a role in weight management.

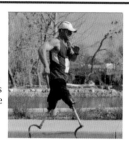

As a high-performance athlete, I am very conscientious of my body weight. As a Paralympic cross-country skier for the US, my sport is all about the athlete's power-to-weight ratio. Ideally, I would like to be as light as possible without sacrificing the specific strength I need to perform. When I first entered the sport, I found that I chronically over-ate. I think the reason behind this was a psychological conditioning process that occurred during my time in the US military—not knowing when the next meal would come caused over-eating for the obvious reason. One of my ski coaches would tell me, "A hungry wolf is a fast wolf", and although I don't think an athlete should be constantly hungry for food throughout the training cycle, I do think that (in the US especially) large portion sizes contribute to this over-eating phenomenon. Not in an obsessive way, but as a matter of routine, I check my body weight first thing in the morning out of bed (before going to the bathroom for consistency). Over time, I started to learn what an ideal training weight is—a few pounds above race weight so as not to get sick; what my race weight is—ideal strength/weight ratio with slight hunger on a daily basis; and what number signifies being underweight—where I get sick easier or am not feeling strong enough to recover from workouts.

When eating a meal, I try to picture what I would naturally want to eat as an over-eater, and try to eat about 2/3–3/4 of that amount. It turns out that this is plenty to keep me going and I'm about 5–10 pounds lighter as a result, with no less power output.

Because of the simple math behind body weight—calories in versus calories out—on recovery weeks or taper weeks as the competition becomes closer the athlete should be consuming less. If I eat the same regardless of the training volume, I will actually gain weight during my taper week, which is the worst thing I could be doing to the strength-to-weight ratio. So, again there must be discipline when it comes to eating. During a high-volume training week, the mind and the stomach become conditioned to higher quantities of food, so during the recovery week or in a taper it can be psychologically difficult to eat a reduced amount of food. I constantly have to tell myself, "Dan, you can eat much less than you think and still be fine!" I have also found that drinking water with a low-sugar dissolved electrolyte tablet helps satiate my stomach and keep it feeling "full" without the need to be snacking as much. Obviously when the blood sugar gets low after a couple hours the athlete should refuel, but not in an excessive way. And again to reiterate, while in the training phase I try to be a few pounds above race weight so as not to get sick, to be able to recover better, and these are typically high volume weeks so I'm eating a lot more and am mentally happy. As the taper starts before the race, I need to have the discipline to eat less and shed a couple pounds to get to that ideal race weight. I tell myself "a hungry wolf is a fast wolf" to keep my mind focused.

—Dan Cnossen, Six-time Paralympic medalist (1 gold, 4 silver, 1 bronze), first American man to win Paralympic gold in biathlon, former US Navy SEAL

Timing

Timing is based off the general rule that eating at ideal times and intervals during the day will keep our metabolism active, and our blood sugar levels stable. As a guideline, we should aim to eat every 2–3 hours, with our first meal, breakfast, coming no more than 1 hour after we wake. Therefore, in addition to a balanced breakfast, lunch, and dinner, grab a balanced mid-morning and mid-afternoon snack (not a full meal), and a small snack before going to bed. When choosing snacks, aim for mostly protein or complex carbohydrates, or both.

So what does that look like in a typical day? First, eat within one hour of waking to kick-start your metabolism and, if you workout early in the morning, fuel yourself based on the duration and type of exercise you will be doing. Supplement each meal with 8–16 ounces of water. Maintain 2–3 hour meal/snack intervals during the day. Then, you may have heard you should not eat after 7:00 p.m., but physiology argues that is not the guideline to follow.

Ideally, we should all aim for our last meal of the night to be 1.5–2 hours before bedtime, because we will spend the next 6–8 hours (or more) fasting. When we sleep, our bodies are repairing cells and tissues and creating new ones. If we do not provide ourselves with the adequate nutrients, our blood sugar levels will drop, and we may burn precious lean tissue for energy, and dampen normal cell/tissue repair and regeneration that happens during sleep. In contrast, eating any closer to bedtime can postpone sleepiness because your body remains alert while it is actively digesting your food. Bottom line: shoot for your last meal or snack to be approximately 2 hours before bedtime. Figure 1–20 outlines how we might plan out a typical day, in three scenarios: weight loss, maintenance, and gain.

Just like quantity should be adjusted based on goals and exertion levels, so should *timing*. For instance, we may need to plan on a pre-workout snack and post-workout meal to assist with muscle recovery. Secondly, the number of meals and snacks you eat in a day depends on how many hours you are awake. Because you should aim to keep your engine continuously fueled, on days when you get up earlier and stay awake later, you would need to eat more meals and snacks. Similarly, you would eat fewer meals and snacks on days you sleep in, or go to bed early.

One thing we would like to note when it comes to timing is the concept of intermittent fasting. There is ample research to support its role in fat burning and longevity and multiple ways to implement it: 24-hour fasting 1–2 days per week (for example every Monday and/or Thursday), or 18-hour fasting 6 days a week, fueling/feeding for 6 hours (only eating from 11:00 a.m. to 5:00 p.m.), with one day off from fasting.[26] As with any topic in this book, you should consult your personal medical professionals before trying a fasting program for yourself. O2X does not endorse intermittent fasting for individuals who participate in a regimented exercise program since it does not allow for proper refueling after exercise.

Meal timing can be challenging, especially with an unpredictable schedule, but there are ways that you can plan ahead and prepare yourself to have food on hand when you need it (fig. 1–20). You may not be able to eat perfectly balanced, nutrient dense meals and snacks like clockwork every 2–3 hours, every day. That's understandable—when you are on the run, or just plain busy, aim to have three main meals made up of real, whole food revolving around maintaining blood sugar levels throughout the day. Grabbing snacks like protein bars or Greek yogurt (watch the added sugar content in both) is a great way to stabilize your blood sugar levels on busy days (fig. 1–21).

MEAL PLANNING: EXAMPLE DAY

	WEIGHT LOSS (-10%)	WEIGHT MAINTENANCE (100%)	WEIGHT GAIN (+10%)
WAKE UP	Protein/Carb/Caffeine (5% calories)	Protein/Carb/Caffeine (10% calories)	Protein/Carb/Caffeine (10% calories)
MORNING WORKOUT	Cardio/Strength	Strength/Cardio	Low Cardio/Strength
POST-WORKOUT/ BREAKFAST	20g Protein/Carb (30% calories)	20g Protein/Carb (30% calories)	20g Protein/Carb (35% calories)
LUNCH	Protein/Carb/Fat (25% calories)	Protein/Carb/Fat (25% calories)	Protein/Carb/Fat (25% calories)
MID-AFTERNOON	Protein (5% calories)	Protein (5% calories)	Protein (5% calories)
DINNER	Protein/Carb/Fat (25% calories)	Protein/Carb/Fat (25% calories)	Protein/Carb/Fat (25% calories)
NIGHTLY SNACK	NONE	Protein (5% calories)	Protein (10% calories)

Figure 1–20. Meal planning: example day

GREAT ON-THE-GO SNACKS

Raw nuts (almonds, cashews)	**Apple slices with almond butter**
Carrot sticks and hummus	**Protein bars (aim for bar that offer at least 10 grams of protein per 150 calories, and 20 g total)**
String cheese	**Greek yogurt**

Figure 1–21. Great on-the-go snacks

Fueling for Exercise

As a tactical athlete, not only is your daily nutrition important, but you must also consider how fueling for exercise can impact your performance and recovery (fig. 1–22). Because of the physical nature of your work, you need to train hard to meet the physical demands of the job. As a result, you need to optimize the impact of your workouts through calibrating the quality, quantity, and timing of your nutrition intake. We will break that down into how to fuel before, during, and after a workout to see maximum impact of your efforts.

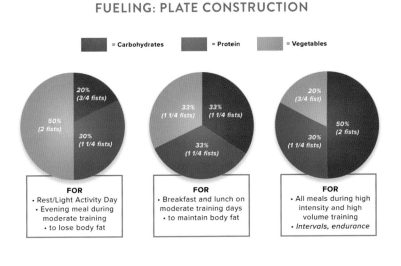

Figure 1–22. Fueling: plate construction

Before exercise

Before we add any fuel to the tank, let's look at what is already in there. People who exercise regularly store almost three times more **glycogen** (i.e., carbohydrates) in their muscles than people who do not exercise regularly.[27] Also, the amount of glycogen that can be stored is dependent on the amount of muscle mass that you have and your body weight. So we can't tell you exactly how much food you should eat before a workout, since it is not a "one size fits all" approach. As a general rule, you should have a larger meal 4–6 hours before your workout (or race)—that will give your body adequate time to digest and store the nutrients. You should aim for about 50 grams of carbohydrates (1 cup of oatmeal or fruit) and at least 10–15 grams of protein (2 eggs or 3 ounces of meat) in this meal.[28]

And, roughly one hour prior to your workout, you should have a meal tailored to accommodate your digestion and your workout.[29] Eat easily digestible foods that are low in fiber and saturated fat. See figure 1–23 for a general guide to when you should eat and what you should eat before a hard workout.

If working out first thing in the morning, focus on hydration beforehand and a complex carb-heavy snack, such as gentle-on-the-stomach oatmeal, whole grain bread with peanut butter, or a bar designed for pre-workout. It is important to note that your pre-workout fuel depends on the intensity and duration of activity you are about to do. For example, for a low-intensity 3-mile walk you may not need a carb-heavy snack as that can reduce your fat utilization during the exercise. On the other hand, if you are participating in a 45-minute high-intensity workout, pre-workout fuel that has complex carbohydrates will help provide the fuel you will need.

During exercise

During your workout, you likely will not need to eat or consume calories, especially if you are trying to lose weight. A 150-pound person burns about 600 calories doing a moderately intense 60-minute cardiovascular workout, and about 250–300 calories during 60 minutes of resistance training. Your glycogen (carbohydrate) stores are sufficient to provide the required energy. However, if you exercise for longer than 90 minutes, or are participating in an endurance event, you will benefit from additional calories during your workout.[30]

After exercise

Post-workout, your primary goals should be to replenish the glycogen that you lost, to hydrate, and to supply your body with enough protein to sustain synthesis and muscle recovery. Aim for up to 40 grams of protein for males and 25 grams of protein for females. And, ideally, you would split this protein equally as follows: half (20 for men, for example) right after the workout, and the other half within the next 2–4 hours. To replenish the glycogen lost from your muscles and liver, you should have a meal with about 30–50 grams of carbohydrates for each hour that you exercised. Your ability to absorb protein will be different in the pre- and post-workout stages. There is evidence that we can process less protein after a workout than just before.[31] Two glasses of 1%–2% chocolate milk (16 ounces) will supply 16 grams of protein and 50 grams of carbohydrate. As a bonus, it is easily digestible and should not cause stomach upset. If you would prefer to avoid milk, a comparable snack is two slices of whole grain bread topped with three eggs or a chicken breast.

Keep in mind that after a very intense workout or prolonged competition, your appetite may increase for hours or days. Continue to eat balanced meals with protein, carbohydrates, and fat, but listen to your cravings. If you are craving salty foods or meat, your body is likely depleted in one of those nutrients (electrolytes or protein). Use your hunger cues to guide what and when you eat, within the parameters of balance we have outlined.

The tips provided for pre-, during-, and post-exercise nutrition will help you to support muscle recovery, optimize glycogen storage, maintain hydration, and stabilize blood sugar. The more you stabilize blood sugar, the better you will perform during workouts. If you skipped meals earlier in the day or ate unbalanced meals, your energy, performance, and results will suffer during and after your workout. Your next workout is only as good as your nutritional strategy from the previous workout (fig. 1–23).

WHEN AND WHAT TO EAT BETWEEN
RIGOROUS PHYSICAL ACTIVITY (Tactical Athlete Specific)

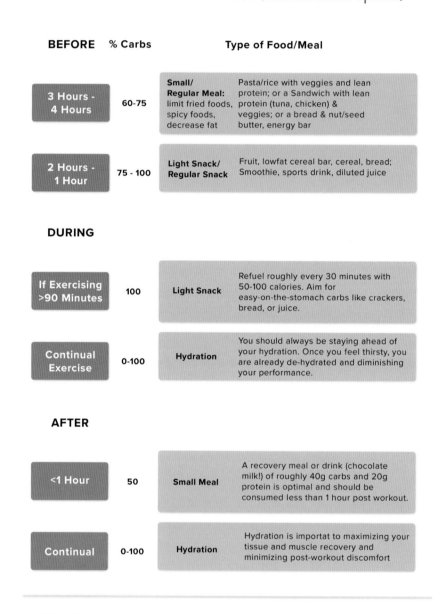

BEFORE	% Carbs	Type of Food/Meal	
3 Hours - 4 Hours	60-75	**Small/ Regular Meal:** limit fried foods, spicy foods, decrease fat	Pasta/rice with veggies and lean protein; or a Sandwich with lean protein (tuna, chicken) & veggies; or a bread & nut/seed butter, energy bar
2 Hours - 1 Hour	75 - 100	**Light Snack/ Regular Snack**	Fruit, lowfat cereal bar, cereal, bread; Smoothie, sports drink, diluted juice

DURING

	% Carbs	Type of Food/Meal	
If Exercising >90 Minutes	100	Light Snack	Refuel roughly every 30 minutes with 50-100 calories. Aim for easy-on-the-stomach carbs like crackers, bread, or juice.
Continual Exercise	0-100	Hydration	You should always be staying ahead of your hydration. Once you feel thirsty, you are already de-hydrated and diminishing your performance.

AFTER

	% Carbs	Type of Food/Meal	
<1 Hour	50	Small Meal	A recovery meal or drink (chocolate milk!) of roughly 40g carbs and 20g protein is optimal and should be consumed less than 1 hour post workout.
Continual	0-100	Hydration	Hydration is importat to maximizing your tissue and muscle recovery and minimizing post-workout discomfort

Figure 1–23. When and what to eat for rigorous physical activity

OTHER CONSIDERATIONS

Supplements

Supplementation is an advanced nutrition strategy, and should be used only when all other aspects of training, rest, and nutrition are at their peak and, ideally, a healthcare provider has been consulted. For example, if you are pregnant, suffering from a chronic illness, or if you eat a restrictive diet that eliminates certain food groups, supplements may benefit you if suggested under the care of your healthcare provider.

The term "supplements" covers a broad spectrum, including vitamins, minerals, herbs, enzymes, organ tissues, glandulars, and metabolites, to name a few. And they come in many forms, including tablets, powders, capsules, gels, and many more. It is important to understand that overconsumption of vitamins or minerals, or both, can result in illness or prevent the absorption of other micronutrients. Remember, this advice is general in nature and you should always consult your healthcare provider before taking any supplemental micronutrients, particularly if you are taking prescription medication.

Because supplements are not FDA approved, their containers cannot represent the product as a conventional "food," or as a sole meal, or diet, item. They are supplementary to a proper diet and should not be relied on as an independent (or sufficient) fuel or nutritional source. Accordingly, rather than seeing "Nutrition Facts" on the label you will see "Supplement Facts."

Among many self-made claims, the most common supplement claims are enhanced hormone secretion, improved muscle recovery, faster and better training response, enhanced exercise performance, and more sustained satiety. Some work, some don't, and some aren't worth the risk.

Supplements are not controlled substances. Sometimes people confuse supplements with substances that are controlled and regulated by the Drug Enforcement Agency—like testosterone, anabolic steroids, and prohormones. These substances require a prescription, and close medical supervision. On the other hand, supplements are not classified, and the FDA does not have the power to stop any potentially dangerous supplement from going on the market; it can only enforce a recall after the supplement has been released to the public. In fact, the FDA has recalled more than 100 dietary supplements for containing unlisted ingredients.[32] A healthcare professional familiar with your daily needs and medical history should review any supplement you are considering using. As a proverbial, baseline "sniff test," look for an NSF- or USP-certified option when researching supplements.

Belying all the extreme caution above, there is consensus that some supplements can be beneficial, but we should remain very careful that the supplements we take are safe and will actually help our specific performance needs. We are not advocating or recommending any of the following, but because they are so prevalent and utilized within the tactical athlete community, and the population in general, we will provide some general background information here.

As mentioned before, a nutrient-rich diet usually provides all that your body needs to function well. But multi-vitamins can be used as a safeguard against unintended or known dietary or metabolic imbalances (fig. 1–24). Similarly, specific supplements like fish oil can boost your omega-3 essential fat levels.

Some other supplements and their purported claims are: Probiotics are live microorganisms that can help digestion and maintain healthy bacteria in your body. Magnesium can help to balance calcium but most importantly promotes muscle relaxation and can aid in pain and stress relief (migraines, back pain, anxiety, constipation) and promote optimal sleep. Turmeric and ginger are powerful anti-inflammatories and can help if you struggle with pain (back pain, for example).

Whey protein is one of the most common supplements for all athletes. In conjunction with strength training, whey improves lean muscle mass, strength, and size. When taken in regulated quantities, whey protein has no known side effects, but look for protein powder products sourced within the USA to reduce the likelihood of contamination with metals. And note that if taken in excess, oversupplementing with whey protein can lead to nausea, cramps, fatigue, and reduced appetite. Whey is also often used as an alternative to milk.

Casein protein is also used to improve lean muscle mass, energy, and stamina. However, unlike whey protein, casein protein can have side effects like rashes, bloating, hives, and gastrointestinal discomfort. If you do not experience side effects from using casein protein, you may choose to use it.

We cannot stress enough: the information contained here is general in nature and should not supplant or override the direct advice of your personal healthcare professional. Please consult your healthcare provider before taking any supplements.

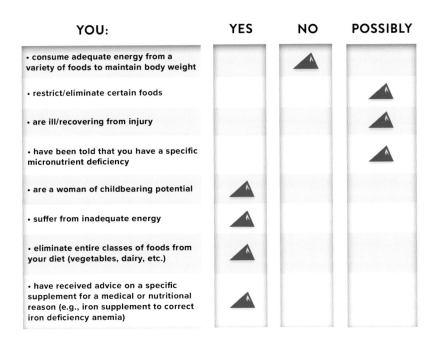

WOULD YOU BENEFIT FROM A VITAMIN/MINERAL SUPPLEMENT?

YOU:	YES	NO	POSSIBLY
• consume adequate energy from a variety of foods to maintain body weight		▲	
• restrict/eliminate certain foods			▲
• are ill/recovering from injury			▲
• have been told that you have a specific micronutrient deficiency			▲
• are a woman of childbearing potential	▲		
• suffer from inadequate energy	▲		
• eliminate entire classes of foods from your diet (vegetables, dairy, etc.)	▲		
• have received advice on a specific supplement for a medical or nutritional reason (e.g., iron supplement to correct iron deficiency anemia)	▲		

Figure 1–24. Would you benefit from a vitamin/mineral supplement?

KEY TAKEAWAYS

Supplements

◇ Always check with your healthcare professionals before taking any supplements

◇ Proper rest, nutrition, training, and hydration should be your first option

◇ Only when your healthcare professionals identify gaps should supplements be taken

◇ Read labels and ingredients very carefully before ingesting any supplement

◇ Vitamins contain zero nutritional value; they improve metabolic efficiency

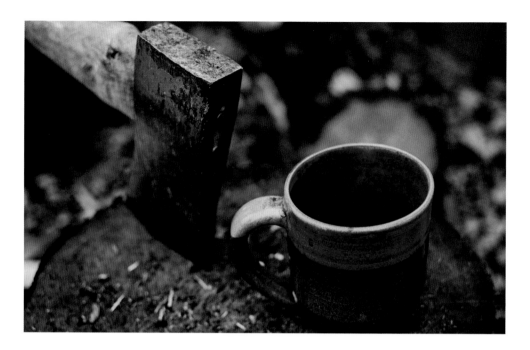

Caffeine

Caffeine
Found primarily in coffee, colas, cocoa, and tea. It is a crystalline compound and a stimulant of the central nervous system.

Good news: in addition to coffee being a morning ritual for many people, consuming the right amount of **caffeine** at the right time can be a performance enhancer, whether you are halfway through a 24-hour shift, gearing up for another pre-dawn raid, or prepping for a training session. Numerous studies have shown consuming caffeine prior to work-outs improves physical performance, and cognitively it increases concentration, focus, reaction time, and decision making.[33]

Specifically, caffeine allows your body to maintain/increase power output, speed, endurance, coordination, agility, and maximum strength capacity.

Quantity *does* matter when it comes to caffeine: you need enough to make a difference, but not so much that it makes you jittery or nervous, and disrupts your sleep. As a rule of thumb, roughly 0.7–1.8 mg of caffeine per lb of body weight creates a helpful differ-ence. For example, anywhere from 100–270 mg of caffeine can positively impact a 150 lb tactical athlete. An 8-ounce cup of coffee contains—depending on roast and preparation—roughly 80–175 mg of caffeine, whereas the same amount of tea contains roughly 40 mg. An 8 oz energy drink contains roughly 80 mg, and a 12 oz soda just under 60 mg. We sug-gest you stick with unsweetened coffee or tea to steer clear of added sugar and artificial ingredients. Like most things in life, moderation is key, so if you overdo caffeine intake, performance enhancements are lost and you may wind up feeling jittery, nauseous, and dizzy (fig. 1–25).[34]

HEALTH EFFECTS OF CAFFEINE

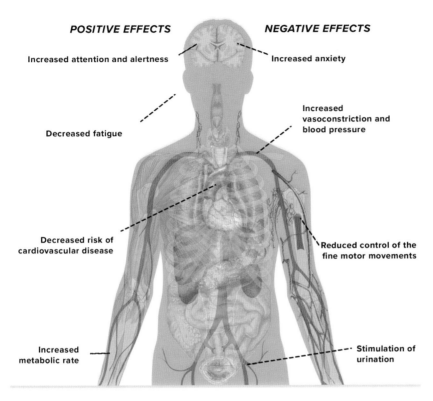

POSITIVE EFFECTS

Increased attention and alertness

Decreased fatigue

Decreased risk of
cardiovascular disease

Increased
metabolic rate

NEGATIVE EFFECTS

Increased anxiety

Increased
vasoconstriction and
blood pressure

Reduced control of the
fine motor movements

Stimulation of
urination

Figure 1–25. Health effects of caffeine[37]

Timing also plays a key role in enhancing performance. Caffeine concentration in the bloodstream peaks in 30–60 minutes and stays high for about 3–4 hours. On average, about half is gone within 4–6 hours and 75% will be cleared within 6–7 hours. In short, your window of opportunity to obtain a performance benefit from caffeine lasts roughly 4 hours from the time you ingest it—so plan accordingly. Consuming caffeine about an hour before you begin a workout or race will help ensure that blood levels are high when you begin.

As an added bonus, coffee can actually help enhance recovery.[35] Beverages with carbohydrates and caffeine rebuild glycogen stores more than drinks that are made of only carbohydrates. Next time you stop for your post-run or post-workout coffee fix, enjoy it and know that you are boosting your body's recovery capabilities.

CONCLUSION

Nutrition fuels human performance. Proper nutrition can raise performance levels to new heights, while poor nutrition can cause sickness, fatigue, and deficits in physical and mental well-being. Although we have been conditioned to think of nutrition in terms of following specific plans that are often written with the goal of weight loss, we should reimagine diet not as the action of restricting what we eat but as the foods we choose to fuel our bodies and minds. By positively reframing how we think about diet and nutrition, we can focus more on how our nutrition can lead to optimizing performance.

To recap some key points covered in this chapter: choosing a meal plan revolving around the quality, quantity, and timing of meals will help stabilize blood sugar levels throughout the day. For tactical athletes, blood sugar stabilization is fundamental to optimal performance as it helps ensure that you can be ready for any call. You have also learned about the importance of getting proper nutrients and hydration to fuel mental performance and build physical strength. As you read the SWEAT and THRIVE chapters think about how your nutrition and hydration habits will align with your conditioning program and mental performance to help you achieve the full benefits of your hard work.

Remember: You can't outwork a bad fork.

CHAPTER QUESTIONS

1. What are the foundational elements of a successful nutrition plan?
2. What are three benefits of developing proper nutrition habits?
3. What is the role of hydration in performance?
4. What are some simple things you can do to improve your hydration?
5. What are macro- and micronutrients and how much do you need each meal?
6. What does "quality" mean when it comes to proper nutrition?
7. What does "quantity" mean when it comes to proper nutrition?
8. What does "timing" mean when it comes to proper nutrition?

CHAPTER NOTES

What are three takeaways from this chapter that you can implement in your everyday life?

1. _____
_____
_____
_____
_____
_____

2. _____
_____
_____
_____
_____
_____

3. _____
_____
_____
_____
_____
_____

ADDENDUM

Reading a Nutrition Label

If you get to the grocery store and cannot remember the detailed guidelines of how to navigate the aisles, don't worry! There are a few key things that will help you make healthy choices so you can fill your cart with foods that will keep you fueled properly. First, remember to keep it simple—fill your cart with whole foods first. The fewer ingredients listed on a nutrition label, generally the better. Work your way from the outside of the grocery store in, and by the time you get to the middle aisles full of processed foods, you will have run out of room in your cart. When in doubt check the ingredients and nutrition label to help guide your choices.

HOW TO READ A LABEL

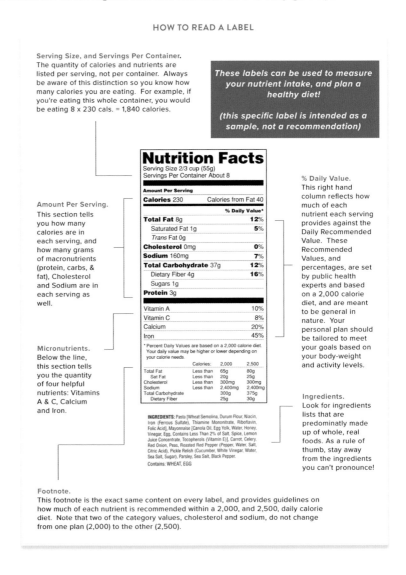

Serving Size, and Servings Per Container. The quantity of calories and nutrients are listed per serving, not per container. Always be aware of this distinction so you know how many calories you are eating. For example, if you're eating this whole container, you would be eating 8 x 230 cals. = 1,840 calories.

These labels can be used to measure your nutrient intake, and plan a healthy diet!

(this specific label is intended as a sample, not a recommendation)

Amount Per Serving. This section tells you how many calories are in each serving, and how many grams of macronutrients (protein, carbs, & fat), Cholesterol and Sodium are in each serving as well.

Micronutrients. Below the line, this section tells you the quantity of four helpful nutrients: Vitamins A & C, Calcium and Iron.

% Daily Value. This right hand column reflects how much of each nutrient each serving provides against the Daily Recommended Value. These Recommended Values, and percentages, are set by public health experts and based on a 2,000 calorie diet, and are meant to be general in nature. Your personal plan should be tailored to meet your goals based on your body-weight and activity levels.

Ingredients. Look for ingredients lists that are predominantly made up of whole, real foods. As a rule of thumb, stay away from the ingredients you can't pronounce!

Nutrition Facts
Serving Size 2/3 cup (55g)
Servings Per Container About 8

Amount Per Serving

Calories 230 — Calories from Fat 40

	% Daily Value*
Total Fat 8g	**12%**
Saturated Fat 1g	**5%**
Trans Fat 0g	
Cholesterol 0mg	**0%**
Sodium 160mg	**7%**
Total Carbohydrate 37g	**12%**
Dietary Fiber 4g	**16%**
Sugars 1g	
Protein 3g	

Vitamin A	10%
Vitamin C	8%
Calcium	20%
Iron	45%

* Percent Daily Values are based on a 2,000 calorie diet. Your daily value may be higher or lower depending on your calorie needs.

		Calories:	2,000	2,500
Total Fat	Less than		65g	80g
Sat Fat	Less than		20g	25g
Cholesterol	Less than		300mg	300mg
Sodium	Less than		2,400mg	2,400mg
Total Carbohydrate			300g	375g
Dietary Fiber			25g	30g

INGREDIENTS: Pasta [Wheat Semolina, Durum Flour, Niacin, Iron (Ferrous Sulfate), Thiamine Mononitrate, Riboflavin, Folic Acid], Mayonnaise [Canola Oil, Egg Yolk, Water, Honey, Vinegar, Egg, Contains Less Than 2% of Salt, Spice, Lemon Juice Concentrate, Tocopherols (Vitamin E)], Carrot, Celery, Red Onion, Peas, Roasted Red Pepper (Pepper, Water, Salt, Citric Acid), Pickle Relish (Cucumber, White Vinegar, Water, Sea Salt, Sugar), Parsley, Sea Salt, Black Pepper.

Contains: WHEAT, EGG

Footnote. This footnote is the exact same content on every label, and provides guidelines on how much of each nutrient is recommended within a 2,000, and 2,500, daily calorie diet. Note that two of the category values, cholesterol and sodium, do not change from one plan (2,000) to the other (2,500).

O2X CALORIC WINDOW CALCULATOR

ACTIVITY LEVEL	GOAL
Not Active = 1 point	Lose Weight = 1 point
Moderately Active = 2 points	Maintain Weight = 2 points
Very Active = 3 points	Gain Weight = 3 points

SCORE	RANGE
2	A
3	A or B (depending on goal)
4	B
5	B or C (depending on goal)
6	C

Activity Level + Goal = Score or Range

Choose your activity level and goal. Add the values of your selections to find what range listed below you should aim for as a daily caloric window. You can use the grams/day listed for Protein, Carbs, and Fats as general guidelines for your plate composition at meals.

Weight	Range A	Range B	Range C	30% Protein (grams/day)	45% Carbs (grams/day)	25% Fat (grams/day)
130	1430 - 1690	1820 - 2080	2080 - 2340	117 / 147 / 166	176 / 220 / 249	44 / 55 / 62
135	1485 - 1755	1890 - 2160	2160 - 2430	122 / 152 / 173	183 / 228 / 259	45 / 57 / 64
140	1540 - 1820	1960 - 2240	2240 - 2520	126 / 158 / 179	189 / 237 / 268	47 / 59 / 67
145	1595 - 1885	2030 - 2320	2320 - 2610	131 / 164 / 185	196 / 245 / 278	49 / 61 / 69
150	1650 - 1950	2100 - 2400	2400 - 2700	135 / 169 / 192	203 / 254 / 287	50 / 63 / 71
155	1705 - 2015	2170 - 2480	2480 - 2790	140 / 175 / 198	210 / 262 / 297	52 / 65 / 74
160	1760 - 2080	2240 - 2560	2560 - 2880	144 / 180 / 204	216 / 270 / 306	54 / 67 / 76
165	1815 - 2145	2310 - 2640	2640 - 2970	149 / 186 / 211	223 / 279 / 316	55 / 69 / 78
170	1870 - 2210	2380 - 2720	2720 - 3060	153 / 192 / 217	230 / 287 / 326	57 / 71 / 81
175	1925 - 2275	2450 - 2800	2800 - 3150	158 / 197 / 224	237 / 296 / 335	59 / 73 / 83
180	1980 - 2340	2520 - 2880	2880 - 3240	162 / 203 / 230	243 / 304 / 345	60 / 75 / 85
185	2035 - 2405	2590 - 2960	2960 - 3330	167 / 209 / 236	250 / 313 / 354	62 / 78 / 88
190	2090 - 2470	2660 - 3040	3040 - 3420	171 / 214 / 243	257 / 321 / 364	64 / 80 / 90
195	2145 - 2535	2730 - 3120	3120 - 3510	176 / 220 / 249	264 / 330 / 373	65 / 82 / 93
200	2200 - 2600	2800 - 3200	3200 - 3600	180 / 225 / 255	270 / 338 / 383	67 / 84 / 95
205	2255 - 2665	2870 - 3280	3280 - 3690	185 / 231 / 262	277 / 346 / 393	69 / 86 / 97
210	2310 - 2730	2940 - 3360	3360 - 3780	189 / 237 / 268	284 / 355 / 402	70 / 88 / 100
215	2365 - 2795	3010 - 3440	3440 - 3870	194 / 242 / 275	291 / 363 / 412	72 / 90 / 102
220	2420 - 2860	3080 - 3520	3520 - 3960	198 / 248 / 281	297 / 372 / 421	74 / 92 / 104
225	2475 - 2925	3150 - 3600	3600 - 4050	203 / 254 / 287	304 / 380 / 431	75 / 94 / 107
230	2530 - 2990	3220 - 3680	3680 - 4140	207 / 259 / 294	311 / 389 / 440	77 / 96 / 109
235	2585 - 3055	3290 - 3760	3760 - 4230	212 / 265 / 300	318 / 397 / 450	79 / 98 / 111
240	2640 - 3120	3360 - 3840	3840 - 4320	216 / 270 / 306	324 / 405 / 459	80 / 100 / 114
245	2695 - 3185	3430 - 3920	3920 - 4410	221 / 276 / 313	331 / 414 / 469	82 / 103 / 116
250	2750 - 3250	3500 - 4000	4000 - 4500	225 / 282 / 319	338 / 422 / 479	84 / 105 / 119
255	2805 - 3315	3570 - 4080	4080 - 4590	230 / 287 / 326	345 / 431 / 488	85 / 107 / 121
260	2860 - 3380	3640 - 4160	4160 - 4680	234 / 293 / 332	351 / 439 / 498	87 / 109 / 123

Figure 1–26. O2X caloric window calculator

2000 CALORIE MEAL PLAN

30% PROTEIN, 45% CARBS, 25% FAT

	BREAKFAST	LUNCH	DINNER
MONDAY	3 Eggs 1 Chicken Sausage 1/2 C Oatmeal 1 TBS Nut Butter 1 C Strawberries	6 Oz. Roasted Chicken 2 C Roasted Spaghetti Squash 1 C Roasted Broccoli	8 Oz. Slow Cooked Pulled Pork 1 C Basmati Rice 1 C Roasted Vegetable
TUESDAY	Protein Smoothie	6 Oz. Roasted Chicken 1 C Roasted Spaghetti Squash 1 C Roasted Vegetable	8 Oz. Carne Asada 1/2 Baked Potato 1/2 T Butter Salad with Avocado
WEDNESDAY	Breakfast Sandwich (3 Eggs, 2 Oz. Carne Asada, English Muffin) 1 Apple with 1 T PB	6 Oz. Sage Mustard Chicken Salad with Avocado	8 Oz. Grilled Salmon 1 C Apple Cinnamon Yams 10-15 Stalks Balsamic Asparagus
THURSDAY	Protein Smoothie	8 Oz. Slow Cooked Pulled Pork 1 Green Smoothie	8 Oz. Roasted Chicken 1/2 Baked Potato (1 T Butter, 1/4 C Salsa, 2 T 2% Greek Yogurt) 2 C Sauteed Peppers and Onions
FRIDAY	3 Eggs 1/2 C Oatmeal 1 TBS Nut Butter 1 C Strawberries	8 Oz. Carne Asada 1 Green Smoothie	9 Oz. Grilled Salmon 1 C Basmati Rice 10-15 Stalks Balsamic Asparagus
SATURDAY	3 Eggs 4 Slices Bacon 1 English Muffin 2 T PB 1 C Raspberries	3 oz. Turkey Breast 1 C Baby Spinach 1/4 Cup Dried Cranberries 1 Serving Feta Cheese 1 Serving Almonds Chopped	6 Oz. Sage Mustard Chicken Super Salad
SUNDAY	3 Eggs 4 Slices Bacon 1 English Muffin 2 T PB 1 C Blueberries	3 oz. Chicken Breast 1 Small Sweet Potato 1 C Broccoli	1 Encrusted Pork Chop 1 C Basmati Rice 1 C Roasted Vegetable

Figure 1–27. 2,000-calorie meal plan

2400 CALORIE MEAL PLAN

30% PROTEIN, 45% CARBS, 25% FAT

	BREAKFAST	LUNCH	PM SNACK	DINNER
MONDAY	3 Eggs 1 Chicken Sausage 1/2 C Oatmeal 1 TBS Nut Butter 1 C Strawberries	9 Oz. Roasted Chicken 2 C Roasted Spaghetti Squash 1 C Roasted Broccoli	5.3 Oz. 2% Fat Greek Yogurt	9 Oz. Slow Cooked Pulled Pork 1 C Basmati Rice 1 C Roasted Vegetable
TUESDAY	Creamy Protein Smoothie	9 Oz. Roasted Chicken 2 C Roasted Spaghetti Squash 1 C Roasted Vegetable	1 Oz. Roasted Salted Almonds 1 Medium Apple	8 Oz. Carne Asada 1/2 Baked Potato 1/2 T Butter Salad with Avocado
WEDNESDAY	Breakfast Sandwich (3 Eggs, 2 Oz. Carne Asada, English Muffin) 1 Apple with 1 T PB	9 Oz. Sage Mustard Chicken Salad with Avocado	2 Oz. Beef Jerky 1 Oz. Roasted Salted Cashews	8 Oz. Grilled Salmon 1 C Apple Cinnamon Yams 10-15 Stalks Balsamic Asparagus
THURSDAY	Creamy Protein Smoothie	9 Oz. Slow Cooked Pulled Pork 1 Green Smoothie	1 Oz. Roasted Salted Almonds 1 Medium Apple	8 Oz. Roasted Chicken 1/2 Baked Potato (1 T Butter, 1/4 C Salsa, 2 T 2% Greek Yogurt) 2 C Sauteed Peppers and Onions
FRIDAY	3 Eggs 1/2 C Oatmeal 1 TBS Nut Butter 1 C Strawberries	9 Oz. Carne Asada 1 Green Smoothie	5.3 Oz. 2% Fat Greek Yogurt	9 Oz. Grilled Salmon 1 C Basmati Rice 10-15 Stalks Balsamic Asparagus
SATURDAY	3 Eggs 4 Slices Bacon 1 English Muffin 2 T PB 1 C Raspberries	1 C of Soup 1 Can of Tuna 2 TBSP of Low-Fat Mayo 1 Whole Wheat Tortilla Tomato and Lettuce	Protein Bar	9 Oz. Sage Mustard Chicken Super Salad
SUNDAY	3 Eggs 4 Slices Bacon 1 English Muffin 2 T PB 1 C Blueberries	4 oz. Lean Hamburger Patty 1 C Baby Spinach 1 Whole Wheat Tortilla 1 Slice Cheese	1 Serving Greek Yogurt 1 Serving Fruit	9 Oz. Encrusted Pork Chops 1 C Basmati Rice 1 C Roasted Vegetable

Figure 1–28. 2,400-calorie meal plan

2000 & 2400 CALORIE FUELING MENU (CONT.)

1 SERVING OF PROTEIN

TIP: Choose lean protein

FISH	**POULTRY**	**BEANS**
3 oz Cod	3 oz Chicken Breast	1/2 c Beans
3 oz Flounder	3 oz Ground Turkey	(black, pinto, lima)
3 oz Halibut	3 oz Turkey Breast	1/2 c Edamame
3 oz Salmon	1.5 oz Turkey Jerky	1/2 c Lentils
3 oz Scallops		1/2 c Soy Milk
3 oz Shrimp		1/2 c Split peas
3 oz Tuna	**DAIRY/EGGS**	1 Tbs Nut Butter

BEEF/PORK

	DAIRY/EGGS
3 oz Beef	8 oz Milk
1.5 oz Beef Jerky	1/2 c Cottage Cheese
3 oz Beef Tenderloin	1/2 c Frozen Yogurt
3 oz London Broil	1/2 c Yogurt
3 oz Pork	1/2 c Greek Yogurt
3 oz Deli Roast Beef	2 Eggs
	4 Egg Whites
	1/4 c Egg Substitute

---

1 SERVING OF VEGETABLES

TIP: Strive for three colors on your plate

RED/PURPLE

Collards	Beets	**GREEN**
Green Beans	Cabbage	Arugula
Kale	Eggplant	Asparagus
Spinach	Radicchio	Broccoli
Zucchini	Radishes	Brussels Sprouts
Green Salad	Red Bell Pepper	Cucumber (raw)
		Cabbage

ORANGE/ YELLOW

Carrots	Red Chilies	**WHITE**
Pumpkin	Red Onion	Cabbage
Rutabagas	Rhubarb	Cauliflower
Yellow Beets	Tomato	Mushrooms
Yellow Squash	Tomato Sauce	Onions
		Turnips

---

1 SERVING OF FIBROUS FRUIT

TIP: Strive for three colors on your plate

RED	**BLUE/ PURPLE**	**ORANGE/ YELLOW**
Cherries	Blackberries	Apricots
Cranberries	Blueberries	Nectarine
Strawberries	Plums	
Raspberries	Purple Figs	
	Mixed Berries	
		GREEN
		Kiwi
WHITE	**MIXED**	Grapes
Apples	Dried Fruit	

Figure 1–29. 2,000- and 2,400-calorie fueling menus

1 SERVING OF CARBS/STARCH

TIP: Aim for 3g Fiber per serving

PASTA/RICE

1/4 c Quinoa
1/3 c Brown rice (cooked)
1/3 c Cous cous (cooked)
1/2 c Whole wheat pasta (cooked)

CEREAL

1/2 c Bran cereal
1/2 c Sugary wheat cereal
1/3 c Granola
1/2 c Whole grain cereal
3/4 c Rice or Corn cereal
1/2 c or 1 Packet oatmeal
1 Instant grits

BREAD

1 Slice whole wheat bread (ww)
1 Slice sourdough bread
1/2 Pita bread (6")
1/2 WW bagel
1/2 WW English Muffin
1/2 Sub bread (6")
1 Small WW roll
2 Corn tortillas (4")

SNACKS

1 Granola bar
2 Graham crackers
5 Wheat crackers
4 Wheat Melba toast
8 Animal crackers
3 c Popcorn
3/4 c Pretzels

PLANT

1 c Squash
1/2 c Peas (cooked)
1/2c Beans
1/2 Baked potato
1/2 c Black eyed peas
1/2 c Corn
1/2 c Sweet potato
1/2 c Mashed potatoes

1 SERVING OF SIMPLE FRUIT

TIP: Strive for three colors on your plate

RED

Blood Oranges
Grapefruit
Papaya
Pomegranate

BLUE/PURPLE

Grapes

WHITE

Banana

ORANGE/YELLOW

Cantaloupe
Mango
Orange
Papaya
Pineapple

MIXED

Fruit Salad
Fruit Cocktail

GREEN

Grapes
Honeydew Melon (cubed)

1 SERVING OF SIMPLE FATS

TIP: Strive for nuts, seeds, avocado, or olive oil daily

PLANT/NUT BASED (Choose more often)

2 tbs Flax seeds
3 tbs Hummus
2 tbs Seeds (pumpkin, sesame, sunflower)
3 tbs Guacamole
1 tbs Coconut oil
1 tbs MCT oil

1 tbs Nut butter
15 to 20 Nuts (almonds, pecans, walnuts)
1/3 Medium avocado
12 Large olives
1 tbs Plant oil (olive, canola, flax)
1 tbs Salad dressing

ANIMAL BASED (Choose less often)

1 tbs Butter (stick)
1 oz Cheese
1 Slice Cheese
2 tbs Cream Cheese
4 tbs Half & Half

Figure 1–30. 2,000- and 2,400-calorie fueling menus (continued)

Meat/Poultry/Seafood
△ Chicken breasts
△ Lean beef (filet)
△ Strip steak
△ Lean beef (patties)
△ Turkey cutlets
△ Eggs
△ White fish (e.g. Tilapia)
△ Salmon
△ Shrimp
△ Lean turkey breast
△ Turkey bacon
△ Pork cutlets (lean)
△ Canned chunk light tuna (in water)

Grains/Bread
△ Whole wheat bread/English muffin
△ Whole wheat tortilla
△ Whole wheat pizza dough (usually found in refrigerator aisle)
△ Oatmeal (whichever type you will eat and enjoy)
△ Brown rice
△ Cous Cous
△ Fiber cereal/granola
△ Whole wheat pasta

Vegetables
△ Sweet potatoes
△ Frozen mixed vegetables (high fiber, try to avoid peas, carrots and corn)
△ Romaine and Arugula lettuce
△ Baby spinach
△ Broccoli
△ Cauliflower
△ Cucumber
△ Tomato
△ Asparagus
△ Avocado
△ Chick peas (canned)
△ Fennel bulbs
△ Peppers (bell, poblano)
△ Scallions/Shallots
△ Black beans and white beans (canned is ok, used in recipes)
△ Garlic
△ Onion

Fruit
△ Frozen blend for smoothies
△ Fresh fruit that you enjoy (bananas, oranges, pears, peaches, nectarines, blueberries etc.)
△ Pomegranate juice (used in recipe)
△ Dried cranberries
△ Raisins
△ Lemon

Dairy/Dairy aisle
△ 1% milk
△ Cottage cheese
△ Greek yogurt
△ Almond milk
△ Cheese: feta, Swiss, mozzarella, cheddar,
△ Parmesan
△ Part-skim ricotta

Spices/Seasonings
△ Thyme
△ Sage
△ Salt
△ Pepper
△ Red pepper flakes
△ Cumin
△ Cilantro
△ Capers
△ Coriander seeds
△ Caraway seeds
△ Garlic powder

Nuts/Condiments
△ Salsa
△ Peanut butter
△ Olive oil (can be used when recipes call for canola oil)
△ Salad dressing (low/ no fat)
△ Balsamic vinegar/vinaigrette
△ Spicy/brown mustard
△ Almonds/Nuts you like
△ Tomato sauce
△ Tabasco sauce
△ Lemon juice
△ Low-fat mayo
△ Horseradish/horseradish spread (low fat, not cream-based)

Baking Aids
△ Chicken broth
△ Beef broth
△ Cornstarch
△ Cider vinegar
△ Bread crumbs
△ All-purpose flour (wheat preferred)

Supplements
△ Protein bars (minimum 20g protein, aim for less than 300 calories)
Protein powder (whey)
△ Healthy snack that you enjoy (for treats throughout the week)

Figure 1–31. Healthy choices grocery list

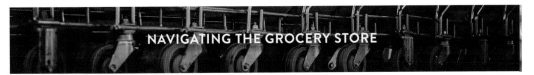

GENERAL TIPS

1. Don't go to the store hungry

2. Make a list based on your goals, meals, and snack planning

3. Focus on consuming the products around the perimeter of the grocery store

4. Aim for whole foods first

5. The fewer the ingredients listed on a nutrition label, generally, the better

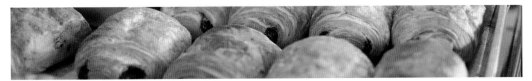

DAIRY AND EGGS

DAIRY: Excellent source of calcium and protein

MILK: Select fat content based on timing. 2% as a snack or meal; 1% after a workout

CHEESE: White cheese is generally lower in fat than yellow cheese.

YOGURT: Aim for yogurts with no or little added sugar. Greek Yogurt is loaded with protein.

EGGS: Excellent complete-protein. Yolks contain healthy cholesterol, fat and micronutrients. If you need to avoid yolks, egg whites or Eggbeaters are an alternative to whole eggs. Egg color is not important: white & brown eggs have the same nutritional value.

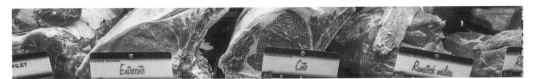

MEAT/SEAFOOD

MEAT: Excellent source of complete protein.

BEEF: is high in saturated fat & cholesterol compared to poultry and seafood

PORK: healthiest options are center cut loin roast, loin chops, and tenderloins.

Because of the high saturated fat and cholesterol, you should limit consumption of bacon, sausage, and ribs. Aim for 95% fat free deli-meats

FISH AND SHELLFISH Leanest meat sources and supply healthy omega-3 fatty acids.

POULTRY: Chicken & turkey are terrific, nutrient dense protein sources, with healthy fat levels. As a general rule, white meat is leaner than dark meat. Boneless, skinless, poultry is best for low fat content.

Generally: With all meat, you can leave on the skin while cooking to add flavor, and remove it while eating to limit fat intake. With ground meats - beef, turkey, chicken - aim for a lean:fat ratio of 90:10.

ALTERNATIVES: Soy-, tempeh-, and seitan-based are alternatives that provide protein with little to no saturated fat or cholesterol.

Figure 1–32.   Navigating the grocery store

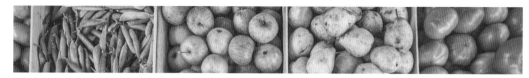

PRODUCE

FRUITS & VEGETABLES: Excellent source of dietary fiber, vitamins, minerals, and complex carbohydrates.

NUTRIENT DENSITY: Darker colors tend to be more nutrient dense than lighter colors. For example, spinach is more nutrient dense than iceberg lettuce.

SWEET POTATOES: Excellent source of complex carbohydrates with vitamins and minerals, especially potassium.

NUTS: Excellent source of fiber, fat and protein, and good for heart health.

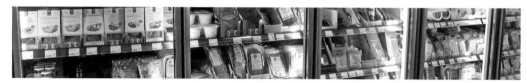

AISLES

RULE OF THUMB: Focus on "no sugar added" options.

BREADS/PASTA: Whole grain options are best. Aim for high fiber (at least 5g/serving) and whole grain options.

DRESSINGS & SAUCES: Often high in saturated fats and sugar, and high in added, non-essential ingredients such as salt & preservatives. Healthy options include oils, vinegar, and yellow or brown mustard.

NUTRITION LABELS: With all 'packaged' and 'wrapped' foods, always monitor the labels for sugars, trans fats, saturated fats, calories per serving, cholesterol, and sodium. These should be minimized, or avoided entirely.

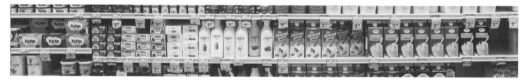

DESSERT/FROZEN

The bakery generally has higher quality ingredients than packaged desserts.

Aim for whole grain options.

For dessert, select low/no sugar added options.

Healthier choices include frozen yogurt, sherbet, and yogurt parfaits. There are 'no sugar added' ice creams available as well.

Frozen fruits and vegetables are still high in vitamins and minerals.

Look for frozen meals that have whole food ingredients and the least amount of sodium, fat, and preservatives.

Figure 1–33. Navigating the grocery store (continued)

BEST SNACKS FOR AVOIDING FOOD EMERGENCIES

The foods below can help you to avoid the five common pitfalls that tend to derail a healthy eating plan:

1. Lack of preparation
2. Skipping breakfast
3. Too busy to plan/prepare a meal
4. Peer pressure
5. Blood sugar crash

Keep these convenience foods in your house, car, gym bag, desk, etc., for when you have food emergencies. Most foods on this list can be purchased at any convenience store.

- Energy bars (aim for ≥ 20 grams of protein
- Raw nuts (recommended: almonds or cashews)
- Beef Jerky and Turkey Jerky (many natural ones available without MSG)
- Oranges/Apples
- Carrot sticks and celery
- Sliced peppers
- Yogurt
- Granola bars (Nature Valley is high in fiber)
- String cheese
- Kale snacks (many come with seasonings and are extremely tasty)
- Flax seed crackers
- Banana
- Hard cheeses
- Pumpkin seeds of sunflower seeds
- Rice cakes and nut butter/peanut butter
- Dried fruit and nuts/trail mix *be wary of portion sizes)
- Vacuum-packed tuna *snack-size portions)
- High-protein breakfast cereals (single serving cups are available)
- High-protein breakfast drink mixes
- Ready-made high-protein shakes (muscle milk, myoplex, svelte, etc.)
- Hard boiled eggs
- Freeze-dried fruits (not high in nutritional value, but low in calories if you are just craving a snack)

Figure 1–34. Best snacks for avoiding cravings

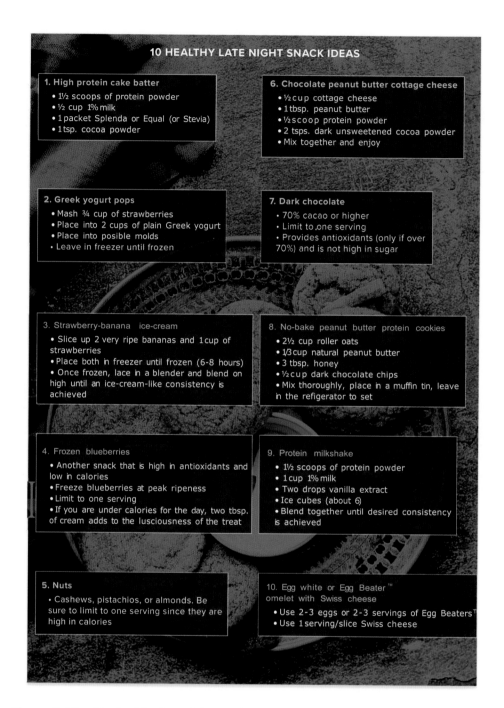

10 HEALTHY LATE NIGHT SNACK IDEAS

1. High protein cake batter
- 1½ scoops of protein powder
- ½ cup 1% milk
- 1 packet Splenda or Equal (or Stevia)
- 1 tsp. cocoa powder

6. Chocolate peanut butter cottage cheese
- ½ cup cottage cheese
- 1 tbsp. peanut butter
- ½ scoop protein powder
- 2 tsps. dark unsweetened cocoa powder
- Mix together and enjoy

2. Greek yogurt pops
- Mash ¾ cup of strawberries
- Place into 2 cups of plain Greek yogurt
- Place into posible molds
- Leave in freezer until frozen

7. Dark chocolate
- 70% cacao or higher
- Limit to one serving
- Provides antioxidants (only if over 70%) and is not high in sugar

3. Strawberry-banana ice-cream
- Slice up 2 very ripe bananas and 1 cup of strawberries
- Place both in freezer until frozen (6-8 hours)
- Once frozen, lace in a blender and blend on high until an ice-cream-like consistency is achieved

8. No-bake peanut butter protein cookies
- 2½ cup roller oats
- 1/3 cup natural peanut butter
- 3 tbsp. honey
- ½ cup dark chocolate chips
- Mix thoroughly, place in a muffin tin, leave in the refrigerator to set

4. Frozen blueberries
- Another snack that is high in antioxidants and low in calories
- Freeze blueberries at peak ripeness
- Limit to one serving
- If you are under calories for the day, two tbsp. of cream adds to the lusciousness of the treat

9. Protein milkshake
- 1½ scoops of protein powder
- 1 cup 1% milk
- Two drops vanilla extract
- Ice cubes (about 6)
- Blend together until desired consistency is achieved

5. Nuts
- Cashews, pistachios, or almonds. Be sure to limit to one serving since they are high in calories

10. Egg white or Egg Beater™ omelet with Swiss cheese
- Use 2-3 eggs or 2-3 servings of Egg Beaters™
- Use 1 serving/slice Swiss cheese

Figure 1–35. Ten healthy late night snacks

RECIPES

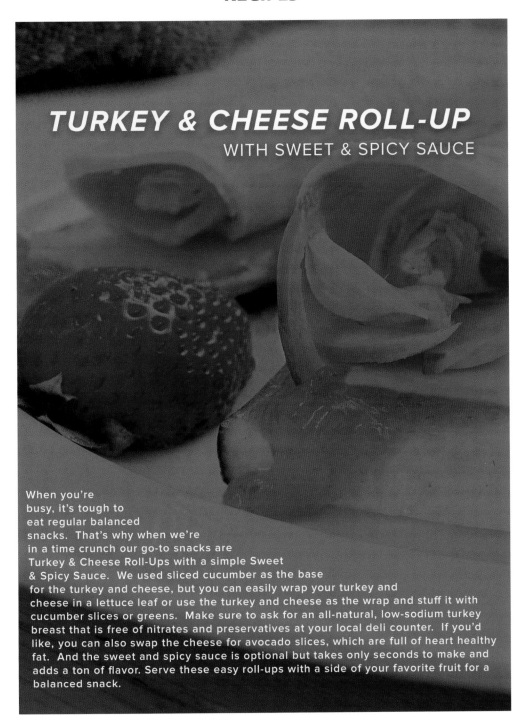

TURKEY & CHEESE ROLL-UP
WITH SWEET & SPICY SAUCE

When you're busy, it's tough to eat regular balanced snacks. That's why when we're in a time crunch our go-to snacks are Turkey & Cheese Roll-Ups with a simple Sweet & Spicy Sauce. We used sliced cucumber as the base for the turkey and cheese, but you can easily wrap your turkey and cheese in a lettuce leaf or use the turkey and cheese as the wrap and stuff it with cucumber slices or greens. Make sure to ask for an all-natural, low-sodium turkey breast that is free of nitrates and preservatives at your local deli counter. If you'd like, you can also swap the cheese for avocado slices, which are full of heart healthy fat. And the sweet and spicy sauce is optional but takes only seconds to make and adds a ton of flavor. Serve these easy roll-ups with a side of your favorite fruit for a balanced snack.

INGREDIENTS

Makes 1 serving

For the sauce:
• 1 tablespoon of apricot fruit spread
• ½ teaspoon Dijon mustard
• 3 drops of Sriracha sauce (depending on spice preference)

For the roll-ups:
• ½ cucumber sliced length-wise
• 3 ounces all-natural sliced turkey breast
• 1 slice of your favorite all-natural cheese
• 1 side of your favorite fruit

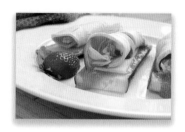

DIRECTIONS

1. In a very small bowl or dish, combine the apricot preserves and Dijon mustard. Add a drop or two of Sriracha sauce at a time until you achieve your desired heat level.

2. Roll up turkey, cheese, and sauce and layer them on the cucumber slices. Serve with your favorite fruit.

NUTRITION PER SERVING

Calories – 268
Fat – 11.1 grams
Saturated Fat – 5.5 grams
Polyunsaturated Fat – 0.4 grams
Monounsaturated Fat – 2.4 grams
Trans Fat – 0.3 grams
Cholesterol – 88.9 grams
Sodium – 338.6 mg
Potassium – 382.5 mg

Carbs – 15.9 grams
Fiber – 0.3 grams
Sugars- 10.5 grams
Protein – 26.3 grams
Vitamin A – 6.6%
Vitamin C – 12%
Calcium – 20.1%
Iron – 4.3%

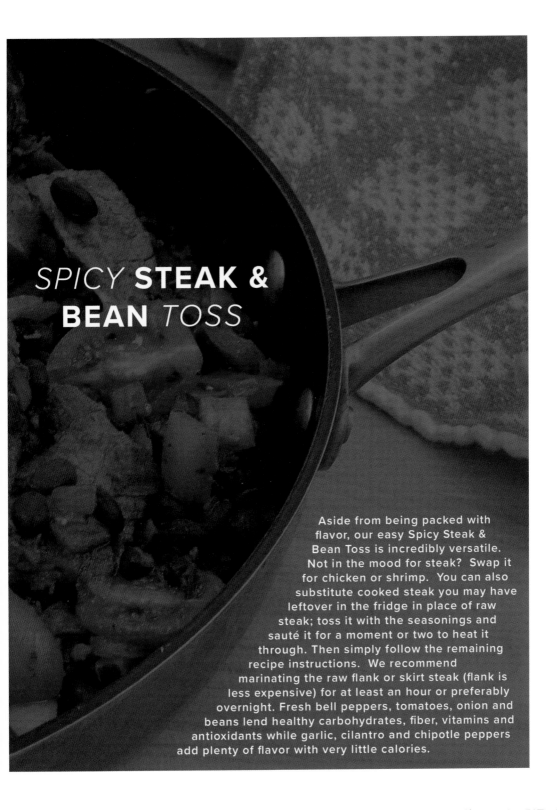

SPICY **STEAK &**
BEAN *TOSS*

Aside from being packed with flavor, our easy Spicy Steak & Bean Toss is incredibly versatile. Not in the mood for steak? Swap it for chicken or shrimp. You can also substitute cooked steak you may have leftover in the fridge in place of raw steak; toss it with the seasonings and sauté it for a moment or two to heat it through. Then simply follow the remaining recipe instructions. We recommend marinating the raw flank or skirt steak (flank is less expensive) for at least an hour or preferably overnight. Fresh bell peppers, tomatoes, onion and beans lend healthy carbohydrates, fiber, vitamins and antioxidants while garlic, cilantro and chipotle peppers add plenty of flavor with very little calories.

INGREDIENTS

Makes 6 servings

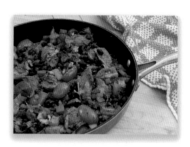

For the marinade:
- 1 lime
- 2 garlic cloves, finely minced
- 2 small handfuls of fresh cilantro, chopped
- 1 tablespoon of extra virgin olive oil
- ½ heaping teaspoon paprika
- ¼ teaspoon sea salt

For the steak:
- 1½ pounds raw flank or skirt steak, cut into three equal size pieces
- 1 bottle of all natural cooking spray
- 2 bell peppers, any color, washed and chopped
- 1 small onion, chopped
- 4 cloves garlic, finely minced
- 1 pint grape or cherry tomatoes, rinsed and halved
- 2 (15 ounce each) cans black beans, washed and drained
- 3 chipotle peppers in the can
- 1 pinch of sea salt

DIRECTIONS

Marinade:
1. Combine ingredients for the marinade in a small bowl.
2. Using your hands rub the marinade on the raw steak until coated and marinate for one hour or preferably overnight.
3. One hour before you're ready to start cooking, let the steak come to room temperature by leaving it on the countertop (steak at room temperature sears best!).
4. You can use that hour to prep and chop the remaining ingredients.

Steak:
1. Heat a large pan over medium heat.
2. Once the pan is hot, coat generously with cooking spray.
3. Let cooking spray get hot.
4. Sear steak in a large pan (pan sear in two batches if necessary to avoid overcrowding the pan) for approximately 3 to 4 minutes per side or until steak is medium rare.*
   * *You can also grill the steak instead of pan sear. Grill until medium rare.*
5. Set steak aside and let rest for 5 to 10 minutes.
6. Slice the steak thin against the grain into bite size pieces.
7. If you used a pan to heat or cook the steak, use that same pan (there is a lot of flavor in there!) and set to medium high heat.
8. Once hot, coat the pan generously with cooking spray.
9. Sauté peppers and onions until slightly charred, about 7 to 8 minutes.
10. Add fresh lime juice to the pan and scrape up the browned bits on the bottom (this is where the flavor is!).
11. Season with salt.
12. Add garlic and sauté an additional minute.
13. Add tomatoes, beans and chipotle peppers and heat through (approximately 3 to 4 minutes).
14. Add cooked steak and fresh chopped cilantro. Season to taste with salt and enjoy.

NUTRITION PER SERVING

Calories – 433
Fat – 14.1 grams
Saturated Fat – 4.7 grams
Polyunsaturated Fat – 0.5 grams
Monounsaturated Fat – 3.3 grams
Trans Fat – 0 grams
Cholesterol – 75 mg
Sodium – 464.4 mg
Potassium – 188.6 mg

Carbs – 33.5 grams
Fiber – 10 grams
Sugars- 10.2 grams
Protein – 36 grams
Vitamin A – 13.6%
Vitamin C – 64%
Calcium – 7.2%
Iron – 26.3%

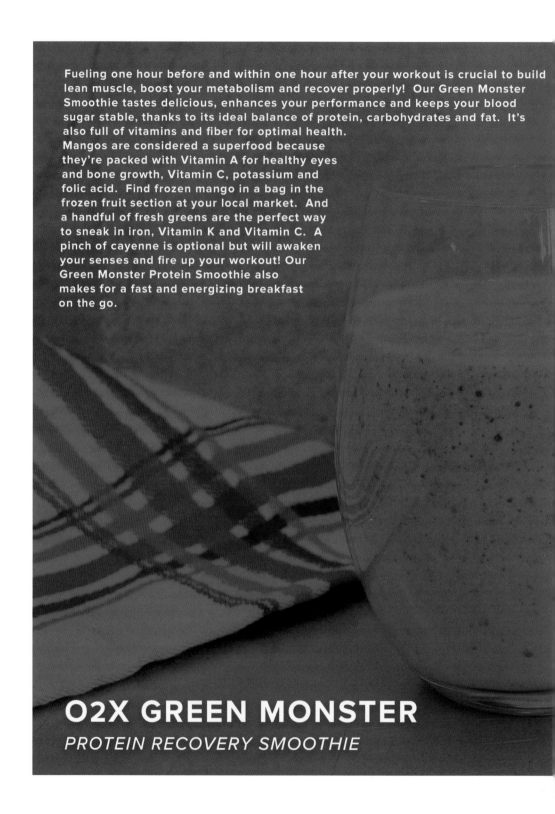

Fueling one hour before and within one hour after your workout is crucial to build lean muscle, boost your metabolism and recover properly! Our Green Monster Smoothie tastes delicious, enhances your performance and keeps your blood sugar stable, thanks to its ideal balance of protein, carbohydrates and fat. It's also full of vitamins and fiber for optimal health. Mangos are considered a superfood because they're packed with Vitamin A for healthy eyes and bone growth, Vitamin C, potassium and folic acid. Find frozen mango in a bag in the frozen fruit section at your local market. And a handful of fresh greens are the perfect way to sneak in iron, Vitamin K and Vitamin C. A pinch of cayenne is optional but will awaken your senses and fire up your workout! Our Green Monster Protein Smoothie also makes for a fast and energizing breakfast on the go.

O2X GREEN MONSTER
PROTEIN RECOVERY SMOOTHIE

INGREDIENTS

Makes 2 servings

- 2 servings of vanilla protein powder
- 2 ½ cups unsweetened coconut milk or almond milk
- 1 heaping cup of chopped frozen mango (if no mango, replace with ice
- 1 handful of spinach or kale
- ½ avocado
- ½ lime juice, freshly squeezed
- 1 pinch dried cayenne pepper (optional)

DIRECTIONS

1. Blend all of the ingredients together until smooth and creamy. If needed, add more ice.

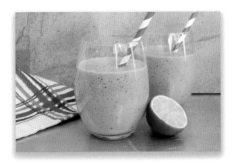

NUTRITION PER SERVING

Calories – 285
Fat – 10.2 grams
Saturated Fat – 2.5 grams
Polyunsaturated Fat – 2 grams
Monounsaturated Fat – 6 grams
Trans Fat – 0 grams
Cholesterol – 15 mg
Sodium – 244.6 mg
Potassium – 1039.1 mg

Carbs – 34.4 grams
Fiber – 8.1 grams
Sugars- 23 grams
Protein – 30.7 grams
Vitamin A – 52.7%
Vitamin C – 77.9%
Calcium – 73.1%
Iron – 12.9%

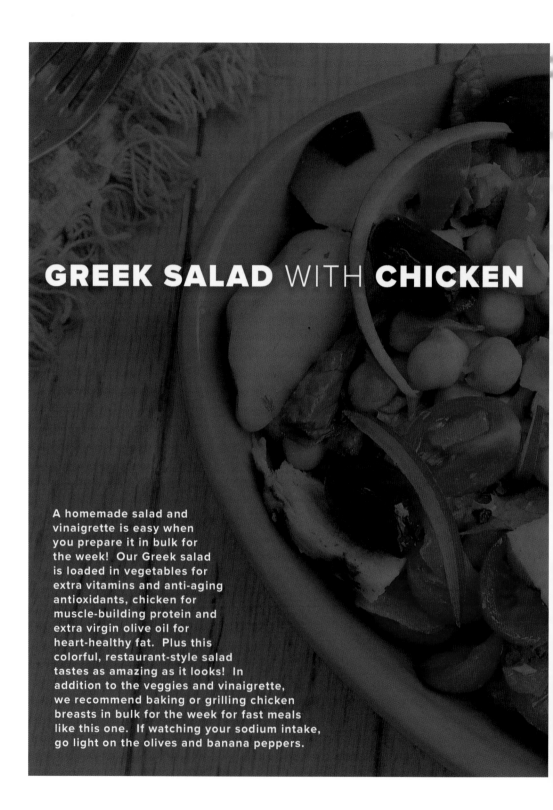

GREEK SALAD WITH CHICKEN

A homemade salad and vinaigrette is easy when you prepare it in bulk for the week! Our Greek salad is loaded in vegetables for extra vitamins and anti-aging antioxidants, chicken for muscle-building protein and extra virgin olive oil for heart-healthy fat. Plus this colorful, restaurant-style salad tastes as amazing as it looks! In addition to the veggies and vinaigrette, we recommend baking or grilling chicken breasts in bulk for the week for fast meals like this one. If watching your sodium intake, go light on the olives and banana peppers.

INGREDIENTS

Makes 5 servings

For the dressing:
- 3 tablespoons red wine vinegar
- ⅓ cup extra virgin olive oil
- 1 large garlic clove, finely minced
- 2 drops of honey
- 1 pinch of sea salt
- 1 pinch of ground black pepper

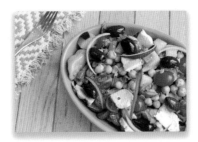

For the salad:
- 5 cooked chicken breasts, chopped or sliced
- 1 can of organic garbanzo beans (or chickpeas)
- 1 pint grape tomatoes, rinsed, dried and sliced in half
- 1 cucumber, chopped
- 1 carrot, peeled and grated on a cheese grater
- 1 small red onion, sliced thin
- 5 big handfuls of your favorite chopped greens
- ½ cup black olives (optional), for garnish
- 1 jar of banana peppers (optional), for garnish

DIRECTIONS

1. Pour red wine vinegar into a small bowl.
2. Slowly stream in the extra virgin olive oil while whisking constantly to form a vinaigrette.
3. Add minced garlic, a few drops of honey and season to taste with salt and pepper.
4. Set aside.
5. Toss all of the salad ingredients together.
6. If serving all five salads immediately, pour the dressing on top and toss to combine.
7. If saving the salad for lunches for the week, don't mix the salad with the dressing until ready to eat.

NUTRITION PER SERVING

Calories – 422
Fat – 19.6 grams
Saturated Fat – 3 grams
Polyunsaturated Fat – 2.8 grams
Monounsaturated Fat – 10 grams
Trans Fat – 0 grams
Cholesterol – 88 mg
Sodium – 459.3 mg
Potassium – 621.2 mg

Carbs – 23.3 grams
Fiber – 6.8 grams
Sugars- 6.5 grams
Protein – 37.8 grams
Vitamin A – 84.2%
Vitamin C – 12.5%
Calcium – 7.1%
Iron – 14.8%

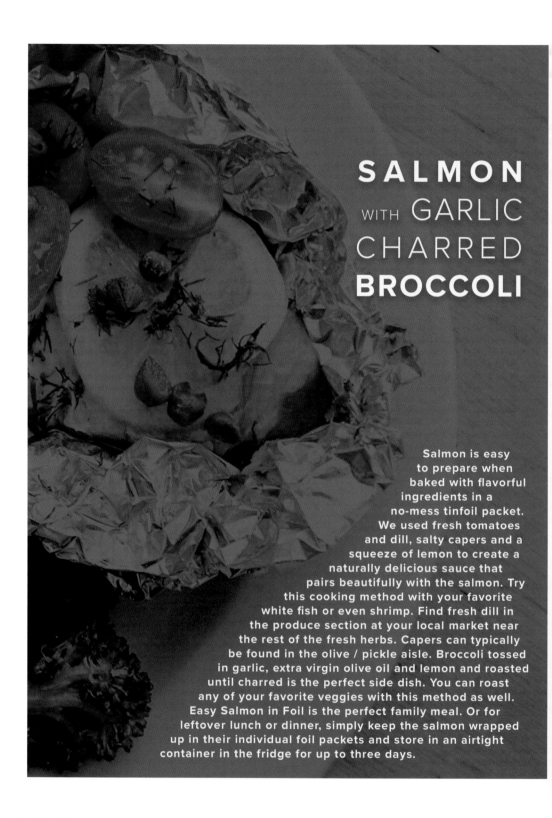

SALMON
WITH GARLIC
CHARRED
BROCCOLI

Salmon is easy to prepare when baked with flavorful ingredients in a no-mess tinfoil packet. We used fresh tomatoes and dill, salty capers and a squeeze of lemon to create a naturally delicious sauce that pairs beautifully with the salmon. Try this cooking method with your favorite white fish or even shrimp. Find fresh dill in the produce section at your local market near the rest of the fresh herbs. Capers can typically be found in the olive / pickle aisle. Broccoli tossed in garlic, extra virgin olive oil and lemon and roasted until charred is the perfect side dish. You can roast any of your favorite veggies with this method as well. Easy Salmon in Foil is the perfect family meal. Or for leftover lunch or dinner, simply keep the salmon wrapped up in their individual foil packets and store in an airtight container in the fridge for up to three days.

INGREDIENTS

Makes 5 servings

For the Garlic Charred Broccoli:
- 2 large heads of broccoli, chopped into florets
- 1 bottle extra virgin olive oil
- Juice from ½ lemon
- 4 garlic cloves, finely minced
- ¼ heaping teaspoon salt
- 1 pinch of fresh ground black pepper

For the Easy Salmon in Foil:
- 1½ pounds of salmon (ask for the skin to be removed and the salmon to be cut into 5 pieces)
- 1 pinch salt
- 1 lemon, halved
- 1 pint grape or cherry tomatoes, sliced in half
- 3 tablespoons chopped fresh dill
- ½ cup capers

DIRECTIONS

1. Preheat oven to 400 degrees.
2. Top a large sheet pan with tinfoil.
3. Toss broccoli with a big drizzle of extra virgin olive oil, lemon, garlic, salt and pepper.
4. Layer broccoli on the sheet pan and roast on the top rack for approximately 20 to 25 minutes or until charred, flipping broccoli half way through.
5. Keep a close eye on the broccoli to make sure it doesn't burn.
6. In the meantime, prepare the salmon.
7. Slice one half of the lemon into 5 slices.
8. Set aside.
9. Place one piece of salmon in the middle of a medium-sized piece of tinfoil.
10. Season the salmon with a touch of salt and the juice from the half of the lemon you didn't slice.
11. Top with one slice of lemon, grape tomatoes, fresh dill and capers.
12. Roll up the sides of the foil to form an air tight packet around the fish.
13. Continue with the remaining pieces of salmon.
14. Place the salmon foil packets on a large sheet pan.
15. Bake in the oven on the middle rack for approximately 20 to 22 minutes, or until salmon is cooked through and no longer translucent.
16. Serve salmon either in or out of the foil with broccoli.

NUTRITION PER SERVING

Calories – 351	Carbs – 11.8 grams
Fat – 20.5 grams	Fiber – 3.9 grams
Saturated Fat – 3.1 grams	Sugars- 2.7 grams
Polyunsaturated Fat – 0.8 grams	Protein – 33.1 grams
Monounsaturated Fat – 5.1 grams	Vitamin A – 42.5%
Trans Fat – 0 grams	Vitamin C – 219.7%
Cholesterol – 84 mg	Calcium – 8.6%
Sodium – 522.2 mg	Iron – 11%
Potassium – 1071.7 mg	

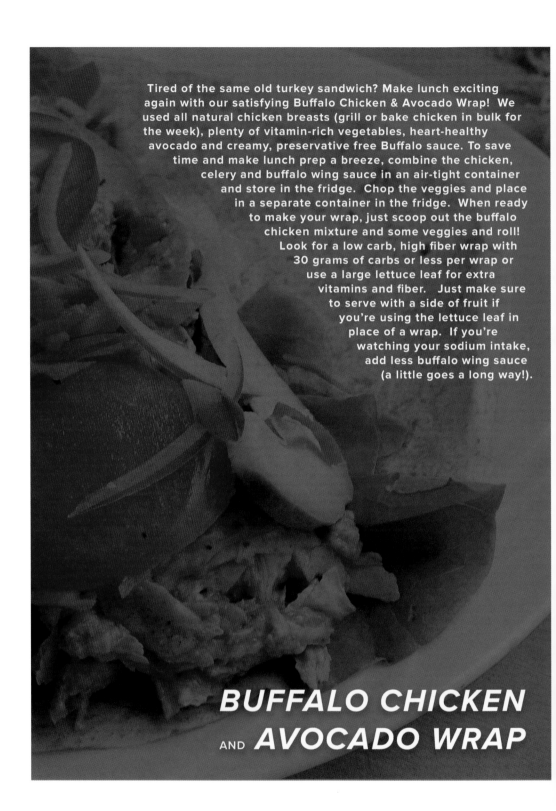

Tired of the same old turkey sandwich? Make lunch exciting again with our satisfying Buffalo Chicken & Avocado Wrap! We used all natural chicken breasts (grill or bake chicken in bulk for the week), plenty of vitamin-rich vegetables, heart-healthy avocado and creamy, preservative free Buffalo sauce. To save time and make lunch prep a breeze, combine the chicken, celery and buffalo wing sauce in an air-tight container and store in the fridge. Chop the veggies and place in a separate container in the fridge. When ready to make your wrap, just scoop out the buffalo chicken mixture and some veggies and roll! Look for a low carb, high fiber wrap with 30 grams of carbs or less per wrap or use a large lettuce leaf for extra vitamins and fiber. Just make sure to serve with a side of fruit if you're using the lettuce leaf in place of a wrap. If you're watching your sodium intake, add less buffalo wing sauce (a little goes a long way!).

BUFFALO CHICKEN
AND AVOCADO WRAP

INGREDIENTS

Makes 4 servings

- 4 large cooked chicken breasts, shredded or chopped
- ⅔ cup buffalo sauce
- 2 stalks celery plus a handful of celery leaves, chopped
- 4 low carb high fiber wraps or tortillas
- 2 handfuls of greens, like chopped romaine lettuce or spinach
- 1 tomato, sliced
- ½ small red onion, sliced thin
- 1 large carrot, peeled and grated
- 1 avocado, sliced

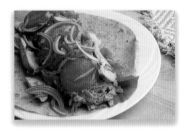

DIRECTIONS

1. Combine the shredded or chopped chicken breasts, Buffalo sauce and celery in a bowl.
2. Fill lettuce leaves with the buffalo chicken mixture or fill the wraps or tortillas with chopped greens and then the buffalo chicken mixture.
3. Layer the remaining ingredients (tomato through avocado) on top. Enjoy!

NUTRITION PER SERVING

Calories – 385
Fat – 13.5 grams
Saturated Fat – 2.5 grams
Polyunsaturated Fat – 1.1 grams
Monounsaturated Fat – 0 grams
Trans Fat – 0 grams
Cholesterol – 87.5 mg
Sodium – 1377.1 mg
Potassium – 263.9 mg

Carbs – 28.5 grams
Fiber – 16.6 grams
Sugars- 2.1 grams
Protein – 34.5 grams
Vitamin A – 83%
Vitamin C – 25%
Calcium – 9%
Iron – 11.4%

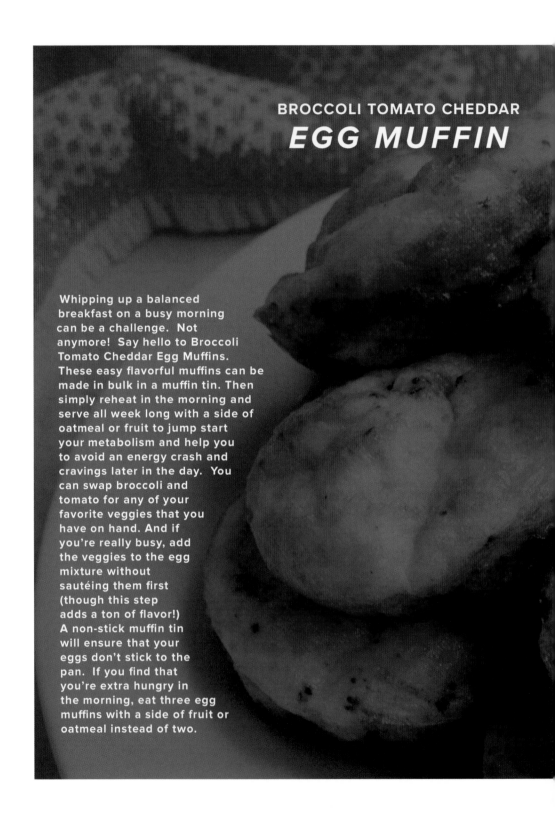

BROCCOLI TOMATO CHEDDAR
EGG MUFFIN

Whipping up a balanced breakfast on a busy morning can be a challenge. Not anymore! Say hello to Broccoli Tomato Cheddar Egg Muffins. These easy flavorful muffins can be made in bulk in a muffin tin. Then simply reheat in the morning and serve all week long with a side of oatmeal or fruit to jump start your metabolism and help you to avoid an energy crash and cravings later in the day. You can swap broccoli and tomato for any of your favorite veggies that you have on hand. And if you're really busy, add the veggies to the egg mixture without sautéing them first (though this step adds a ton of flavor!) A non-stick muffin tin will ensure that your eggs don't stick to the pan. If you find that you're extra hungry in the morning, eat three egg muffins with a side of fruit or oatmeal instead of two.

INGREDIENTS

Makes 12 egg muffins or 6 servings (2 muffins per serving)

- 1 drizzle of extra virgin olive oil
- 1½ cups frozen broccoli florets, defrosted and drained very well
- 1 tomato
- ½ onion, chopped
- 1 handful of fresh or dried thyme, basil, cilantro or parsley
- 1 garlic clove, minced or grated on a microplane
- 1 pinch of salt
- 1 pinch of pepper
- 12 extra large eggs
- all natural, propellant-free cooking spray (preferably organic)
- 1 heaping cup of shredded cheddar cheese

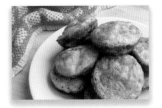

DIRECTIONS

1. Preheat the oven to 350 degrees. Generously coat a non-stick muffin tin with cooking spray.
2. Press the broccoli florets with paper towels or a clean dish towel to remove as much moisture as possible.
3. Chop florets very small and press again with paper towels or dish towel to remove any remaining moisture.
4. Cut the tomato in quarters, remove the seeds with your thumb and chop small.
5. Heat a large frying pan over medium high heat.
6. Once the pan is hot, add a drizzle of extra virgin olive oil and swirl to coat pan.
7. Once the oil is hot, add onion and herbs and sauté until onions are slightly softened (about 5 to 6 minutes).
8. Add the broccoli and sauté for about another 5 minutes.
9. Stir in tomato and garlic and sauté only one minute (you don't want the tomatoes to get mushy).
10. Season with salt and pepper and remove from heat.
11. Set aside 6 whole eggs.
12. With the remaining 6, crack the eggs, separate the yolks from the whites and save the yolks for another time.
13. Whisk together the egg whites plus the 6 whole eggs until combined.
14. Season with salt and pepper.
15. Gently stir the veggies into the whisked eggs.
16. Using a measuring cup, distribute the egg and veggie mixture evenly into the muffin tin.
17. Add shredded cheese to each egg muffin and press into the egg and veggie mixture with a spoon.
18. Bake at 350 degrees for approximately 18 to 20 minutes or until the eggs are set.
19. Broil for one minute until the cheese is slightly browned on top, if desired.
20. Store in the fridge in an airtight container for a fast breakfast all week long.
21. Serve with your favorite fruit or oatmeal for a balanced meal.

NUTRITION PER SERVING

Calories – 216
Fat – 14.1 grams
Saturated Fat – 6 grams
Polyunsaturated Fat – 0.3 grams
Monounsaturated Fat – 1.6 grams
Trans Fat – 0.2 grams
Cholesterol – 229.2 mg
Sodium – 341.4 mg
Potassium – 233.5 mg

Carbs – 4.3 grams
Fiber – 1.5 grams
Sugars- 1.5 grams
Protein – 16.2 grams
Vitamin A – 14.1%
Vitamin C – 46.6%
Calcium – 18.1%
Iron – 7.6%

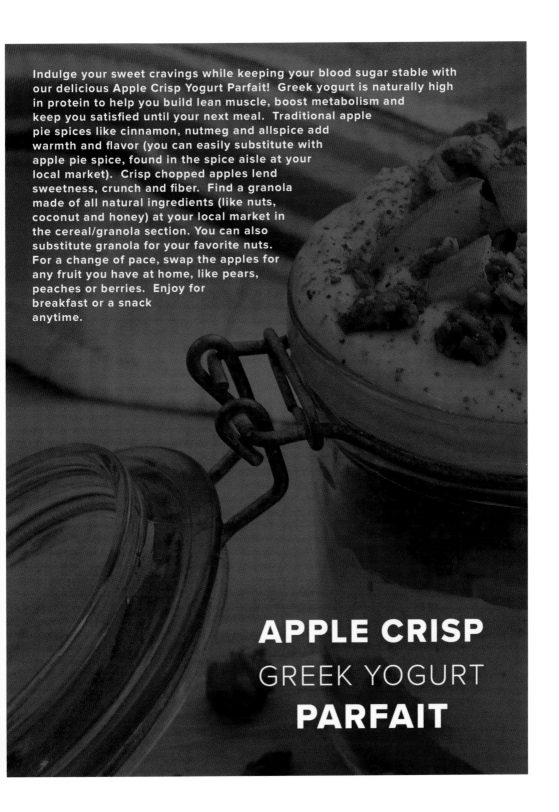

Indulge your sweet cravings while keeping your blood sugar stable with our delicious Apple Crisp Yogurt Parfait! Greek yogurt is naturally high in protein to help you build lean muscle, boost metabolism and keep you satisfied until your next meal. Traditional apple pie spices like cinnamon, nutmeg and allspice add warmth and flavor (you can easily substitute with apple pie spice, found in the spice aisle at your local market). Crisp chopped apples lend sweetness, crunch and fiber. Find a granola made of all natural ingredients (like nuts, coconut and honey) at your local market in the cereal/granola section. You can also substitute granola for your favorite nuts. For a change of pace, swap the apples for any fruit you have at home, like pears, peaches or berries. Enjoy for breakfast or a snack anytime.

APPLE CRISP
GREEK YOGURT
PARFAIT

INGREDIENTS

Makes 1 serving:

- 1 heaping cup of plain 1% or 2% Greek yogurt
- ½ teaspoon of pure vanilla extract
- 2 pinches cinnamon
- 1 pinch allspice
- 1 dash nutmeg
- 1 pinch of stevia for sweetener
- 1 apple, chopped (skin on)
- ⅓ cup of all natural granola, or your favorite nuts like pecans or walnuts

DIRECTIONS

1. Combine Greek yogurt, vanilla and spices.
2. Sweeten to taste with stevia.
3. Add additional spices, if desired.
4. Layer with chopped apple and granola or nuts. Enjoy!

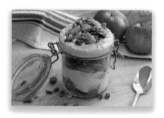

NUTRITION PER SERVING

Calories – 315	Carbs – 30.3 grams
Fat – 12.2 grams	Fiber – 4.3 grams
Saturated Fat – 7.2 grams	Sugars- 21.4 grams
Polyunsaturated Fat – 0 grams	Protein - 23.4 grams
Monounsaturated Fat – 0 grams	Vitamin A - 2.5%
Trans Fat – 0 grams	Vitamin C – 11.2%
Cholesterol – 18.8 mg	Calcium – 25.2%
Sodium – 101.7 mg	Iron - 3.4%
Potassium – 389.5 mg	

According to Duke University research, 45% of what people do is habitual. Five elements need to be in place:

1. **"A reason"** – You need a motive for changing behavior

2. **"A trigger"** – You must know what triggers your previous behavior. Without this understanding, your current trigger will lead into your old behavior without conscious thought on your part. Be as specific as possible when identifying your triggers. Try to note when you generally default to a negative reaction.

3. **"A micro-habit"** – Make sure your new habit "takes less than 60 seconds to implement." For nutrition, make sure it does not disrupt your day or routine too much. If it does, it will not be sustainable.

4. **"Effective practice"** – Break down your new habit/nutritional practice into small segments and practice each one for a few days or weeks (depending on how big of a change it is) before making it more substantial. This requires "repetition in a variety of circumstances." Sure it might work at the office, but does it work at home? Does it work on Tuesdays? Does it work on Saturdays and Sundays? Does it work during happy hour? Does it work on vacation? Does it work when you are stressed? What about when you are sick or sleep deprived? Keep repeating until you do not have to think about it, and your choices become commonplace.

5. **"A plan"**– Don't give up when you accidentally revert to an old habit of eating. Remember the saying "that's why pencils have erasers". Start fresh tomorrow (or at the next meal) by creating a plan that will work. Know your trigger, know you might not stick to the plan, know you can revise your plan and 'start fresh' at any meal or any day.

Work on creating plans so that you have a long-term (six month) plan with many short-term milestones.

The purpose of completing the 3-Day Recall is to determine the balance of caloric input and output. Caloric output is the number of calories your body "burns" daily for energy, and caloric input refers to the number of calories consumed. Providing your activity level below will aid in calculating the number of calories you burn from physical activity.

Please record the date and time of your activity. This should be done for three (3) days. Since food intake and physical activity often change over the course of the weekend, it would be best to have one (1) of the three (3) days recorded be one (1) weekend day.

DIRECTIONS FOR 3-DAY RECALL

To determine the amount of calories you consume, please record everything you have eaten over a three-day period.

1. Begin the food journal with documenting the time that you ate.

2. In the column labeled "Type of Food," record what food you ate. This includes any snack items or unconscious eating such as accepting a piece of candy from a friend. Please be specific in describing the food. For example, rather than writing down milk, please indicate whether it was whole, skim, 1%, 2%, or chocolate; or if you consumed bread, whether it was whole wheat, white, rye, etc. If necessary, break food items down into smaller groups. For instance, if you ate a turkey sandwich, write down wheat bread, turkey breast, American cheese, mustard, and lettuce. Also, include foods such as mayonnaise, salad dressing, butter, sugar, or salt. Remember to record beverages such as water, alcohol, coffee, tea, soda, and fruit juices.

3. In the column labeled "Amount," write the quantity of each food consumed. Try to do your best to approximate the serving amount.

4. In the column labeled "Method of Preparation," document how the food was cooked (e.g., frying, braising, grilling, microwaving, steamed, etc.). Please indicate the name of the restaurant if you ate out.

5. In the last two columns write down how hungry you were prior to eating (0 = not hungry to 5 = extremely hungry) and how full you were at the end of eating (0 = not full to 5 = extremely full).

3-DAY DIETARY RECALL FORM

DAY 1 RECALL: DATE____/____/____   **DAY OF THE WEEK:** _____

TIME	TYPE OF FOOD	AMOUNT	WHERE	PREPARATION	HUNGER (0-5)	FULLNESS (0-5)

DAY 1 ACTIVITY

TIME	TYPE OF ACTIVITY	DURATION	INTENSITY

Is this a typical day? Yes_____ No _____ If no, please describe why:

Please rate your energy level 0-5 (low-high):

DAY 2 RECALL: DATE ____ / ____ / ____   **DAY OF THE WEEK:** _____

TIME	TYPE OF FOOD	AMOUNT	WHERE	PREPARATION	HUNGER (0-5)	FULLNESS (0-5)

DAY 2 ACTIVITY

TIME	TYPE OF ACTIVITY	DURATION	INTENSITY

Is this a typical day? Yes _____ No _____ If no, please describe why:

Please rate your energy level 0-5 (low-high):

DAY 3 RECALL: DATE___/___/___   **DAY OF THE WEEK:** _____

TIME	TYPE OF FOOD	AMOUNT	WHERE	PREPARATION	HUNGER (0-5)	FULLNESS (0-5)

DAY 3 ACTIVITY

TIME	TYPE OF ACTIVITY	DURATION	INTENSITY

Is this a typical day? Yes_____ No_____ If no, please describe why:
Please rate your energy level 0-5 (low-high):

Part of this exercise is to create an individual challenge to 'change things up' for the next six months. You may have mastered your nutrition program, or you may not have made any sustainable changes, but there is always room for creating a goal to reach a new level of fitness.

Think of something that you would like to accomplish from a nutritional perspective in the next six months. Lose weight? Gain weight? Increase lean muscle? Eat more nutrient dense foods with the family? Avoid the weekend junk food binge? Use the worksheet below (and tips from the book) to create a main goal. We will then work together to break it up into several smaller goals that are easy to achieve.

If you are happy with your current nutrition program and do not wish to make any changes, please create a goal that can be incorporated into your daily life, on and off the job.

Step 1: List your **Overall Goal**. This goal needs to be attainable in the next six months.

_____

_____

Step 2: Break that goal down into six smaller milestones that you can achieve every 2-6 weeks. List them below:

• Milestone 1: Weeks 1-2

_____

_____

_____

    • What are you going to do to achieve this goal?

    _____

    _____

    _____

• Milestone 2: Weeks 2-4

_____

_____

    • What are you going to do to achieve this goal?

    _____

    _____

    _____

• Milestone 3: Weeks 4-6

_____

_____

_____

• What are you going to do to achieve this goal?

_____

_____

_____

• Milestone 4: Weeks 6-12

_____

_____

_____

• What are you going to do to achieve this goal?

_____

_____

_____

• Milestone 5: Weeks 12-18

_____

_____

_____

• What are you going to do to achieve this goal?

_____

_____

_____

• Milestone 6: Weeks 18-24

_____

_____

_____

• What are you going to do to achieve this goal?

_____

_____

_____

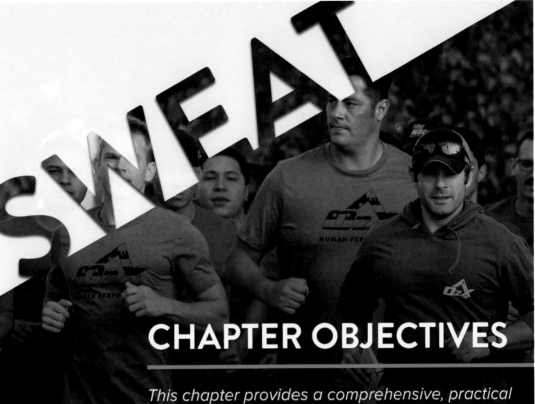

CHAPTER OBJECTIVES

This chapter provides a comprehensive, practical overview of strength and conditioning, with the perspective of maximizing conditioning and minimizing injuries for tactical athletes.
You will learn a number of key takeaways, including:

- Why training for performance is more effective than general fitness

- Why training for job specific performance will keep you healthier

- How properly calibrated stress will enhance your readiness

- How to maximize your conditioning gains through job-specific training

- How understanding pain will reduce your injuries and improve recovery

- Why proper warm up and cool down is essential to minimizing injury

- How to PREPARE and RECOVER to maximize longevity and durability

WELCOME TO SWEAT

This section is dedicated to helping you understand and incorporate performance training into your daily life and routine.

As I sit down to write this, I am reminded of a day in my own journey. I was finishing a tough session of working on my speed, strength, and endurance, and I was tired, sweaty, and ready for a shower and food. As I was walking out of the gym, someone stopped me to ask, "What are you training so hard for?" I looked up at them and replied, "Life."

I've been a strength and conditioning professional for almost 20 years now, but I'm also a practitioner. I've not only trained athletes, warriors, and first responders to achieve their goals, but I've also used myself as a guinea pig over the years. I do this because I love what I do; I love the science and theory of training and I love what it does for the people I work with. At the end of the day, physical training is about preparation. It's about preparing for life.

Life is a gift. And each of us has been given a calling to pursue within that gift.

For tactical athletes, their calling revolves around helping others, which is what some may say is the noblest cause of all. The gift of life does not come without challenges, however, and it is our job to be prepared to overcome obstacles so that we can fulfill our purpose of serving others. Preparation comes through targeted, well-planned training. It is not easy and it requires determination and hard work, but training is the only path to growth.

My hope for this chapter is that you will walk away with tools to improve your effectiveness in your calling. I hope that you'll see the importance of physical training and see that there is a difference between training for fitness and training for performance. I hope to open your eyes to the many different types of strength, endurance, and injury prevention. I want you to learn new ways to improve each of these physiological factors. In short, my goal is to help you view your own physical training differently and to help you take away techniques and theory to better improve yourself physically.

My ultimate goal is to give you the tools you'll need to help you achieve the calling of your life: to protect those that are unable to protect themselves. Happy learning and training!

—Mike Sanders, MA, CSCS, SOCOM Human
Performance Specialist, and O2X SWEAT
Specialist

INTRODUCTION

A tactical athlete is someone whose occupation includes a great deal of both mental *and* physical challenges. This chapter—SWEAT—focuses on the physical elements of training, exploring the scientific and practical elements of conditioning and how it helps keep tactical athletes healthy, and durable.

Proper conditioning will help you optimize your daily performance by keeping you strong, flexible, and prepared for unpredictable physical demands. *Proper* conditioning will also increase your daily job readiness and prolong your career by decreasing injuries, enhancing your metabolism, improving your sleep and mental health, and reducing the long-term effects of pain. In contrast, *poor* conditioning will lead to injuries and corrosive pain, and it will have negative ripple effects on your job performance, sleep, metabolism, and mental health. Accordingly, as a tactical athlete, proper conditioning habits will keep you safer, stronger, and more resilient so you can finish your career as strong as you started.

The foundational elements of a successful conditioning plan are (1) planning for your occupational and individualized needs, (2) conducting personal screenings and analyses to identify weaknesses, (3) calibrating stress and training levels to minimize injury, and (4) following the proven O2X PREPARE SWEAT RECOVER methodology. In this chapter, as in the previous one, we will begin with science, explain the foundational elements, and then provide you practical tools on injury prevention, pain management, alignment, and the importance of proper execution. First, let's consider a key concept in the proven, science-backed O2X approach for tactical athletes: training for general fitness versus training for performance.

> *Fitness*
> General health and wellness

Fitness and **performance**, although closely related, are not the same thing. *Fitness* should be thought of as overall, general physical ability attained through non-task-specific training programs (indoor cycling or boutique fitness classes, for example). This is not a criticism; someone engaging in a fitness program will improve his or her general health and well-being. However, we are aiming to do more here. This book is written for tactical athletes who must train to *perform* with specific goals in mind. For example, a firefighter who is tasked with moving injured people, wearing heavy bunker gear, dragging hoses, and lifting equipment needs to train specifically to *perform* those duties. Bottom line: job-specific training will reduce injury rates, improve productivity, and improve efficiency and morale.

> *Performance*
> Specific, task-related aptitude

One final, critical note on the tactical athletes trained by O2X, who are the subject of this book: they are asked to be perpetually ready, through their entire careers. *Tactical athletes do not have the luxury of an off-season or preseason training camp.* Firefighters, law enforcement officers, and military personnel, for example, must maintain perpetual readiness, 12 months per year—*for decades*—and any and every shift can be game day. This raises unique questions around sustainability, burnout, periodicity, injury prevention, and longevity. We will address these concerns for you in this chapter. First, let's examine a little physiology and science to help us understand the *why*, which will make the *what* and the *how* much easier to implement.

TISSUE AND MUSCLE TISSUE

Adaptation
The body's increase in its resistance to stress.[32]

To better understand conditioning, **adaptation**, and our bodies, we must first understand tissue and blood supply and how they impact adaptation. Tissue is, at the simplest level, a group or layer of cells that perform specific functions.[1] We have a vast range of tissue types in our bodies: bones, muscles, ligaments, tendons, nerves, bones, cartilage, and discs (fig. 2–1). Blood is, technically, also a tissue and plays a key role in adaptation.

COMMON TISSUES IN THE BODY

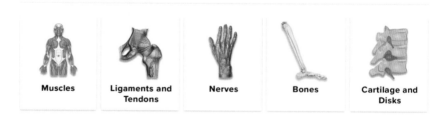

| Muscles | Ligaments and Tendons | Nerves | Bones | Cartilage and Disks |

Figure 2–1. Common tissues in the body

Let's start with the connection between blood supply and adaptation. Later, we will discuss how muscle tissue (or any tissue, for that matter) experiences stress, suffers microtraumas, and then adapts, emerging stronger through proper recovery (nutrition, hydration, and rest).

Next, let's consider that blood, and blood flow, is the transport vehicle for nutrients, hydration, and even hormones that promote cellular growth and recovery. Therefore, it follows that tissues with *ample* blood flow (e.g., muscle) can experience more significant adaptation gains than tissue with lower blood flow (e.g., cartilage, ligaments, and nerves).

Stated another way: blood supply is essentially a food-delivery service for recovering tissue. Why is this connection between blood supply and adaptation important? Because it helps us understand that (1) muscles have a very high capacity for strength adaptation (as compared with, say, ligaments, which play a secondary role) and therefore (2) conditioning our muscles to be strong (through gradual adaptation) is critical to reduce injury. Keep in mind that this very same blood-nutrient-muscle connection also plays a vital role in injury recovery as well. This will come into play later in the chapter.

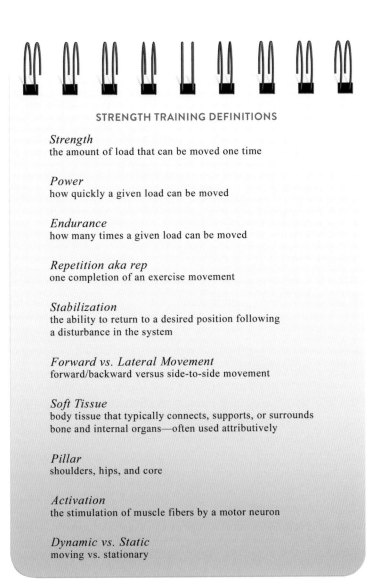

STRENGTH TRAINING DEFINITIONS

Strength
the amount of load that can be moved one time

Power
how quickly a given load can be moved

Endurance
how many times a given load can be moved

Repetition aka rep
one completion of an exercise movement

Stabilization
the ability to return to a desired position following a disturbance in the system

Forward vs. Lateral Movement
forward/backward versus side-to-side movement

Soft Tissue
body tissue that typically connects, supports, or surrounds bone and internal organs—often used attributively

Pillar
shoulders, hips, and core

Activation
the stimulation of muscle fibers by a motor neuron

Dynamic vs. Static
moving vs. stationary

Figure 2–2. Strength-training definitions

General Physiology of Conditioning

As discussed in the introduction, the range of physical demands on tactical athletes runs the gamut. A law enforcement officer, for example, may be required to chase a suspect for miles on foot, make life-and-death decisions under extreme stress, and then patiently investigate an active crime scene for hours. A firefighter may have to wait inside the firehouse for hours and then—on a moment's notice—rapidly climb a 60 ft ladder while wearing bunker gear, equipment, and a mask. For military personnel on deployments lasting several months or more, the range can be even more dramatic.

The possible situations are as infinite as the variety of physical demands that tactical athletes put on their bodies. To better understand how to prepare for these diverse physical demands, let's first study the basic scientific framework of our bodies' different energy and strength systems, taking a look at overall movement strategies and body structure.

Alignment
How the head, shoulders, spine, hips, knees, and ankles relate and line up with each other. Proper alignment of the body puts less stress on the spine and helps you have good posture.

Physiological Systems and Movement

As with our discussion of fueling, the car analogy remains relevant. Just as a car has mechanical, electrical, and fuel systems, so too do our bodies. And just as cars measure output in torque, horsepower, speed, and MPG, we have measurements for our strength and endurance systems. Finally, just as cars require balanced wheels and axles along with proper alignment to avoid accidents and uneven driving, we need to have bodily symmetry, balance, and **alignment** to minimize injury. With that said, let's look under the hood at our various physiological systems.

Intensity
The effort expended during a training session.[33]

Energy systems

As tactical athletes (in fact, as humans), we have a number of different energy systems. To begin understanding our energy system framework, let's first look at the controlling factors of intensity and duration.[2] Regarding intensity: on any given day, a tactical athlete may find himself working at maximum intensity (high-speed foot pursuit), moderate intensity (working a vehicle extrication), or minimum intensity (completing a long-distance foot patrol under a heavy ruck). Similarly, let's consider duration: the sprint of a high-speed foot pursuit will (and could only) last a matter of seconds, the extrication could continue intensely for 2–3 min. before requiring a break, and the foot patrol might go on for hours. Why is this important? The specific **intensity** and **duration** of an activity are the main factors determining which energy system our body uses.

Duration
The amount of time spent during exercise. Determining the ideal duration of exercise varies based on an individual's fitness goals and the intensity of a given exercise session.

In physiological terms (organized in fig. 2–3) we use our **immediate energy system** to perform activities of maximum intensity (90%–100%) and minimum duration. Next in line, we use our **anaerobic energy system** for activities of moderate to just under full intensity (75%–90%) that last a little longer (0.5–3 min.). Finally, we use our **aerobic energy system** for minimum-intensity activities, like walking or running slowly, that last longer than a few minutes.

Immediate Energy System
The short-duration, high-intensity energy system, also called the phosphagen system, that lasts about 5–10 sec. This system generates great power and speed but is not very efficient—like a high-end sports car.

ENERGY SYSTEMS

	Immediate Energy System (Phosphagen)	Anaerobic (Fast/Slow Glycolysis)	Aerobic (Oxidative)
Intensity	*100% - 90%*	*75% - 30%*	*30% - 20%*
Duration	*5 - 10 seconds*	*1 - 3 minutes*	*more than 3 minutes*
Work-Rest Ratio	*1:20 - 1:5*	*1:4 - 1:2*	*1:3 to none at all*

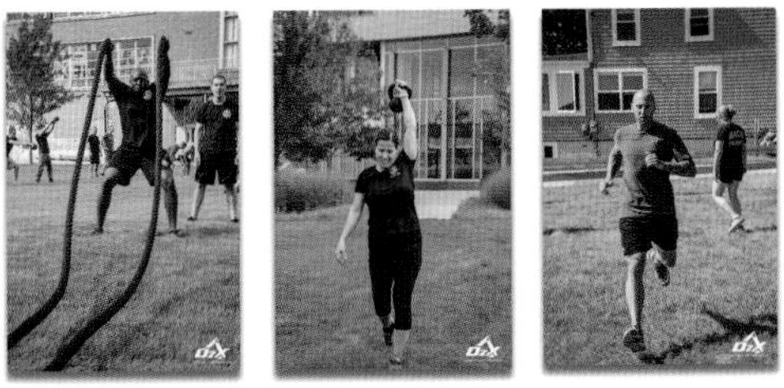

Figure 2–3. Energy systems

Why are we covering technical physiology? This deeper dive helps us understand why you may need a diverse conditioning program to (a) train your various energy systems so that you can (b) perform the various duties of your job safely and efficiently.

One more piece of helpful science: let's make the physiological connection between intensity and duration. Said another way, let's explain why we can only do the most intense activities (90%–100% effort) for a very short period of time (a few seconds) yet we can do the less intense activities for a much longer period (hours). The answer is fuel, and more specifically the *amount* of fuel we can store in our tank (i.e., our muscles and cells) for each energy system (fig. 2–4).

As you can see in the diagram, our immediate energy system (max intensity, on the left) requires a muscle fuel called **adenosine triphosphate (ATP)**. Bodies can only store a very small amount of ATP in our muscle cells, so we can only perform an intense activity for a few brief seconds before we need to rest and recover and let those energy levels replenish. At the other end of the spectrum, our aerobic (oxidative) energy system (minimal intensity, on the right) uses glycogen (simple sugar) and fatty acid (fat) as fuels. As we know, even the most fit among us have sugars and decent levels of fat in our bodies, allowing us to perform minimal-intensity activities for hours (maybe even days) on end. Bottom line: learning about these energy/fuel systems will help you understand how your body works, thereby improving your training and motivation.

Anaerobic Energy System
Also called fast/ slow glycolysis, this is not as fast as the immediate energy system but very capable of high performance.

Aerobic Energy System
The energy system, also called the oxidative system, that requires oxygen and is activated for long-duration, low-intensity exercise like walking or running slowly for an extended time.

ATP
The molecule within cells used for energy reactions.

ENERGY SYSTEMS AND FUEL SOURCE

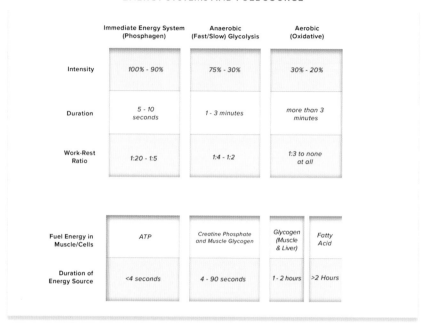

	Immediate Energy System (Phosphagen)	Anaerobic (Fast/Slow) Glycolysis	Aerobic (Oxidative)	
Intensity	100% - 90%	75% - 30%	30% - 20%	
Duration	5 - 10 seconds	1 - 3 minutes	more than 3 minutes	
Work-Rest Ratio	1:20 - 1:5	1:4 - 1:2	1:3 to none at all	
Fuel Energy in Muscle/Cells	ATP	Creatine Phosphate and Muscle Glycogen	Glycogen (Muscle & Liver)	Fatty Acid
Duration of Energy Source	<4 seconds	4 - 90 seconds	1 - 2 hours	>2 Hours

Figure 2–4. Energy systems and fuel source

KEY TAKEAWAYS

Energy Systems

◇ Work intensity and duration dictate the energy system required for specific tasks.

◇ Short-duration activities at max intensity tap into anaerobic energy systems.

◇ Long-duration activities at lower intensity levels use aerobic energy systems.

◇ Cells and muscles store different amounts of fuel used for each energy system.

◇ Understanding energy systems and fuel helps you determine an appropriate training program for performance.

Strength systems

As a concept, strength is defined as the body's "ability to exert force";[3] and developing strength goes hand in hand with energy system basics. The three general components of strength along the strength–endurance continuum are strength, power, and muscular endurance[4] (as detailed in the strength systems diagram, fig. 2–5). Each category helps us perform different tasks and, like energy systems, must be developed systematically.

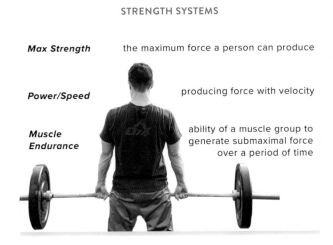

STRENGTH SYSTEMS

Max Strength   the maximum force a person can produce

Power/Speed   producing force with velocity

Muscle Endurance   ability of a muscle group to generate submaximal force over a period of time

Figure 2–5. Strength systems

When building **strength**, there are three types of movements you can incorporate into your routine: concentric (shortening), eccentric (lengthening), and isometric (holding). In practice, strength is helpful in lifting things, lowering things, and holding a position steady. Take the example of a pull-up. When you pull your body up, you are lifting and contracting your muscles concentrically. As you lower back down, you are yielding to the resistance with control, which is an eccentric movement. And if you hold your arm at 90 degrees and pause there, you are maintaining a static, or isometric, hold. Take a look at the second strength systems chart (fig. 2–6) to get a better understanding of the range of strength and endurance and their respective intensity and durations (i.e., in the form of repetitions).

You develop maximum strength by combining two physiological adaptations: increased muscle fiber diameter (**hypertrophy**) and increased neural recruitment of muscle fibers (central nervous system, CNS, development). Put simply, bigger muscles and the ability to use them. When you perform an activity that pushes you beyond homeostasis, two adaptations can occur. First, the muscle fibers increase their diameter, which in turn sets the stage for strength gains. Specifically, the fibers suffer microtrauma, and your body then sends out a signal (alarm response) in the area to repair the damaged tissue. The tissue is

Strength
The ability to exert force.

Hypertrophy
Enlargement of muscle fiber cross sectional area following training.[34]

repaired, your muscle fibers enlarge, and your body adapts, becoming more resistant to microtrauma[5] and therefore better equipped to handle future increased loads.

The second adaptation involves increasing *neural recruitment* of muscle fibers. Think of your muscle fibers as cylinders in a car: if you have an eight-cylinder engine but your electrical system is hitting only six of the spark plugs, then your car is utilizing (or recruiting) only 75% of its available power potential. A similar dynamic happens in your muscles. At the outset of training, your nerve fibers may be trained and configured to recruit power from only your larger muscle fibers. Through time and training, your nerves can learn to recruit power (i.e., neural recruitment) from more of your muscle fibers.

STRENGTH SYSTEMS CONT.

	Max Strength	Power	Endurance
Intensity	*100% - 85%*	*100% - 85%*	*Bodyweight - 70%*
Repetition Range	*1 - 5*	*1 - 5*	*10 to max*
Work-Rest Ratio	*1:20 to 1:5*	*1:20 to 1:5*	*1:2 to 1:3*
Example Exercises	• *Presses* • *Squats* • *Deadlifts*	• *Cleans* • *Jerks* • *Plyometrics*	• *Push Ups* • *Pull Ups*

Figure 2–6. Strength systems (continued)

Each of these adaptations can be trained with specific protocols that should both be included in any well-rounded program. Hypertrophy training is typically identified by moderate-intensity loading (67%–85% of 1RM, one-rep max) with moderate volume (6–12 reps for 3–6 sets) and limited recovery between sets (30–90 sec). CNS development involves higher-intensity loads (85% or more) lifted fewer times (<6 reps for 2–6 sets) but with greater rest between sets (2–5 min.).[6] While not mutually exclusive, meaning that adaptations in both size and neural recruitment can occur simultaneously and some training protocols do a decent job of targeting both, the above-listed assignments maximize the potential for adaptation in each.

Maximum strength is important for tactical athletes as their jobs often require moving tremendous loads. For firefighters, this could be lifting a down firefighter in gear out a window. A law enforcement officer may need to restrain a suspect who outweighs him by 100 lb. One effort, maximum force. Our next topic, power, is closely related to strength, but it includes one extra dimension: time.

Similar to strength, **power** is a measure of maximum effort, although power also factors in time. If strength is the amount you can lift, power is how fast you can lift it. To generate power, your body needs to refine the ability to quickly activate muscle fibers into a single explosive movement. For tactical athletes, this could be to swing an axe, take down a suspect, or jump up to climb over a wall—tasks that require great force to be applied quickly.

Power
The rapid development of force.

All tactical athletes require power, so developing it in programming is a must. Adaptations in power are most commonly trained with dynamic barbell movements (clean, snatch, jerk) and plyometrics (leaps, jumps, bounds, slams). As power is a function of CNS development, training protocols are very similar to those for maximum strength. The energy systems utilized to rapidly apply force are taxed best with high-intensity (85% or more of 1RM) low-volume (1–5 reps for 3–5 sets) movements with long recovery times between sets (2–5 min.). Remember that the goal of power and plyometric training is to cultivate the ability to develop force quickly, so repetitions should be executed with maximum energy; you get out of it what you put in. To be successful, a tactical athlete requires not only great strength but also the ability to use that strength to generate force quickly. Next we'll discuss how strength is applied over a much greater period of time.

Muscular Endurance
The ability to exert force over an extended time.[35]

The final piece of this puzzle is **muscular endurance**. As the name suggests, this concept also relates to the development of force, but specifically the body's ability to sustain that force over a longer period of time. For tactical athletes, these are the tasks like carrying tools and hose to the 20th floor of an apartment building or a lengthy infiltration under a heavy ruck—long slogs that require the strength to move under a load and the *endurance* to do it for a long time.

Like strength and power, there are specific protocols to best train endurance. Training muscular endurance is accomplished with relatively light loading (<67% of 1RM) at a high volume (12-plus reps for 2–3 sets) with little to no rest between sets (<30 sec). The key to individual success is to pair the requirements of your job with the design of your training. For example, the muscular endurance requirements for a truck company firefighter in New York City are vastly different from those of a smoke jumper in Wyoming, and their training programs should reflect those differences.

You can see that as a tactical athlete, you have unique and diverse strength training requirements. You need **strength** to lift heavy objects (picking up a patient), you need **power** to generate force quickly (manually breach a door), and you need **endurance** to operate under load for a long time (foot patrol in kit). Successful resistance training requires a balance among the three and a clear focus on job-related performance.

Again, it is worth asking: why are we learning this? The strength–endurance continuum (fig. 2–7) is an important physiological concept that allows you to understand and categorize the physical demands of your job, which will in turn allow you to design a specific program. Secondly, proper strength training increases stability, reduces overuse injuries, improves body composition, and lowers injury rates.[7] These benefits occur because strengthened bodies are prepared—thereby making us better able to perform—when impacted by outside resistance.

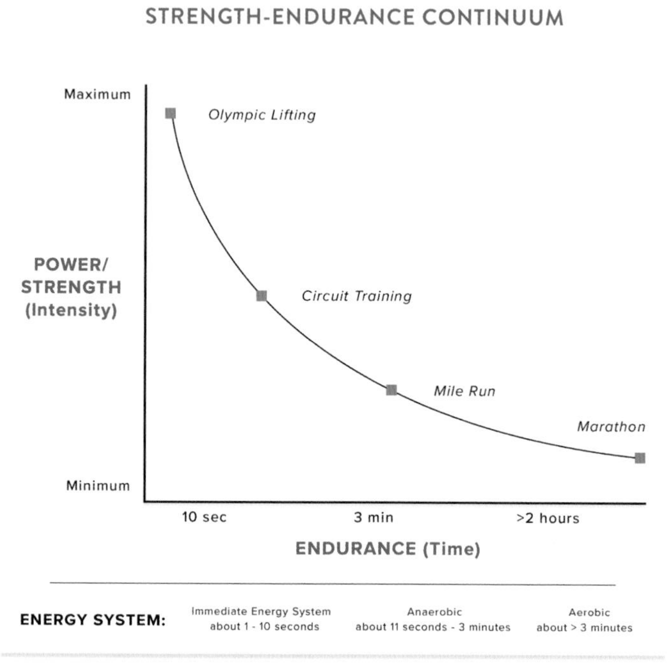

STRENGTH-ENDURANCE CONTINUUM

Figure 2–7.   Strength–endurance continuum

KEY TAKEAWAYS

Strength Systems

⬦ Strength is the body's ability to exert force.

⬦ Different types of strength fall along a strength–endurance continuum.

⬦ Resistance, repetitions, and intensity of movements determine which part of the strength–endurance continuum is targeted by exercise.

⬦ You need strength, power, and endurance for your job as a tactical athlete.

Adaptation

Now that we have a better understanding of our energy and strength systems, let's examine how working out results in physical conditioning gains. Here's a hint: the body is an expert when it comes to adapting and making incremental gains when faced with stress and adversity.

Good stress vs. bad stress

While "stress" usually has negative connotations, not all stress is bad for us (fig. 2–8). In fact, some levels of stress are *necessary* to heighten our mental and physical acuity in the face of adversity. Stress on our muscle tissue and the resulting incremental adaptation gains allow our physiological systems to grow. For example, lifting weights stresses our muscles and leads to strength, and sprinting stresses the heart and leads to cardiovascular gains. This good stress is called **eustress**.

Eustress
A constructive amount of stress that can lead to positive growth and adaptation. It does not become overwhelming and detrimental like distress. Instead, it is a form of good stress that promotes growth.

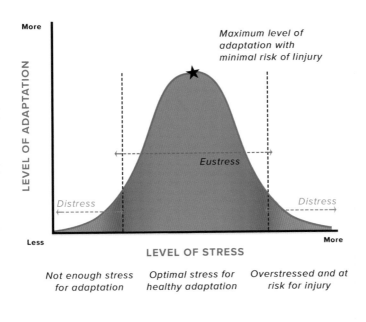

Figure 2–8. Stress vs. physical adaptation

Distress, on the other hand, occurs when we experience more frequent or extreme levels of stress and our bodies and minds get overloaded. In some cases, we may experience burnout and persistent fatigue for a few days. In more severe cases when distress continues and accumulates over an extended period, we may suffer a physical or mental breakdown—or both.[8] Physical signs of distress that accumulate over time include exhaustion, injury, pain, and muscle degradation. Alternatively, eustress can be anything that stimulates the body to adapt positively.[9]

Homeostasis

Another important concept behind understanding adaptation is **homeostasis**, which is the body's tendency to seek and maintain equilibrium in our physiological systems. A terrific example is body temperature: no matter the external circumstances, our bodies work (i.e., adapt) to maintain an internal temperature of 98.6°F. For example, when our bodies are stressed by being in a warmer environment, they generate sweat to cool us off. And when our bodies are stressed by being exposed to a colder environment, they shiver to generate warmth. This is an example of our bodies adapting to maintain equilibrium when the homeostatic condition is challenged.[10]

One final thought on homeostasis, adaptation, and burnout: our bodies like consistent, balanced internal states. Adaptation is our bodies' protective response to remain balanced. That's why stress that pushes us out of homeostatic equilibrium is usually uncomfortable; our bodies are uncomfortable being outside homeostasis. Listening to your body is critical, as you should be able to assess whether the stress you are enduring is creating a positive adaptation (eustress) or having decremental effects (distress). If you are able to identify distress in the early stages, you can prevent yourself from entering a chronic state of both physical and mental burnout.

General adaptation syndrome

As we started to discuss above, we must seek out challenges that trigger eustress to push the body to adapt into a better version: stronger, smarter, and more resilient. Let's look at the smallest, quickest example of this. Our bodies react to a physical challenge (e.g., lifting a 300 lb barbell) by adapting and preparing for a returning challenge. That way, when we encounter that challenge for a second time, our bodies are better prepared to deal with it efficiently and with less negative effects. You can then increase the challenge load (e.g., lifting a 315 lb barbell) and make incremental gains over time.

This concept of growth and adaptation was labeled general adaptation syndrome, or GAS, and was scientifically documented in the 1950s by a pioneering endocrinologist, Dr. Hans Selye. His GAS theory outlines three stages of how people deal with and adapt to stressors (fig. 2–10).

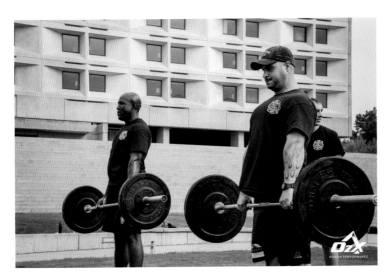

Figure 2–9. Adapting to stressors

The following explanation of each stage applies Selye's theory to conditioning, (i.e., physical training):[11]

1. **Alarm Reaction:** The demands of a workout push the homeostatic condition. To compensate, the body relies on lean mass (muscle) and energy stores (liver and muscle glycogen) to sustain function. In turn, this triggers secretion of stress hormones such as cortisol. Cortisol may trigger the body to break down muscle tissue, also known as a catabolic response (vs. an anabolic response, which is building up muscle tissue).

2. **Resistance:** The body begins to repair the damage caused by overload placed on the tissues; *muscles adapt*, and energy is restored. Stated again, incremental adaptations lead to incremental gains. Over time, these incremental adaptations accumulate and bring about increased strength.

3. **Supercompensation:** When training is well designed with the proper nutrition and rest to support positive adaptation, the body will begin to adjust to a new, improved normal state. Athletes become bigger, faster, and stronger as a result of their bodies' reactions to stress. This is known as supercompensation and is the goal of training.

   or

   Exhaustion: When work and stress levels are too high, hard, or frequent and you do not allow for sufficient rest and recovery, performance drops. This may lead to overload, burnout, or adrenal fatigue. Overall health may suffer, injury rates may increase, stagnation sets in, and you may have a *decrease* in performance. In short, stress does in fact become negative at this stage.

To put this concept in more relatable terms, think of doing manual labor around your house. Maybe you had to cut, split, and stack firewood. You woke up sore the next day thinking, "Wow, I worked muscles yesterday I've never used before." In reality, you may have used those muscles before, but just not recently and under such high stress. The resulting soreness is your body's adaptation against the challenge to its homeostasis.[12] Specifically, your body was not familiar with providing nutrients for such intense work, and the muscles were not strong enough to support such intense work. Therefore, your body triggered an alarm response, releasing energy stores (anabolic response in fig. 2–10) to fuel the repair effort. Finally, the pain that you feel the next day is a result of microtrauma on the muscles that you used and also your body's attempt to repair and strengthen those muscles. Bottom line: our bodies are amazing at adaptation in the right conditions. If pushed through a challenge, we will adapt, and our performance will improve.[13]

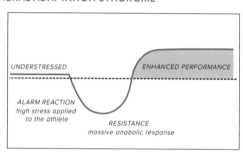

GENERAL ADAPTATION SYNDROME

PROPERLY STRESSED

The correct aplication of high-grade stress causing an alarm reaction and hormonal release within the athlete. This then signals a massive resistance stage response, leading to positive adaptation.

UNDERSTRESSED

ENHANCED PERFORMANCE

ALARM REACTION
high stress applied
to the athlete

RESISTANCE
massive anabolic response

Figure 2–10. General adaptation syndrome

Training for *maximum* adaptation has three primary components: determining the needs and demands of your job, tailoring a specific conditioning program to meet those needs, and implementing proper rest and recovery techniques. We will address these three key components next.

Calibration Levels that Maximize Adaptation

Day-to-day, short-term calibration

On a day-to-day level, we need to make sure our repetitions (reps) and workouts are strenuous enough to induce a positive adaptation. Thinking back to the GAS: the first requirement of adaptation is to trigger an alarm reaction. Undertraining is insufficient to generate any positive adaptation. Properly stressing and training is optimal and generates positive, *incremental* adaptation, which in turn sets a new, higher level of homeostasis. This prepares us positively for the next time we face the same stress and is an incremental building block. Finally, overtraining for an extended period of time without proper recovery leads to negative adaptation *decrements*, setting us back in our development. The following three examples (fig. 2–11) illustrate what happens when you (in order): undertrain, properly train, or overtrain.

3 ADAPTATION SCENARIOS

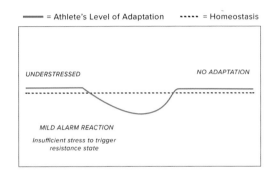

UNDERTRAINED/ UNDERSTRESSED

Low-grade stress that produces a mild alarm reaction response. This response does not result in any positive adaptation because the stimuli were not enough to disrupt the athlete's homeostatic balance.

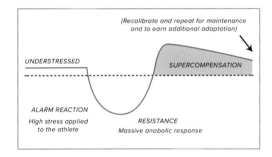

PROPERLY STRESSED

The correct application of high-grade stress causing an alarm reaction and hormonal release within the athlete. This then signals a massive resistance stage response, leading to positive adaptation.

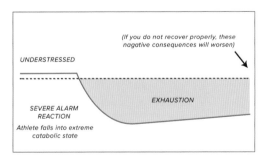

OVERTRAINED/ OVERSTRESSED

Too much stress leading to a severe alarm reaction that pushes the athlete into an extreme catabolic state meaning exhaustion, slow recovery, and loss of positive adaptation, thus decreased performance.

Figure 2–11. Three adaptation scenarios

Longer-term calibration

As a tactical athlete, you have no off-season and are expected to sustain high levels of performance for decades. Unlike a professional sport cycle, there is no preseason training time allotted to prepare and no postseason to rest and recover from the previous season. As a result, you need to learn how to adjust to your ongoing schedule and develop a performance plan designed with career longevity in mind.

Because of that, there are two important training-calibration symptoms to watch for in your training and in your actual work demands: **overreaching** and **overtraining**. Overreaching is training to a point of fatigue that results in short-term performance losses (decrements) and mental and physical fatigue that may last for days, or even several weeks. However, if you take adequate time to recover from overreaching, you can enjoy delayed training gains because you'll be giving your muscle tissue time to recover and your depleted energy levels time to replenish, and both can recover above and beyond previous levels.

Overtraining, on the other hand, is when you put yourself through extended instances and periods of overreaching without allowing for proper recovery time. When this happens, usually over the course of a few months or even years, the stress of workouts from which you haven't recovered accumulate, and the body never has a chance to build itself back up to prepare for the next workout. This pushes the body into a state of deep fatigue.

KEY TAKEAWAYS

Calibration Variables that Affect Adaptation

◇ Day to day, your workouts need to generate enough stress to provoke and stimulate an alarm reaction. Simply: you need to push yourself enough to "make a difference" but not so much to cause injury.

◇ The resistance phase leads to supercompensation (good) or exhaustion (bad) dependent on quality of training programming, rest, and nutrition.

◇ Be mindful of experiencing any long-term fatigue. If this builds up or accumulates for weeks or months without proper recovery, you can suffer a breakdown: physically or mentally, or both.

Bottom line: recovery and calibration is extremely important to adaptation gains.

Recovery Variables that Maximize Performance

Maximizing conditioning requires attention in the planning stages of programming (a needs analysis, specific design), during your actual workouts (proper calibration), and after each workout (optimal recovery). Specifically, proper nutrition, sleep, rest, and various forms of therapy can help tactical athletes get the hard-earned benefit from their workouts.

Nutrition

As we covered in the first chapter, just as your car needs fuel to run, the body also needs food and hydration to perform. It takes some time to learn how to eat properly. Energy is only restored if you have eaten and hydrated enough to replenish what you expended during your last workout, working fire, or gunfight. Rather than repeat everything in the last chapter, just remember that if are looking for results from a conditioning program, then you need the right fuel to see the full gains and benefits of your effort. Eating the right things, in the right amounts, at the right time (quality, quantity, and timing) will do that for you.

Rest and recovery

In addition to nutrition, physical rest and recovery are also essential to maximizing the benefits of your workouts (fig. 2–12). Consider this important fact: you do not get stronger *during* a workout. It is only *after* a workout that you can see gains or adaptation. As you work out, you use energy (stored fuel) to support your efforts, then fatigue sets in and your performance begins to decline. This happens because when the body realizes fuel levels are diminishing, it will restrict how much power or speed you can generate. Therefore, if you're working out effectively, you get tired at the end of a set or a run and cannot lift as much or run as fast. This is our bodies' way of maintaining homeostasis. Consider this a workout at the cellular level; your muscle fibers are being exhausted to the point of failure. The only way for your muscles to get *stronger* from that particular workout is for them to rest and recover *afterward*. In the next chapter, THRIVE, we will spend more time on the specifics of sleep and recovery and how to optimize them.

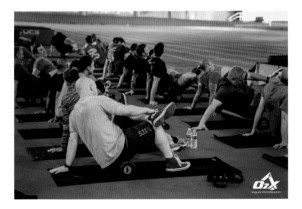

Figure 2–12. Foam roll

Therapeutic modalities

In addition to sleep and nutrition, there are a number of recovery methods, or **therapeutic modalities**, you can employ to optimize and accelerate recovery. There are a great number of different theories and products with varying degrees of scientific data to support their efficacy. Consistent benefits have been found with figure 2–13.

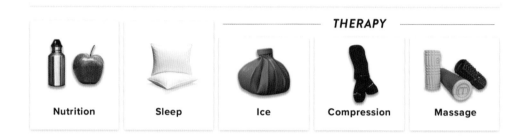

Figure 2–13. Recovery methods

Ice baths

Cool water to about 55°F–60°F and submerge the affected limb or limbs for 15–20 min. once or several times per day.[14] This relieves inflammation, constricts your blood vessels, and it simply feels refreshing.

Compression garments worn post-exercise

Stockings, tights, and armbands that deliver compression (about 10–30 mmHg) aid in preventing post-exercise muscle soreness and swelling while decreasing time to recovery. Be careful to replace compression garments frequently—after several washings, a 10–20 mmHg garment will lose its ability to compress effectively.[15]

Sports massage/foam rolling

Manipulation of the affected muscle post-exercise with massage or foam rolling can make the muscle *feel* better. There are no consistent data to support that massage or foam rolling will enhance performance during subsequent exercise sessions, as compared to no massage/foam rolling, but athletes report feeling better when massage therapy was used post-exercise.[16]

PRIORITY: NEEDS ANALYSIS—MATT CADY

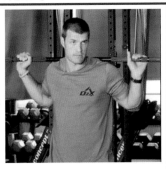

During my tenure as a Tactical Human Performance Specialist I had the pleasure to train Special Forces Operators. I had an operator come to me stating that he wanted to gain muscle mass and improve his strength but was having difficulty. He said that he had also been having problems sleeping and that in general he just felt tired all the time.

We started discussing his lifestyle, training, and nutrition. He was running about 50–70 miles per week, lived a vegetarian lifestyle, and had a high-stress job as a Green Beret. The vocation he chose and his work schedule were variables that could not be adjusted, so we focused on his training and nutrition. The two challenges we faced in designing a program that would work with his schedule were his lifestyle as a vegetarian and the distance he ran each week. Gaining muscle as a vegetarian and an endurance athlete is challenging. His program was designed to include foods that would provide adequate amounts of protein and macronutrients as well as workouts that would properly train him for strength and mass gains.

Because this operator was a natural runner, the biggest hurdle I faced was helping him understand and be willing to lower the mileage he was running each week. We had to discuss muscle physiology, muscle fiber types, and how the body needs rest and recovery in order to gain strength and mass. Based on his goals of gaining muscle mass and strength we discussed the importance of training the energy systems of his body differently. One change we identified was for him to increase his caloric intake by consuming more protein-dense foods. We also discussed the importance of spacing out his food intake throughout the day, ideally eating protein every 2–3 hours.

The process was slow because these were some drastic lifestyle changes for him. After 6–12 months we had changed his running regime to predominately shorter sprints and high-intensity interval training with only one or two 5-mile runs per week. His weight training workouts evolved from basic push-ups and sit-ups to more advanced techniques. These techniques included strength lifts such as bench, squat, and deadlift; Olympic lifts such as cleans and snatches; and plyometric exercises.

As we progressed through his new training regimen, he saw improvements in his strength numbers, overall body composition, and explosiveness. An example of his strength gains is his ability to bench-press. When we first began training he was able to bench-press 50 lb dumbbells for five repetitions; through his program, he was able to increase the weight of the dumbbells to 100 lb for five repetitions. His body composition changed by increasing muscle mass and decreasing fat mass. He became more explosive from the plyometric exercises and Olympic lifts he was completing. The addition of sprints to his training helped lower the time it took to complete the 2-mile run for the Army Physical Fitness Test (APFT).

— *Matt Cady, Human Performance Coordinator, 7th Special Forces Group FL, Total Performance Hockey Director, Division I Hockey Player at Miami University (OH), CSCS*

Adaptation in Practice

Energy system development (ESD) and residual training effects (RTE)

Because you train with the intention of becoming better than you were yesterday, it makes sense that you need to deliberately develop the strength and energy systems covered above. For example, if you want to increase your maximum strength, you need to follow a training program designed for that purpose. This aspect of training is called energy system development, or ESD, and it applies to all of the strength and energy systems. In figure 2–14, ESD is on the left (and ends, to state the obvious, when the workout phase ends). The moment the workout phase ends (see centerline of fig. 2–14), the residual training effects, or RTE, concept kicks in.

Residual training effects are the measurement of how long (in days) you retain the benefits of training.[17] For example, if you follow a three-week training (i.e., development) phase to develop maximum strength and peak at the end of the phase, then you can expect the residual training effects (i.e., the benefits) of that phase to last for approximately 30 days, give or take 5 days. One final concept: maintenance phases. A maintenance phase involves working an energy system to simply sustain a certain level of conditioning, as compared to developing an energy system. You would perform a maintenance phase between developmental phases in a use-it-or-lose-it context. Maintenance phases are critical to properly periodized plans, which we will cover in a moment.

> **RTE**
> The measurement of how long you retain the benefits of training.

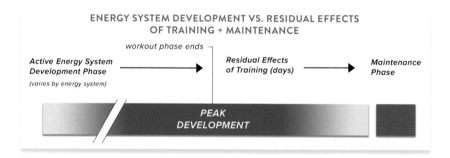

Figure 2–14. Energy system development vs. residual effects of training: maintenance

You can refer to the chart (fig. 2–15) to see residual training effects for all the energy and strength systems.

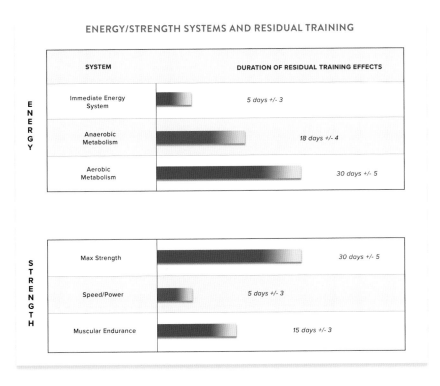

Figure 2–15. Energy and strength systems and residual training

As you look at the RTE chart, pay particular attention to how some systems have similar residual durations. In other words, aerobic and max strength have the same 30-day residual time frame (±5 days). The same could be said for anaerobic and muscular endurance, and immediate energy and speed/power, respectively. It would make sense then to pair these different aspects together first for development, and second for the residual period. A basic example of layering three different energy-system-development plans into a simple, periodized block is laid in the next section.

The next step is to learn how periodization works and helps lay the foundation for building training programs with energy and strength system development in mind.

Periodization

Armed with knowledge of the various energy systems and their respective residual durations, the logical next question is how to design an optimized training schedule. Enter periodization, which is the long-term cyclic structuring of a training program to maximize adaptation relative to a particular event or goal. In the peak performance diagram (fig. 2–16),[18] the peak performance star represents the event or goal, and the programming (i.e., reps and intensity) would be the training schedule designed to peak at the right time. This is an important concept in conditioning, and the peak performance diagram represents what an Olympic athlete would conceptually follow.

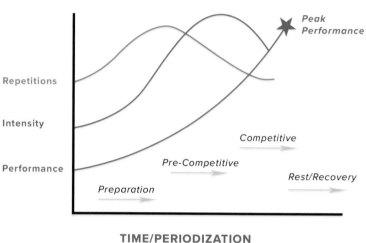

PEAK PERFORMANCE

Repetitions

Intensity

Performance

Peak
Performance

Competitive

Pre-Competitive

Rest/Recovery

Preparation

TIME/PERIODIZATION

Figure 2–16. Peak performance

For most tactical athletes, however—particularly first responders—this peaking, single-goal-oriented periodization is not possible. As discussed throughout this book, tactical athletes must maintain perpetual readiness, day after day, month after month—even *decade after decade.* And as a further challenge, which we will detail below, on any given day they may call on multiple diverse energy and strength systems, requiring adequate readiness in all systems.

Despite these unique challenges, there is an effective way to design conditioning programs for tactical athletes. A periodized plan for these circumstances involves cyclical, perpetual blocks of programming hitting all of the energy systems in a structured rotation; and of course it includes transitional phases for maintenance, rest, and recovery. This way, while it is impossible to anticipate when the next extreme call will happen, you can maintain a consistent level of conditioning and readiness in every energy and strength system.

We will provide more guidance on this toward the end of this chapter. As a practical example of periodization for tactical athletes, please review the example 9-week periodized programming block (fig. 2–17). In week 1, this plan calls for development workouts in A (aerobic and max strength), and maintenance workouts in C (immediate and speed/power). Week 2 has those same elements, but also adds in maintenance work in B (anaerobic fast/slow glycolysis and strength/endurance).

One final helpful point: this is a 9-week program, and when you get to the end you would start back at the beginning, with planned rest and recovery included. To maintain interest, you can and should be picking different exercises within these various categories. For your benefit, there are some completely developed 9- and 12-week block training plans, built specifically for tactical athletes, in the addendum.

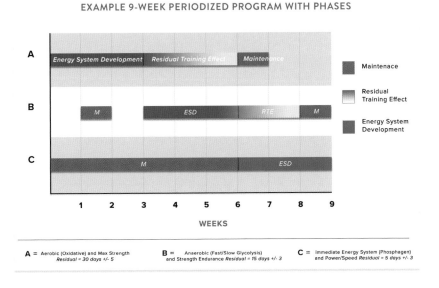

EXAMPLE 9-WEEK PERIODIZED PROGRAM WITH PHASES

Figure 2-17. Nine-week periodized program template

One-rep max, extrapolation

Within periodization there is still the element of planning individual workout sessions. To do this, you will need to calibrate and determine the volume (reps) and intensity (weight load) of your exercises *to achieve your desired adaptation.*

A fundamental building block of this calibration is the one-rep max (1RM) concept. In plain English, your one-rep max is the maximum amount of weight you can push or pull for one repetition, in any given exercise movement, before failure. You can also calculate your one-rep max by a method called extrapolation.[19] Here's how: select a weight you reasonably estimate to be less than your max (but at least roughly 50% of your estimated max) and do repetitions to failure. Using figure 2-19, you can calculate your 1RM. For example: if you put 200 lb on the bar and can bench-press that weight 10 times before failure, then you know from the chart that 200 lb is roughly 75% of your 1RM. Therefore your 1RM is (200 lb / 0.75), or 266 lb. Armed with this knowledge, you can design volume (reps) and intensity (load weight) for that movement—bench-press—inside a program.

Resistance and rate of perceived exertion

One-rep max is a fundamentally sound and precise way to calibrate reps and load. However, if you do not have a calculator or scratch pad handy, or you do not have access to a structured program, you may need to estimate on the fly. The practical resistance guidelines laid out in figures 2–18 and 2–19 provide a very good estimation of reps and loads, matching them to the various strength systems goals you could be pursuing.

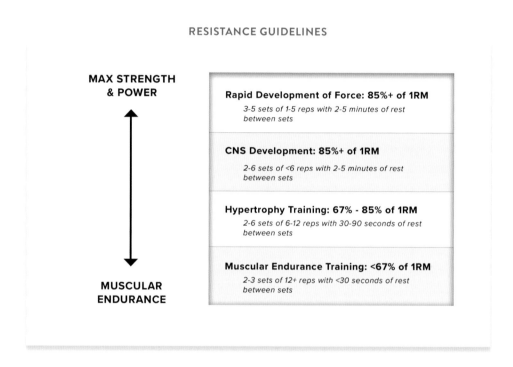

RESISTANCE GUIDELINES

MAX STRENGTH & POWER

Rapid Development of Force: 85%+ of 1RM
3-5 sets of 1-5 reps with 2-5 minutes of rest between sets

CNS Development: 85%+ of 1RM
2-6 sets of <6 reps with 2-5 minutes of rest between sets

Hypertrophy Training: 67% - 85% of 1RM
2-6 sets of 6-12 reps with 30-90 seconds of rest between sets

Muscular Endurance Training: <67% of 1RM
2-3 sets of 12+ reps with <30 seconds of rest between sets

MUSCULAR ENDURANCE

Figure 2–18. Resistance guidelines

To help you understand this chart, please think about the age-old gym wisdom: high reps with lower weight help produce strength *endurance*, and lower reps with higher weight help produce *max strength*.

Finally, one very practical tool to help you maximize adaptation and achieve your specific physiological goals (i.e., energy and strength system goals) is evaluating your rate of perceived exertion, or RPE. As with many 1–10 scales, 1 is the least amount of exertion, and 10 is the max amount of exertion you can deliver before failure. You can use this chart any number of ways, including recalibrating the reps and loads prescribed in a plan any particular day, depending on how you're feeling that day. For example: if your program calls for you to do 1 set of 6 reps at 250 lb (and that is something you can normally do), yet you can only complete 4 reps before failure, then something that is normally an 8 RPE is actually a 10 RPE on that day. Therefore, to avoid overtraining and increasing your injury risk, you should recalibrate your workout for that day. Figure 2–20 provides a practical method for assessing your RPE.

REPS AND % RANGE

REPS	% RANGE
1	100 (max)
2	95
3	93
4	90
5	87
6	85
7	83
8	80
9	77
10	75
11	73
12	70
13	67
14	65
15	63
16	60
17	57
18	55
19	53
20	50

Figure 2–19. Reps and percent range

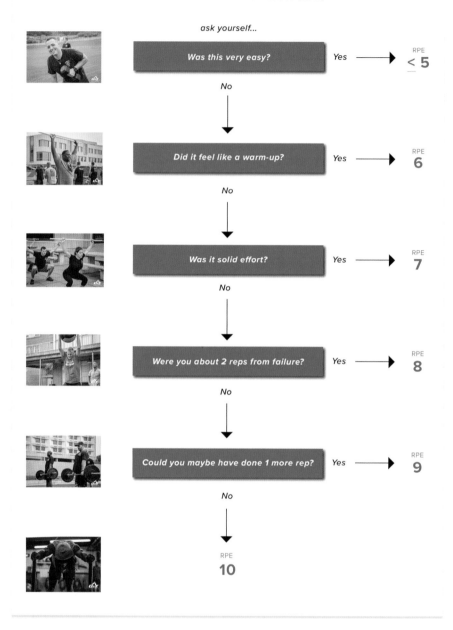

RATE OF PERCEIVED EXERTION (RPE)

ask yourself...

Was this very easy? — Yes → RPE < 5

No ↓

Did it feel like a warm-up? — Yes → RPE 6

No ↓

Was it solid effort? — Yes → RPE 7

No ↓

Were you about 2 reps from failure? — Yes → RPE 8

No ↓

Could you maybe have done 1 more rep? — Yes → RPE 9

No ↓

RPE 10

Figure 2–20. Rate of perceived exertion (RPE)

MAXIMIZING ADAPTATION

We now know that properly calibrated stress (eustress) is what leads to incremental gains in strength and conditioning; we also understand that planning a program methodically and purposefully to target residual training effects is critical to tactical athlete longevity. The question then becomes, What variables can we control to *maximize* the effectiveness of our training, minimizing our injuries and maximizing our performance? Well, let's break out the framework into training variables and recovery variables.[20]

Training Variables

Within the actual training, we must identify our individual needs, then design a job-specific program to meet those needs. We also need to calibrate the amount of stress (training) to make sure we put ourselves through (a) enough to move past the useless, very low levels of stress, (b) enough so we experience the positive supercompensation reaction, but (c) not so much that we experience overreaching and overtraining. Let's start with the needs analysis.

Needs Analysis
The process of assessing the demands of a job, sport, or task as well as the ability of the tactical athlete.

Needs analysis
Needs analysis is just like it sounds—we start by analyzing our specific needs. We will share a more detailed and specific example of needs analysis later in the chapter when we talk about program design, but prior to that we will share the importance of the information. At its core, completing a needs analysis allows you to think critically about what your job requires of you and how you can plan for common obstacles and potential job-related injuries. In addition, a complete needs analysis also takes your individual

experience and fitness level into consideration, so you can design a program specific to your needs, not the general needs of a person in your role.

A comprehensive needs analysis includes four main categories: assessment of job-specific tasks, the physiological profile of those tasks, injuries commonly sustained in your profession, and your personal, training experience (also called "training age"). This allows you to consider the types of movements, strength, and energy systems your job requires and sets the foundation for building your conditioning program. Examples of those needs as they relate to firefighters (and other tactical athletes) are shown in figure 2–21 comparing a firefighter to a decathlete.

Ask questions like (1) What physical tasks are required in your line of work? (2) What types of energy systems and physical strengths are necessary to complete these tasks? (3) Have you sustained any previous injury that could impact your performance? And what types of injuries are common within your industry? (4) What is your training age? This refers not to your experience with general fitness and conditioning, but more specifically to the amount of time and experience you have training in the right way. For example, if you have spent years training as a runner with limited to no experience resistance training and decide to start a strength training plan, your training age for strength training would start at zero. This information allows you to develop an individualized training program geared to the unique performance needs of a tactical athlete.

Specificity of training

Specificity of training—the second training variable we can control to help maximize performance—is, in many ways, a recap of everything we have learned so far. Basically, if we have taken the time to identify the needs of our job, matched those needs with a physiological profile, identified the common injuries in our profession, and have taken an honest look at our own training age and experience, then . . . we should be able to design a smart, specific training program.

For example, if your job regularly requires 30–90 min. of sustained movement, with moderate upper-body lifting and pulling, then that means you may need to develop your aerobic oxidative energy system, strength, and power. And because you know your profession commonly suffers shoulder tears and cardiac events, and you're a 37-year-old who runs once a week and hasn't had time to lift weights since your mid-20s, then you have a framework for designing a conditioning plan, with *specificity*.

Here is a helpful example to keep in mind when considering the importance of specificity. Let's compare a strongman competitor with a triathlete. Both of these individuals are athletes, and both are in top physical shape. The strongman lifts and moves heavy objects. The triathlete, on the other hand, is able to swim, run, and bike extreme distances. While each is well conditioned for the specific needs of their event, it is not likely that either could easily trade places and compete well in the other's discipline. Additionally, while each may use a variety of training and cross-training methods, they would not prepare for their events using general group-fitness classes or non-task-specific training sessions.

They each have different goals, call on different energy and strength systems, are prone to different injuries, and have different levels of experience and fitness. Therefore, just as athletes need specificity of training, so do tactical athletes. A special operations soldier is different from a firefighter, they are both different from a patrol officer, and all three are certainly different from an investigator. If you follow this concept, it will help you minimize your injuries, increase your overall mental and physical health, and prolong your career.

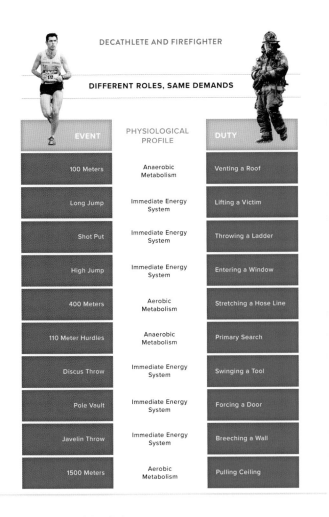

Figure 2–21. Decathlete and firefighter

EQUIPMENT, GEAR, AND TACTICAL ATHLETES

Finally, it's worth noting that for tactical athletes, on the job performance and physical training to prepare for it often look very different. A firefighter may accomplish resistance training wearing shorts, a t-shirt, and athletic footwear, while on a level gym floor in a climate-controlled space. He or she may then utilize the strength adaptations of that training session in a dynamic environment, loaded with heavy turnouts, SCBA, and structural firefighting boots. This is the same for law enforcement officers who carry heavy equipment and wear body armor as well as military members who often are burdened with even more cumbersome gear.

It is vital to understand the tremendous strain that extra loads and restrictive protective gear place upon tactical athletes. Beyond making you sweat more and requiring more energy to move around, heavy loads place extreme strain on your body's structure and connective tissues. Your body moves itself through your environment using a complex series of levers in which muscles contract to move bones around joints. Most of the time, these levers are operating at a mechanical disadvantage, meaning that your muscles are fighting an uphill battle nearly every time you move. Add to this lever system an SCBA, a ruck, body armor, a rifle, an axe, a duty belt, turnout gear, or a helmet—most likely more than one—and your body is faced with a much greater challenge. Having an appreciation for this change and adjusting your training and movement to account for that is necessary not only for maximum performance, but also for avoiding injuries and improving durability.

Good movement patterns outside of gear will translate into good ones when loaded, and if you do not move well in PT clothes, you cannot expect to do so in any sort of gear. Effective physical training, PREPARE, RECOVER, and prehab are essential elements of learning to move well and are covered elsewhere in this chapter. It is imperative to both understand the added strain placed on your body by heavy equipment and prepare for it accordingly.

In addition to a well-structured physical training program, there are times in the training cycle of tactical athletes when training in gear is appropriate. This is a complex topic that can be the subject of an infinite line of "what if?" questioning, but we will summarize a few key points here.

Training in Your Gear

The first step is to consider the goal of each training session and determine whether gear will help or hurt your ability to reach that goal. If the goal of the training is to develop power through a dynamic barbell movement or address mobility weaknesses or stability asymmetries, it is best to skip the gear and focus on movement patterns. If the goal of the training is to condition yourself for job-performance activities, such as advancing a hoseline into a burning building or practicing respond-to-contact drills, then training in gear is probably a good idea.

When to Train in Gear

Tactical skills training should be conducted in gear frequently, like players training for game day in football pads. This practice should be initiated steadily and gradually increased, especially in untrained populations of new tactical athletes. This acclimates the body to operating conditions and practices job functions under real-world loading. The purpose is job-specific practice: practice doing your job under load, with limited range of motion, when overheated, and so on. This also has a mental performance application of assimilating to tough conditions like being out of breath wearing a respirator, working while hot and tired in full kit, and so on. Additionally, training is the best time to test new equipment, adjust how you carry your kit, or break in new gear. As a rule, avoid attempting complex movements in gear where the impaired range of motion could lead to serious injury. Also be careful to hydrate well before, during, and after any training in gear. Training in gear can lead to increased heat acclimation that has been repeatedly shown to improve cardiovascular performance.[21]

Considerations for Not Training in Gear

As mentioned above, gear can limit range of motion and hinder body position awareness, which further increases the loading on your joints and the risk of injury when executing some movements. It is important to train under conditions that maximize the potential for adaptation, so since physical training while wearing gear limits range of motion, it may reduce your potential for maximum adaptation. This is why you do not see NFL players wearing their pads in the weight room; training should match the goals for the session, and bulky protective gear will limit range of motion. In the case of firefighters (or any tactical athletes with contaminated gear), it should be noted that it is incredibly unhealthy to expose yourself to the toxins unnecessarily, especially when you are sweating and your pores are wide open.

This section does not address all of the possible nuances when determining when and how to train in gear. Striving to match your training with your abilities and goals will allow you to train safely while maximizing your ability to excel in your job.

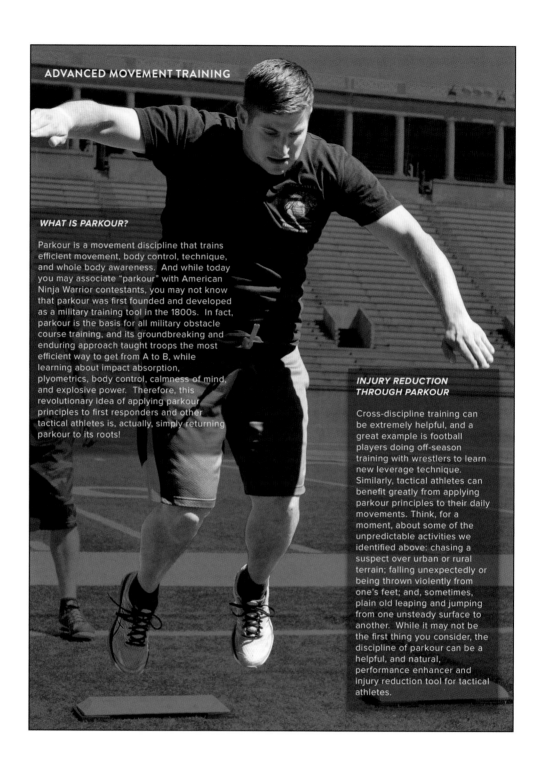

ADVANCED MOVEMENT TRAINING

WHAT IS PARKOUR?

Parkour is a movement discipline that trains efficient movement, body control, technique, and whole body awareness. And while today you may associate "parkour" with American Ninja Warrior contestants, you may not know that parkour was first founded and developed as a military training tool in the 1800s. In fact, parkour is the basis for all military obstacle course training, and its groundbreaking and enduring approach taught troops the most efficient way to get from A to B, while learning about impact absorption, plyometrics, body control, calmness of mind, and explosive power. Therefore, this revolutionary idea of applying parkour principles to first responders and other tactical athletes is, actually, simply returning parkour to its roots!

INJURY REDUCTION THROUGH PARKOUR

Cross-discipline training can be extremely helpful, and a great example is football players doing off-season training with wrestlers to learn new leverage technique. Similarly, tactical athletes can benefit greatly from applying parkour principles to their daily movements. Think, for a moment, about some of the unpredictable activities we identified above: chasing a suspect over urban or rural terrain; falling unexpectedly or being thrown violently from one's feet; and, sometimes, plain old leaping and jumping from one unsteady surface to another. While it may not be the first thing you consider, the discipline of parkour can be a helpful, and natural, performance enhancer and injury reduction tool for tactical athletes.

EXAMPLES OF APPLICABLE MOVEMENTS

FUNDAMENTAL LANDINGS AND FOOTWORK

Most every tactical athlete deals with daily steps, drops and awkward and uneven walking. By training in parkour, tactical athletes can learn fundamental mindfulness of movement, proper jumping and landing techniques, and generate muscle memory and strength for navigating situations in which you face unsure, unpredictable footing.

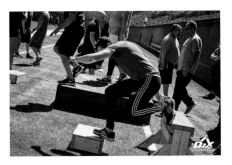

VAULTING AND JUMPING

Plenty of first responder and military situations involve vaulting or jumping. And because obstacles come in all shapes and sizes, being able to efficiently clear and pass these obstacles with speed and stability will lower the risk of dangerous impacts, and thus lower injury rates.

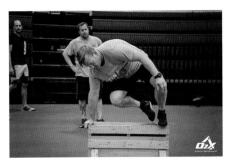

BALANCE

Inherent in every movement, whether by a tactical athlete or not, is the need for balance. Interestingly, balance is a "use it or lose it" skill that needs to be cultivated and maintained: the opposite of balance is total body unawareness and instability. Parkour offers excellent balance drills and exercises, which in turn will strengthen your core, stabilize your legs and core, reduce falls, and therefore reduce injuries.

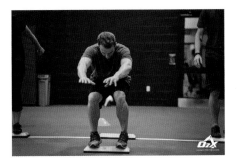

ASCENDING/DESCENDING

Unfortunately, first responders and other tactical athletes sometimes find themselves at a large height and the only path to safety is down, and quickly. Using parkour training to learn momentum absorption techniques, rolling skills, and proper landing technique can mean the difference between a broken ankle (or worse) and walking away slightly sore, but intact.

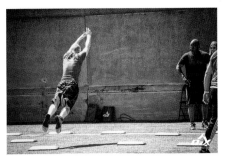

THE COMEBACK—MIKE SANDERS

A needs analysis is extremely important when designing a sound strength and conditioning program for yourself or others. The goal behind all strength and conditioning training should be to 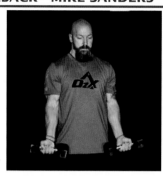 bring out the full physical potential of the athlete. As we've talked about, anyone that engages in a strength and conditioning program aimed at increasing performance will have certain needs based off physiological profiles, job tasks, injuries, and training age. These are discovered through performing a needs analysis. We need to have answers for questions like the following: What are the physiological tools the athlete needs to perform at his or her highest potential? What injury does the individual have that needs attention? How well is the individual trained at conception of the training protocol?

A good needs analysis gives us the blueprint for intelligent, responsible training. Moreover, it's also important to understand that the needs of the athlete can change based off the same factors that brought you to your original needs analysis. For example, physiological needs may change—an athlete may need to improve strength because it's not been well developed. Other examples may be that the individual's job tasks have changed slightly and need to be addressed, or they have been injured and need to work to rehabilitate the injury.

Many years ago, I learned the lesson of needing to shift the strength and conditioning program for one of my hockey players. This particular athlete is one of the hardest working athletes I've ever worked with and used the strength and conditioning program as a resource for achieving his personal goals in hockey. Interestingly, he had been brought on as a walk-on; he knew he would have to work super hard to make the lineup. You'll have to believe me when I tell you that athletes like this are the guys and gals that strength and conditioning coaches love to work with. These athletes give the coach their best, day in and day out, without skipping a beat—a strength coach's dream. He would do just about anything I asked of him. Bottom line: this guy just plain wanted to play and knew he didn't have the same talent as some of his teammates, so we trained and trained to produce more speed, strength, and endurance to make up for the lack of hockey skill.

Not long into his collegiate career, he became very ill and ended up being hospitalized. I can't remember exactly how long he was in the hospital, but I can tell you that his health became dire and he ended up losing 35 lb while there. The good news is that he fought the illness off and was able to return back to the hockey program, although he had missed most of the season in the process.

I can still remember the first day he came back into the weight room. In short, he looked terrible; he was pale, gaunt, skinny, and looked incredibly fragile and weak. I also still remember his question to me that day. He asked, with his head hanging down, "I'm never going to get back to where I was, am I?" I responded, "Yes! We're going to get you back. Your body remembers what it was and it wants to get back there. You stay with me this summer and we'll get you back."

He agreed to stay with me throughout the summer and we promptly got to work. The first thing I had to do was rethink his needs analysis. Physiologically he was a wreck. Everything we'd worked on before was gone. His strength and power were gone because he had lost a lot of muscle mass. He was weak and unstable, and he'd get tired walking across the street. His training age wasn't even close to what it had been just a few months before. We had to redesign his program because his old program would have killed him.

The next thing we did was start training. As you can imagine, we began below the level I had started with him when he came on campus. I used easier, less stressful exercises. We rode a stationary bike a lot to bring up his conditioning a little bit. We didn't perform any Olympic weightlifting because his body just wasn't ready for it. We started from the very basic level and then began to make improvements. Over time, we would rethink and redesign his needs and his program as he developed. This process kept going for weeks until one day something really satisfying happened, and I can still remember it like it was yesterday.

It was early September in Denver. We were on the turf field and I remember it was hot. We were doing a conditioning session in the middle of the day and had just finished plyometric, agility, and conditioning training. We were about a month or so away from hockey season being in full swing, and we were coming to the end of the off-season training for this athlete. We'd been working together all summer, and he had been growing out his hair and beard as his body was slowly coming back to its former athletic self.

I distinctly remember looking at him as he was just finishing up, and I said to myself, "Now that is a man that I would not want to mess with." He had gotten all and more of his muscle back, he was moving like a cheetah, and his endurance was through the roof. He was in a better state than he was before being hospitalized. It was an amazing transformation and extremely satisfying to the both of us.

The best part about this guy is that shortly after, he became the alternate captain of the team and then the captain his senior year. During those two years, we won national championships in Division I men's ice hockey, and it was led by a walk-on who almost lost it all early in his career.

PAIN, INJURY, AND INJURY PREVENTION

Minimizing injury is essential to *maximizing* tactical athlete performance. If you're out on disability, working at less-than-optimal strength, or operating with pain, then your life and your job performance will both suffer. This will impact your livelihood, your happiness, your longevity, and your overall well-being. As with most concepts in this book, we will begin with some science and physiology to help understand the role of pain and why injuries happen. Next we'll look at how they happen, then we'll get into the practical injury-reduction habits you can use right away. Finally, we will wrap up this section with some additional discussion of pain—both acute and chronic. First, let's delve into some background physiology.

At the most basic level, an injury is defined as tissue (muscle, bone, ligament, etc.) breaking down from being overstressed, whether through repeated small stresses (tendonitis in runners) or a larger, individual stress (broken bone from a fall). And while *overstressed* is a technically accurate term, it doesn't tell the whole story. There are many reasons a tissue could become overstressed, as detailed in figure 2–22.

We will share a number of personal screening methods to help you identify, and mitigate, the root cause (poor alignment, imbalance, etc.) of many injuries. But first, let's learn about the more *immediate* injury-reduction methodology: pain as protection. In other words, let's look at when pain becomes a signal for distress and how our body is activated to respond to it.

COMMON INJURY CAUSES

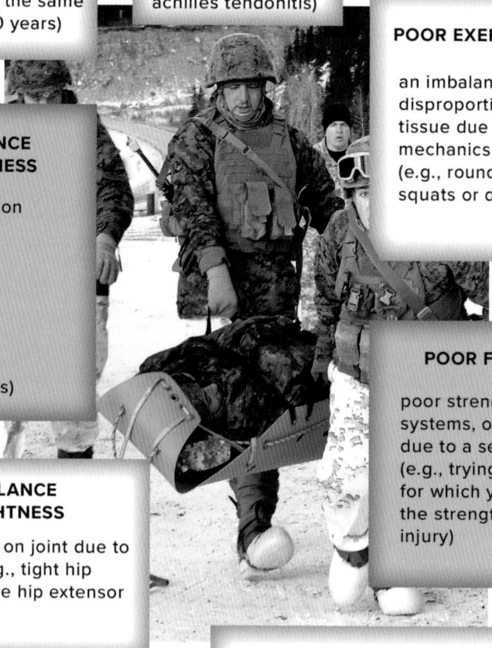

SINGLE IMPACT

a large force placed suddenly on tissue (e.g., fall resulting in broken bone)

INADEQUATE RECOVERY

dangerous fatigue, or weakness, due to improper periodization (covered later in Chapter) or recovery resulting in injury (e.g., running a race too soon after a marathon, causing achilles tendonitis)

POOR NUTRITION HABITS

improper prepatory nutrition (fueling up for performance) or recovery nutrition (refueling for growth) resulting in lack of tissue readiness, resulting in injury

REPETITIVE STRESS

a small stress placed repetitively on tissue (e.g., carrying an EMS bag the same way every shift for 10 years)

POOR EXERCISE TECHNIQUE

an imbalanced or disproportionate force on tissue due to poor body mechanics (e.g., rounded back during squats or deadlifts)

JOINT IMBALANCE DUE TO WEAKNESS

an imbalanced force on joint due to muscle imbalance (e.g., strong pectoral and weak rotator cuff resulting in anterior tissue structure stress)

POOR FITNESS LEVEL

poor strength or endurance systems, or excess weight, due to a sedentary lifestyle (e.g., trying to lift something for which you do not have the strength, resulting in an injury)

JOINT IMBALANCE DUE TO TIGHTNESS

an imbalanced force on joint due to muscle tightness (e.g., tight hip flexors requiring more hip extensor strength)

POOR MOVEMENT PATTERNS

an improper or imbalanced movement (or pattern of movements) causes asymmetric load absorption and load distribution (e.g., repeatedly lifting a ladder on only one arm/shoulder, resulting in strained shoulder)

POOR SLEEP QUALITY

poor sleep quality resulting in poor movement patterns (see box to the right)

Figure 2–22. Common injury causes

Pain as Protection

Pain plays a productive and important role as a protective warning signal (fig. 2–23).

Just as dashboard tachometers warn against revving RPMs too high, pain is a very accurate warning signal to our brain: "you are in danger of a potential injury, so *stop!* or *slow down!* before the injury occurs or worsens." The diagram shows how pain serves as a warning buffer (yellow zone) between healthy effort levels (white), and an effort level that will cause injury (red).

To some extent, *pain protects you from yourself.* For example, have you ever been on a run, felt knee pain, stopped running, and then felt the knee pain go away? In that case, as you were approaching—and about to cross—the injury tolerance of your knee tissue, the warning buffer of pain caused a change in your behavior, which stopped you from becoming injured. If you had ignored the pain, you very likely would have caused tissue damage.

As with many concepts, there is nuance, and the process of distinguishing between normal soreness and pain that is indicative of an injury can be different for everyone. Here are a few key indicators that you should seek medical attention right away:[22]

- The injury causes severe pain, swelling, or numbness.
- You can't put any weight on the area.
- An old injury hurts or aches.
- An old injury swells.
- The joint doesn't feel normal or feels unstable.

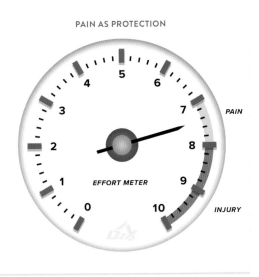

Figure 2–23. Pain as protection

Acute versus Chronic Pain

We talked about the positive role that pain plays in warning us against injury. Here, let's explore a little background neurology and physiology to better understand how pain works.

Most people associate pain with the site on their body where they are experiencing it. However, pain is triggered by messages sent to the brain. As seen in the nervous system diagram (fig. 2–24), your brain maps to every part of your body. If a pin pricked your finger, for example, a series of nerves in your hand would release chemicals that would travel and communicate with nerves through your arm, through your spinal cord, and up to the part of brain that represents that finger.

NERVOUS SYSTEM

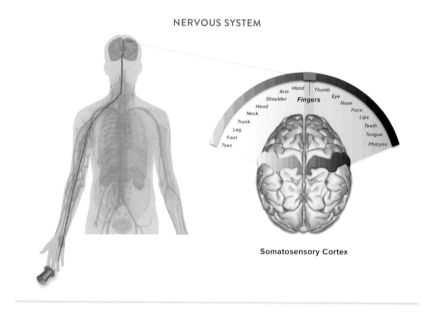

Somatosensory Cortex

Figure 2–24. Nervous system

Naturally, over time, if this area of the brain is not receiving communication on a regular basis, the brain will adapt and those nerves will be redistributed. *The main point is that everything you feel occurs in your brain, not where you feel it.* Why is this important? Well, for a few reasons.

First, the pain signals may be originating from a contained area (think: strained knee, or a cut on your arm). Or the source can be more diffuse, as in disorders like lower back pain.[23] In either case, our brains process the sensation of pain.

Secondly, our brains put pain "in context." In other words, when pain is communicated to the brain, your mind reconciles that pain with your memories and past experiences. This helps us make sense of the present sensation. For example, when you feel pain for the first time, your brain is unsure of the sensation, resulting in a more intense feeling. As a result, you receive a more severe warning signal. When kids fall off a bike and scrape their knee the first time, it most often results in screaming and tears. But as you go through life and experience new things, the brain can put the various experiences into perspective (context) and modulate the pain you feel. This is where the misconception of tolerance originates.

Thirdly, most people tend to believe that the intensity of their pain is always directly related to the intensity of the damage. This is true for acute (short term) pain, but not true for its more complicated sibling: chronic pain. The acute pain diagram (fig. 2–25) highlights some of the keys differences between acute and chronic pain.

To understand how pain levels can be greater than the actual tissue damage (i.e., chronic pain), we need to take a deeper dive into each type of pain.

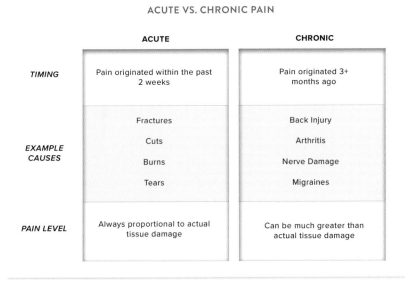

ACUTE VS. CHRONIC PAIN

	ACUTE	CHRONIC
TIMING	Pain originated within the past 2 weeks	Pain originated 3+ months ago
EXAMPLE CAUSES	Fractures Cuts Burns Tears	Back Injury Arthritis Nerve Damage Migraines
PAIN LEVEL	Always proportional to actual tissue damage	Can be much greater than actual tissue damage

Figure 2–25. Acute vs. chronic pain

Acute pain

Acute pain (fig. 2–26) follows a predictable pattern: Tissue is damaged, and pain (often sharp) is immediately produced to alert you to the damage. As the damage heals, pain decreases. In other words, the damage and pain signals are directly connected and proportional. After acute pain goes away, you can go on with life as usual. It sounds simple, and it is, *but only with acute pain.* Chronic pain is more complicated.

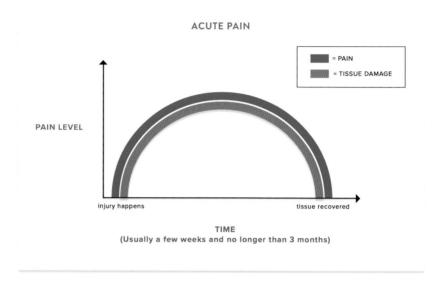

Figure 2–26. Acute pain

Chronic pain

Chronic pain is pain that is ongoing and usually lasts longer than 6 months. Unfortunately, this type of pain can continue even after the injury or illness that caused it has healed or gone away. Pain signals remain active in the nervous system for weeks, months, or years. While it makes sense that chronic conditions, such as arthritis and back pain, can cause chronic pain for months or years, why does chronic pain remain even after the underlying cause has been remedied? It is because during the extended time you suffered from the chronic injury, you built up months of negative memories, emotions, and experiences connected with the chronic pain, and those neural pain pathways became deep enough "ruts" to remain after the cause was eliminated. The longer the initial pain lasts, the more intense and persistent the chronic pain (i.e., pain not related to the actual tissue damage) can be. Figure 2–27 illustrates the ongoing persistence of pain *after* the tissue damage has subsided.

Another conceptual and visual explanation of chronic pain is illustrated on the classic 0 (no pain) to 10 (intense pain) scale. If you experience an injury and you rank the immediate pain an 8 out of 10, then all 8 points are correlated to actual damage. As figure 2–28 shows, that is acute pain. If, after that, the damage has mostly healed but the pain persists at an 8 (out of 10), then it is likely that only 2 of those points are correlated to actual remaining damage and the other 6 points are from the negative pathways built up during the initial injury. As illustrated, that is chronic pain.

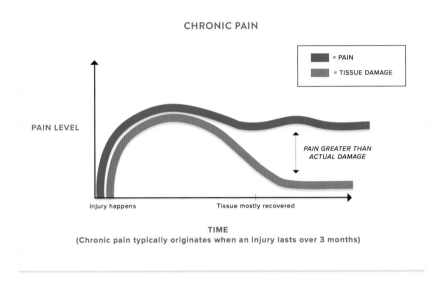

Figure 2–27. Chronic pain

Application for tactical athletes

Because of the physical nature of tactical athletes' professions, and the recurring, relentless nature of those demands, chronic pain is a pervasive issue with firefighters, police, and military personnel. This can cause significant physical effects including tense muscles, limited ability to move around, lack of energy, and appetite changes. If that weren't enough, the emotional effects of chronic pain include depression, anger, anxiety, and fear of reinjury. These physical and emotional impacts can, and do, affect performance. Because of this, it is critical that you actively manage and seek medical assistance for pain. The toll can be both physical and emotional, and recent science suggests that the emotional management may be even more important.[24]

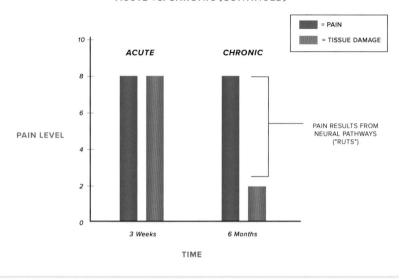

Figure 2–28. Acute vs. chronic pain (continued)

KEY TAKEAWAYS

Pain, Acute and Chronic

◇ Although pain originates at the source of the injury or provocation, it is experienced and processed in our brains.

◇ Acute pain levels are directly correlated to actual tissue damage, and are tied to injuries occurring within the past 3 weeks, roughly.

◇ Listen to your body! It is not advisable to work through acute pain.

◇ Chronic pain levels can be higher than the actual tissue damage would justify. Chronic pain is tied to extended periods of actual pain that build negative neural pathways lasting beyond the actual injury.

◇ The longer you are in pain, the deeper the neural pathways become.

PUSHING TOO FAR—JOHN HALL

"Pain is weakness leaving the body." "You're not injured, you're just hurt." "Rub some dirt on it."

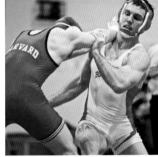

These are just a few of the classic maxims that many of us are all too familiar with. We have heard these words in moments of pain, exhaustion, or injury, from our coaches, teammates, and supervisors alike. Chances are these words became so ingrained in us that we learned to accept pain as a norm.

Throughout my youth, much of my life revolved around organized sports and athletics. By the time I graduated high school and went on to continue my athletic career as a Division I wrestler at Boston University, I had heard the gamut of "Suck it up" phrases a thousand times over. Whether it is in athletics as a competitor, our occupation as a tactical athlete, or our personal endeavors in human performance, we are told to persevere and push ourselves beyond our own limits. While I strongly believe that this is one of the greatest lessons that one can learn in life, we must also understand that we each have physical limits. It is imperative that we acknowledge and understand what those limits are. If we don't, we run the risk of exceeding our own physical threshold to the point of no return.

I am too familiar with never wanting to give in to pain. In athletics, I felt the responsibility to my family, teammates, coaches, and myself to perform—irrespective of my own physical health. This mentality reached an apex during my junior season of competition, when I suffered a broken rib in the first match of the season. In spite of my broken rib, I refused to quit and continued the competition, disregarding my physical trainer's warnings that my efforts would likely lead to further damage. In turn, this is exactly what happened. With 5 days until our next competition, and 20 lb to lose before weigh-in, I resorted to strictly using a stationary bike to lose the weight because I was not able to wrestle due to my broken rib. In the subsequent days, this led to overexertion of my shoulder. I worked my shoulder beyond its capacity to the point of what seemed at the time to be a career-ending injury: long thoracic nerve palsy.

In the following 12 months, as I trained through my rehabilitation program to reteach my arm and shoulder to do basic functions—such as raising my arm above my head or opening a door—I was constantly reminded of the importance of recognizing the difference between eustress and distress. I was reminded of the lasting impact that we can have on our bodies when we do not properly program our exercises or when we do not appropriately recognize the signals that our bodies send us. In sustaining this injury, it became clear to me that the age-old rule that increased input directly equates to increased output has a few very important exceptions. Thankfully, through the support and diligence of the staff that guided me through my intensive rehabilitation program, I was able to condense a 2–3 year recovery process into just less than 12 months. In doing so, my rehabilitation team was able to reintroduce me into competition against all odds.

The adage "work smarter, not harder" comes to mind, and it rings truer now more than ever in my training. Prehabilitation exercises, effective warm-ups, accurately programmed training, and post-workout recovery are imperative, not only to increase our performance but also to mitigate debilitating injuries.

—*John Hall, NCAA Division I Wrestler, O2X Operations*

Injury Reduction Through Personal Analysis

As laid out in the common injury causes diagram (fig. 2–22), we know that multiple biomechanical factors can cause injury: poor technique, inflexibility, imbalances due to tightness and weakness, dysfunctional movement patterns, asymmetric load absorption, and poor overall fitness. And therefore, if we can improve our technique, become more flexible, reduce imbalances, correct our movement patterns, and improve our overall fitness, then we can reduce the occurrence of injury. The questions then become: How can we effectively and accurately identify these weaknesses and imbalances? And how can we improve them?

Leveraging years of scientific research, empirical data, and good old-fashioned proven results, O2X has identified and provides three screening techniques that, if administered properly and followed up with professionally designed corrective programming, will dramatically reduce your risk of injury. Like taking an X-ray or CT scan to see what is happening *inside* your body, or drawing blood to evaluate your biometrics, these three physical tests help you evaluate your baseline fitness and biomechanics. Specifically, these are (1) physical testing (PFT assessments), (2) movement screening, and (3) gait analyses. Let's look at them in order.

Physical fitness tests (PFTs)

PFTs are a quick and efficient method for measuring fitness levels, identifying macro weaknesses and imbalances, and setting baselines against which future improvements can be measured. The O2X Scotty Salman Physical Performance Test (fig. 2–29) seeks to measure all the major physical performance systems in our bodies: upper body, push; upper body, pull; lower body, push; core stability; and cardiovascular capacity. Again, this test is not meant to be a comprehensive body analysis, but the results help identify strengths and weaknesses in your conditioning and endurance and provide an excellent, standardized way to measure progress over time. More specifically, the diagram details the activities, sequence, and timing of the O2X PFT. Age- and gender-specific PFT standards are included in the Appendix.

TRIBUTE—SCOTTY SALMAN, BOSTON FIRE

A US Army veteran and a Boston firefighter for 21 years, Scotty Salman embodied health, wellness, and performance. Scotty was a model of fitness, exuded mental toughness, and had a natural ability to lead by positive example.

In April 2015, Scotty attended the Boston Fire Department's *first* O2X Human Performance Workshop.

During the PT test portion of this first O2X HP Workshop, Scotty held a plank for over 5 min., outlasting every other participant in the group, including those years younger than him. As he held his plank, the entire class surrounded and cheered him on. It was clear: Scotty's

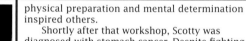

physical preparation and mental determination inspired others.

Shortly after that workshop, Scotty was diagnosed with stomach cancer. Despite fighting hard and refusing to give up, Scotty Salman lost his battle with the disease 5 weeks later, on June 4, 2015. As a tribute, we have named the O2X physical baseline assessment in Scotty's honor. Through this tribute, we want to demonstrate what it means to be a tactical athlete and we want to memorialize the legacy of a hero. Scotty is why we at O2X do what we do—at age 59, he took health and wellness seriously. And as a Boston Fire Academy trainer, he truly led by example.

Scotty remains a constant reminder of the health crisis that firefighters and other tactical athletes face to serve others and keep their communities and country safe. He set the human performance standard for O2X, and his spirit pushes us to do better and be better every day. Scotty made the ultimate sacrifice in service of others and his legacy is woven into the fabric of O2X.

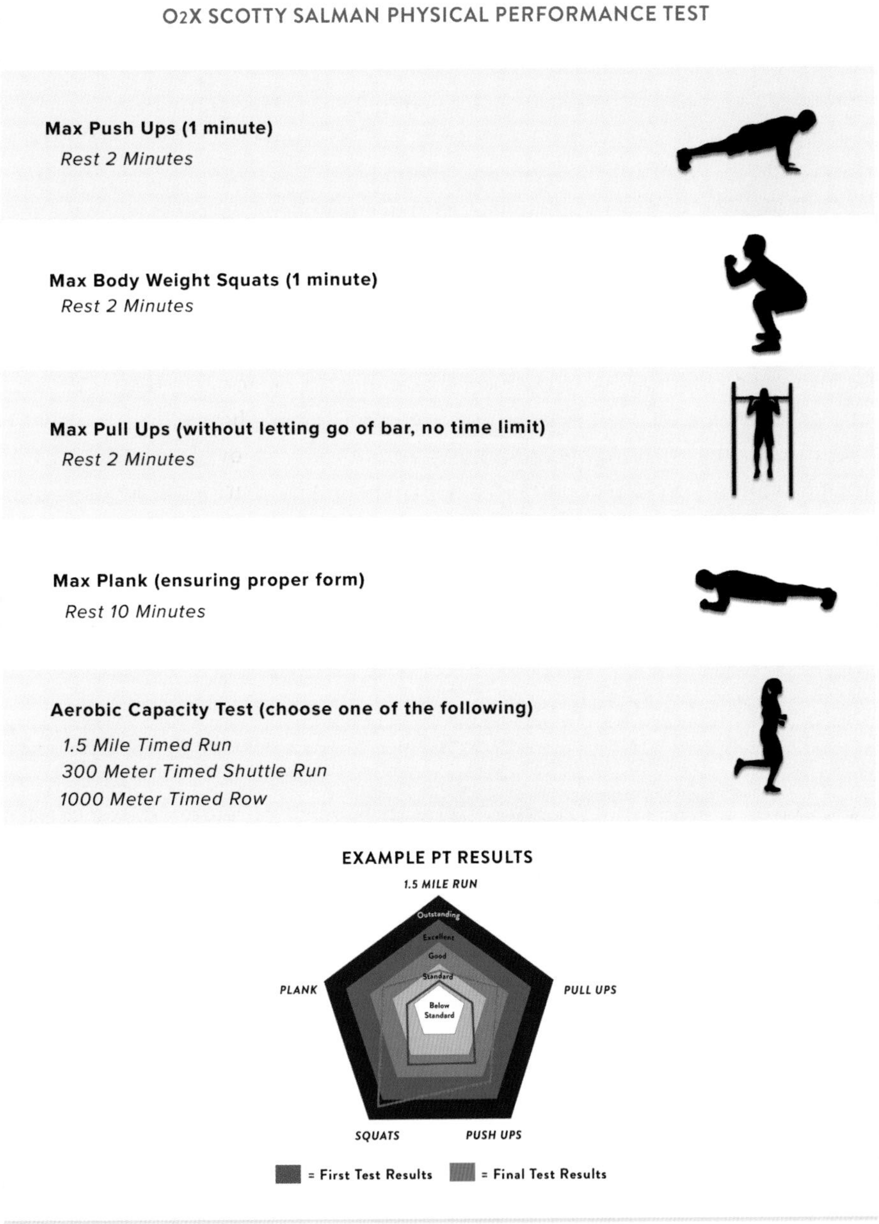

O2X SCOTTY SALMAN PHYSICAL PERFORMANCE TEST

Max Push Ups (1 minute)
Rest 2 Minutes

Max Body Weight Squats (1 minute)
Rest 2 Minutes

Max Pull Ups (without letting go of bar, no time limit)
Rest 2 Minutes

Max Plank (ensuring proper form)
Rest 10 Minutes

Aerobic Capacity Test (choose one of the following)
1.5 Mile Timed Run
300 Meter Timed Shuttle Run
1000 Meter Timed Row

EXAMPLE PT RESULTS

1.5 MILE RUN

Outstanding
Excellent
Good
Standard
Below Standard

PLANK

PULL UPS

SQUATS   PUSH UPS

■ = First Test Results   ▨ = Final Test Results

Figure 2–29. PT standards

Movement screening

If you've seen an athlete with multiple sensors attached to his or her body, with cameras and motion sensors tracking their every movement for the creation of video games, then you understand the concept of the O2X movement screening assessment. Back to our car analogy: the PT test above measures *macro* strength systems (torque and horsepower), and the objective of O2X movement screening is to measure our bodies' mobility, alignment, and stability (a car's turn radius and alignment).

More specifically, a properly administered movement screening test will have motion-capture technology that accurately and objectively measures the biomechanics and kinematics of tactical athletes. Figure 2–30 identifies the four areas we screen and evaluate.

These tests identify ranges of motion, flexion angles, symmetry variances, limb length and other biomechanical criteria. These results are then measured against normative, healthy neuromuscular ranges, which allows us to flag asymmetries and joint imbalances. Ultimately, this helps tactical athletes identify predispositions to injury so they can be dealt with *before* they mature into an injury.

Targeted strength exercises, often called prehabilitation or *prehab* (instead of the after-the-fact *rehab*), increase strength, stability, mobility, and balance. In turn, this advances our ultimate goal for tactical athletes: reducing—or even totally avoiding—injuries that keep you from performing at your maximum levels.

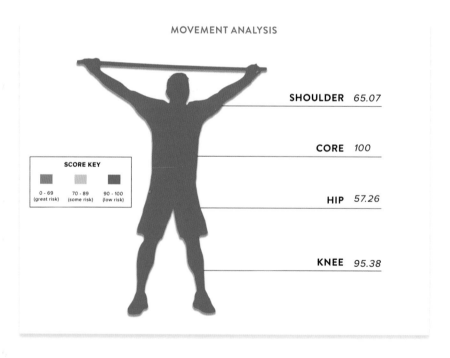

Figure 2–30. Movement analysis

Gait and footwear analysis

Finally, another major strategy toward reducing tactical athletes' injuries is identifying proper footwear. It stands to reason that almost every movement tactical athletes make—all day, every day—originates from their feet, gait, and footwear. Similar to the movement screening above, gait analysis looks at the **biomechanics** of your foot and the biomechanics of your walking and running gait. Overall, the O2X footwear process focuses on four stages: intelligence gathering, gait analysis, footwear selection, and proper fit. Let's look at these stages in order.

As with any task, you need the right equipment for the job. SWAT teams wear different helmets than firefighters because their jobs are inherently different. This applies to footwear as well, and proper footwear selection depends on your job function, training age (experience, skill level), injury history, gear brand history, and frequency of use. The best boots for patrolling the desert under a ruck will probably not be the same choice for walking a beat in a big city. Similarly, the right shoes for a distance run aren't the best for deadlifts. You need to find the right shoes for your work and your training. These are self-evident factors, and the range of answers here is almost infinite. By identifying your needs at the outset of the process, you will greatly help narrow the field of options as you seek to find the right pair.

Next, you should find a footwear specialist (including an athletic trainer, physical therapist, or podiatrist) to perform a gait analysis. Most reputable running-shoe stores have qualified footwear specialists and treadmills with slow-motion video replay systems to help them analyze your gait. At its most basic level, gait analysis establishes the way your body moves. This includes three basic foot strike patterns—neutral, overpronation, and supination—and your arch type (typical or flat).

Once you know your arch type and foot strike pattern, you can narrow down your shoe selection: 90% of screenings identify either a normal or overpronated arch, thereby recommending a neutral or stability shoe style (see fig. 2–31). In the event you're outside these two gait types, your specialist can, and should, recommend a stabilizing or corrective orthotic shoe. Or, depending on the severity of your pronation or supination (i.e., arch) issues, you may need to consult an orthopedic physician to get an appropriate shoe or orthotic insert.

Next, a qualified footwear specialist should determine your strike pattern: either midfoot, heel strike, or forefoot (i.e., how you land when walking or running), which dictates the appropriate level of cushioning and proper shoe structure type for you. Your workhorse shoe (i.e., your high-mileage, everyday shoe or boot) should also err on the side of having more cushioning than less. Different job factors will dictate various construction and design features: zippers for quick doffing, metal shanks and safety toes for protection, or ultralightweight construction for ease of movement. But it's of utmost importance that your shoes or boots are matched to your personal and professional needs while being as comfortable and supportive as possible.

Biomechanics
The use of principles of mechanics as it relates to movement. It refers to how our bodies work and move in a variety of conditions. At its core, biomechanics is how the body moves through space.

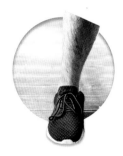 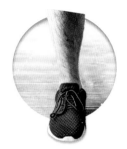 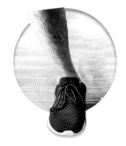

PRONATION
(arch collapses,
ankle rolls in)

NEUTRAL
(arch flexes within range,
ankle is relatively stable)

SUPINATION
(arch does not flex and
ankles roll out)

ARCH TYPE

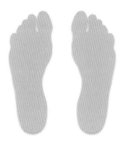 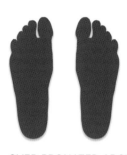

TYPICAL ARCH

OVER-PRONATED ARCH

STRIKE PATTERNS

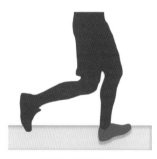 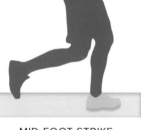 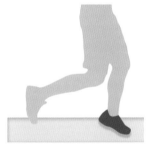

HEEL STRIKE
(most common pattern;
common in long distance
running

MID-FOOT STRIKE
(classically taught
pattern; most common in
athletes)

FOREFOOT STRIKE
(high intensity strike;
common in sprinters and
hill running)

Figure 2–31. Gait analysis

Finally, "fit" is not any more complicated than it sounds: your shoe should match the length, width, and volume of your foot, with allowances according to the chart.

It is important to note that there are ways to strengthen your foot and your foot strike pattern. This can include strengthening the muscles involved in movement like hamstrings, quadriceps, glutes, adductors, and abductors. You can also spend time walking barefoot, when it's appropriate and safe to do so. And there are ways you can work on foot and ankle mobility that will help strengthen your foot and prevent injuries.[25]

If you wander into a shoe store and are picking out shoes without the help of an expert footwear specialist, there are a few things you can test to ensure that you leave with a stable shoe or boot (fig. 2–32). The first thing to test is the heel, also called the heel counter. To do this, make sure the heel is stiff and not flimsy; when you squeeze the heel, it should not fold or compress. Second, check the flexion stability by grabbing the shoe at each side, heel and toe, and bend the toe of the shoe back toward the heel. The shoe should flex where your toes bend, but not in the middle of the shoe. Third, rather than bending the shoe, twist it to see how much torsional stability there is. Finally, upper stability is a component most critical for shoes that will be used for sports or activities that involve a lot of lateral movement. To test this, put one hand on top of the shoe and one hand on the sole and move your top hand left and right to see if it moves around significantly. If it does move, it's a sign that the shoe lacks stability for side-to-side movement.

The key thing to remember is that a stable shoe or boot can help mitigate the risk of placing unnecessary stress on your body.

If you're in the shoe store and cannot remember all of the technical jargon above, you can remember that the O2X shoe-selection process can be reduced to the three Fs: Fit, Feel, and Function. Fit: the length, width, and volume detailed above. Feel: the arch support and cushioning make up the vast majority of a shoe's "feel." Finally, function: the right shoe for the right job.

Ideally, these three personal analyses will help you identify imbalances and asymmetries *before* they cause an injury. O2X administers these three screening techniques for tactical athletes and provides tailored, professionally designed corrective programming to help you dramatically reduce your risk of injury.[26]

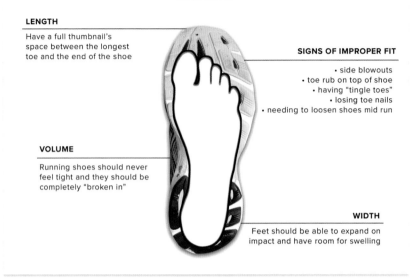

PROPER FIT

LENGTH
Have a full thumbnail's space between the longest toe and the end of the shoe

SIGNS OF IMPROPER FIT
• side blowouts
• toe rub on top of shoe
• having "tingle toes"
• losing toe nails
• needing to loosen shoes mid run

VOLUME
Running shoes should never feel tight and they should be completely "broken in"

WIDTH
Feet should be able to expand on impact and have room for swelling

Figure 2–32. Proper fit

KEY TAKEAWAYS

Personal Analyses to Minimize Injury

◇ Most injuries occur because of poor biomechanics, imbalances (muscular and tightness-induced), asymmetrical movement, and repetition of poor movement patterns.

◇ Identifying and correcting these causes is proven to reduce injury.

◇ PT test, movement screening, and gait analysis are three proven methods to help identify areas for improvement.

◇ Success only occurs if you follow up the knowledge with corrective measures.

THE O₂X PREPARE SWEAT RECOVER METHODOLOGY

We have covered a lot of physiology and neuroscience, and now it is time to begin apply-ing the principles we have shared. When properly applied in your specific conditioning program, the proven, fundamental principles developed by O₂X will help you and other tactical athletes minimize injuries, enhance longevity and durability, and therefore come even closer to maximizing performance. Let's begin with the O₂X tactical athlete workout formula of PREPARE SWEAT RECOVER.

PREPARE, in more general terms, is the warm-up introduced in the injury-prevention section: PREPARE readies your body for exercise and reduces the potential for injury. Below, we include movements *specific* to the physical demands facing first responders and other tactical athletes. The O₂X PREPARE step is largely synonymous with **prehab**, short for prehabilitation. Medical researchers define prehab as "the process of enhancing functional capacity of the individual to enable him or her to withstand [a] stressor."[27]

For tactical athletes, O₂X prehab includes strengthening hips, knees, back, core, and shoulders—areas that absorb a lot of stress. **SWEAT** is the conditioning—running, lifting, rowing, tactical training, and the like—and is where the muscle adaptation (i.e., strength-ening and growth) is activated. Finally, **RECOVER** is what we refer to as "cool down." And while many of the recovery methods are general and beneficial to most everyone involved in a conditioning program, we tailor and contextualize the recovery methods that are ideal for tactical athletes. With that introduction, let's look at some specifics.

> *Prehab (Prehabili-tation)*
> The process of enhancing func-tional capacity of the individual to enable him or her to withstand the stressor of inac-tivity associated with an orthope-dic procedure. A generic prehabil-itation program incorporates the components of warm-up, a cardiovascular component, re-sistance training, flexibility train-ing, and practic-ing functional tasks.[36]

An Optimal Workout Formula

PREPARE (10 min.)

Align and Prehab: The goal of this step is to align the body and activate the muscles that help with posture and stabilization across the joints of the body. The exercises in **PREPARE** are chosen to improve flexibility and to target commonly weak muscles that create imbalances that lead to injury; the exercises add *mobility* and *stability*. Because of our sedentary habits, the backsides of our hips and shoulders tend to be weak and the front sides tend to be tight (figs. 2–33 and 2–34).

This is why these exercises are focused on strengthening the backside and loosen-ing the front. The objective is to get the body as symmetrical and balanced as possi-ble (fig. 2–35). You will also note a strong emphasis on core strength and spine flexibility (fig. 2–36). The core connects our shoulders and hips and is a force transmitter (fig. 2–37). If it is weak and inflexible, then forces are not transmitted effectively and injury risk increases.

POSTURE

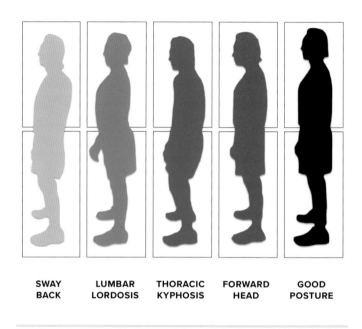

SWAY BACK | LUMBAR LORDOSIS | THORACIC KYPHOSIS | FORWARD HEAD | GOOD POSTURE

Figure 2–33. Posture

ALIGNMENT

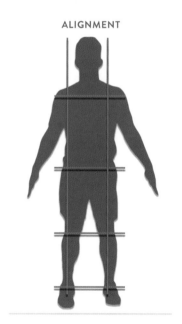

Figure 2–34. Alignment

PREPARE AND RECOVER

PREPARE

ACTIVATION (Reps/Time listed below)	**PREHAB** (As needed)
Glute Activation Glute Bridge: DL or SL: 2x10 Band Walk: Forward/Lateral: 2x10 steps *(band below knees or around ankles/toes)* Hip ER Against Band: 2x10 each leg	**Spine Mobility** Thoracic Up and Overs: 5 each side Cat/Camels/C-Curves: 5 each side
Pillar Activation Front Plank: 2x30 sec Side Plank: 2x30 sec Crab Plank: 2x30 sec	**Shoulder Mobility** Shoulder Arcs: 5 each side Shoulder Stretch with Strap: 5 each side **Hip Mobility** Kneeling Quad/Hip Flexor Stretch: 5 each side Hip CARs: 5 each leg
DYNAMIC STRETCHES (5-10 each side per exercise) Knee Hug Hip Cradle/Figure 4 Hip Flexor/Quad Lunge with Rotation Inch Worm Lateral Lunge Single Leg Deadlift High Knees/Butt Kick	**Spine Stability** Dead Bugs: 10 each side Stationary Bear Crawls: 10 **Shoulder Stability** Sidelying ER with Weight: 10 Prone Swimmers: 10 **Hip Stability** Split Squat Lunge: 5 each leg Single Leg Balance: 30 seconds

RECOVER

SOFT TISSUE WORK + STATIC STRETCHING (20-30 SECONDS EACH EXERCISE)

Piriformis (sit on ball)	Lat (roller)
Hip Flexor (ball or roller)	Spine (roller or peanut)
Calves (ball or roller)	Upper Trap (ball)
Hamstrings (ball or roller)	Posterior Shoulder (ball or roller)
IT Band (roller)	Forearms (golf ball or ball)
Groin/Adductors (roller)	Plantar & Palmar Fascia (golf ball)
Quad (roller)	

Figure 2–35. PREPARE and RECOVER

ACTIVATION

1. PILLAR ACTIVATION
▼

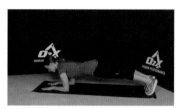

Front Plank
2 x 30 sec

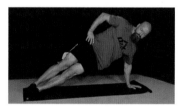

Side Plank
2 x 30 sec

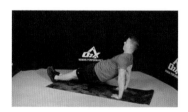

Crab Plank
2 x 30 sec

2. GLUTE ACTIVATION
▼

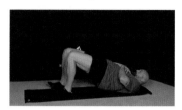

Glute Bridge (Double Leg or Single Leg)
2 x 10

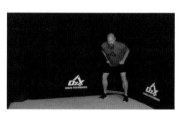

Band Walk (Forward or Lateral)
2 x 10

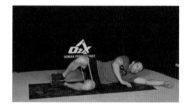

Hip External Rotation Against Band
2 x 10

Figure 2–36. Activate

PREHAB

Complete 2 sets of the following exercises as needed

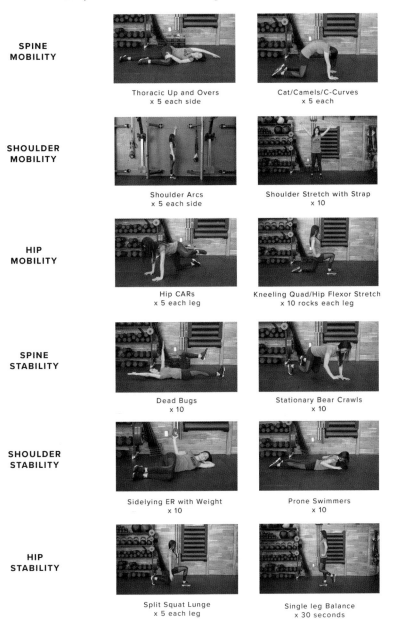

SPINE MOBILITY

Thoracic Up and Overs
x 5 each side

Cat/Camels/C-Curves
x 5 each

SHOULDER MOBILITY

Shoulder Arcs
x 5 each side

Shoulder Stretch with Strap
x 10

HIP MOBILITY

Hip CARs
x 5 each leg

Kneeling Quad/Hip Flexor Stretch
x 10 rocks each leg

SPINE STABILITY

Dead Bugs
x 10

Stationary Bear Crawls
x 10

SHOULDER STABILITY

Sidelying ER with Weight
x 10

Prone Swimmers
x 10

HIP STABILITY

Split Squat Lunge
x 5 each leg

Single leg Balance
x 30 seconds

Figure 2–37. Prehab

Movement Prep: This portion of **PREPARE** is a dynamic warm-up (e.g., jumping rope, a brief run) to simply get the blood circulating to warm your muscles and raise your body temperature. It not only serves as a warm-up but also reinforces good movement patterns, elongates muscles, and increases dynamic flexibility. A dynamic warm-up (fig. 2–38) simulates what is about to be asked of the muscles in the workout, preparing them for the load or forces that you will place on them. (Save the static stretching for step 3, **RECOVER.**)

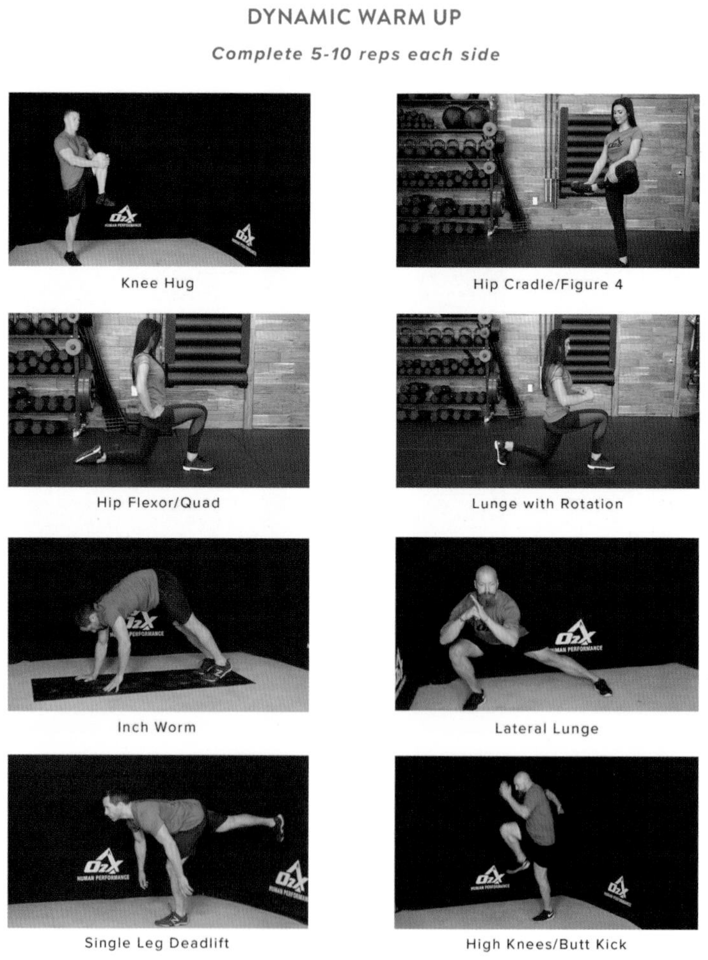

DYNAMIC WARM UP

Complete 5-10 reps each side

Knee Hug	Hip Cradle/Figure 4
Hip Flexor/Quad	Lunge with Rotation
Inch Worm	Lateral Lunge
Single Leg Deadlift	High Knees/Butt Kick

Figure 2–38. Dynamic warm-up

SWEAT

This is the conditioning portion of the workout that triggers adaptation: it puts positive stress on the bones, muscles, ligaments, and tendons to increase their capacity to handle future stress loads. While we will get into how to design a specific conditioning program later, for now please know that you should challenge yourself to keep things exciting by incorporating variety. There are so many exercises and cardiovascular activities that you can do, and the more you incorporate, the lower your risk of repetitive or overuse injuries and boredom. Varying your workouts will also ensure that you get maximum benefit with minimal risk. Be sure to incorporate exercises that increase your heart rate at least 40–60 beats above your resting heart rate (e.g., if your resting heart rate is 70 beats per minute, you should be including exercises that get your heart rate up to 110–130 beats per minute). And, of course, be sure to incorporate exercise movements that mimic or best approximate what you do on the job. At the end of this chapter, we will walk you through how to create a thoughtfully designed, periodized conditioning program that will help you achieve your performance goals.

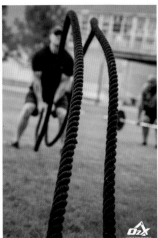 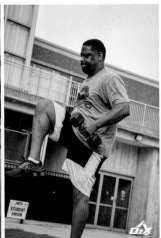 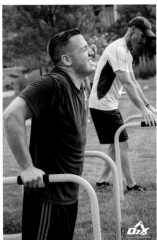

RECOVER

The purpose of this step is to cool down, elongate, and restore the tissue that you have just stressed in order to maximize recovery, healing, and . . . *adaptation*. Remember that when we discussed maximizing adaptation through recovery techniques, we learned that adaptation does *not* occur during the workout; it happens *afterward*. Specifically, growth happens through effective recovery techniques, including nutrition (rehydration, nutrient replenishment), rest, and therapeutic modalities. For this reason, this step is integral and should be performed whenever possible, for as long as possible. These recovery methods enhance blood flow to the recently exhausted areas. And blood flow, as discussed above, is the delivery mechanism for recuperative nutrients, oxygen, and hydration (figs. 2–39a and 2–39b).

RECOVER (Part 1)

Perform each stretch for 20-30 seconds

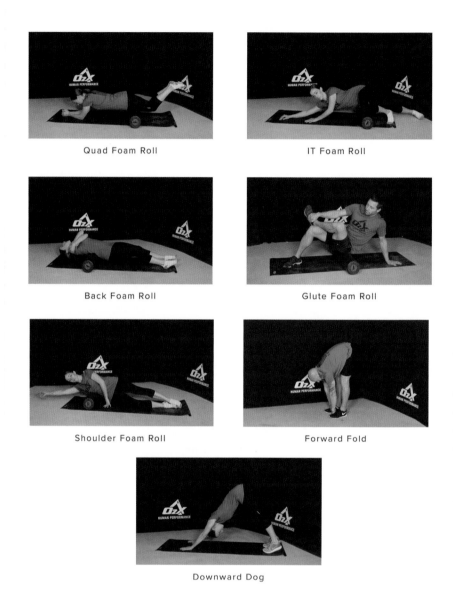

Quad Foam Roll

IT Foam Roll

Back Foam Roll

Glute Foam Roll

Shoulder Foam Roll

Forward Fold

Downward Dog

Figure 2–39a. RECOVER (Part 1)

RECOVER (Part 2)

Perform each stretch for 20-30 seconds

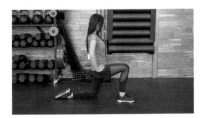

Hip Stretch

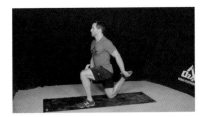

Quad Stretch

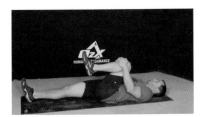

Knee to Chest Stretch

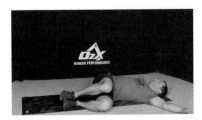

Spinal Twist Stretch

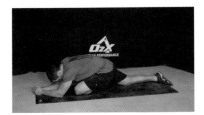

Prone Glute Stretch

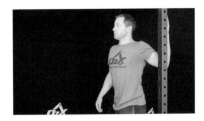

Bent Arm Chest Stretch

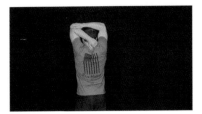

Tricep Stretch

Figure 2–39b. RECOVER (Part 2)

One note about static stretching: the old-school approach was to do static stretching (toe touches, hamstring stretches, etc.) *before* a workout. Through advances in physiology and exercise science, we know that static stretching should only be done *after* a workout.[28] The American College of Sports Medicine (ACSM) guidelines suggest that you should hold each static stretch for about 30 sec and do two to four repetitions (for a total time of 120 sec for each stretch) in order to increase overall flexibility and joint range of motion.[29]

Static stretches are best performed right after your workout, when your muscles are warm. Spend more time on areas that feel tight and less time on those that have good flexibility. Try to be efficient with static stretching. For example, if you only have 10 min. to stretch, it is better to spend 5 min. stretching your tight hamstrings and hip flexors rather than spending 30 sec on each muscle in your body.

The previous sections should have given you an understanding of the importance of training for performance and new ways in which you can approach your training.

Injury-Prevention Techniques

One final, and very important, way to reduce injury during conditioning exercises is preparing for your sessions. Properly warming up *before* a workout, isolating and strengthening problem areas susceptible to injury during your workout, and fully cooling down *after* a workout are three important injury-prevention techniques you can adopt immediately.[30] Adding certain activities into your daily workout helps keep injury, particularly overuse injury, to a minimum.

1. **PREPARE: Warm up**—Never begin your workout without properly preparing the body for work. Always remember to perform a dynamic warm-up (e.g., walk at a fast pace, run in place, do jumping jacks) and work on your trigger points (those muscles and joints that tend to feel tight or restrictive during and after exercise). The goals of warming up are:
   a. Raising your core temperature,
   b. Increasing your blood flow to soon-to-be-activated muscles, and
   c. Central nervous system (CNS) activation—basically letting your nerves warm up by telling your brain that something is about to happen.

2. **PREPARE: Isolation Exercises**—Seek out and perform exercises that strengthen problem areas that are more susceptible to injury. For firefighters, for example, these would include the following, though other tactical athletes would be different:
   a. Shoulders
   b. Hips
   c. Low back

3. **RECOVER: Cool down**—You should always finish your workout with a series of exercises that are designed to let your heart rate return to normal (or close to it) and let your muscles and joints cool off. For example:

    a. Perform a static stretch (hold a muscle still in an extended position for about 30 sec).[31]

    b. Work on your trigger points.

    c. Foam roll.

KEY TAKEAWAYS

PREPARE SWEAT RECOVER

◇ **PREPARE** readies your body for exercise by raising your body temperature by a degree, and it reduces the incidence of injury while promoting balance and symmetry.

◇ **Prehab**, a component of **Prepare**, involves movements specifically designed to strengthen overly stressed areas (hips, knees, back, shoulder).

◇ **SWEAT** is a properly designed conditioning program to help you achieve your performance goals.

◇ **RECOVER**—foam rolling, static stretching, and therapy, for example—is critical because this is where the actual growth and adaptation happens.

CONDITIONING PROGRAM DESIGN

Now that you know the basics of physiology, adaptation, energy systems, **periodization**, conditioning, and injury prevention, the next step is using a framework to tie all those elements together to understand how to build a conditioning program. Keep in mind that designing programs is an art and science that experts can help you create. Recall the first concept we discussed here in **SWEAT**: fitness and performance are related, but significantly different, concepts. Fitness is a general state, achieved through nonspecific training activities. It is a good goal, but we want more for our tactical athletes. Performance training is inherently specific to your particular profession and even more dialed in for the specific demands of you, your experience, and your role in your profession. Every training variable can be maximized to obtain an optimal outcome.

    Before beginning the process of building a workout program, it is important to set a goal. Choosing a specific performance-related goal will guide your programming. Once you have set your goal, program design has five defined elements discussed throughout this chapter and laid out in the program design diagram (fig. 2–40).

Periodization
A long-term cyclical structure of training that is designed to maximize performance coinciding with important events such as a race or duty-specific tasks.

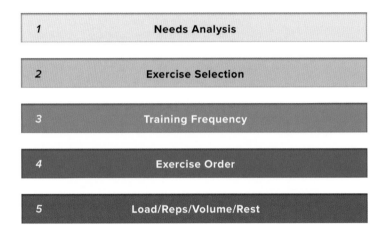

Figure 2–40. Program design

We will define all five steps and show you how to apply them using a hypothetical scenario. This plan will be for Roger, a 39-year-old firefighter who hasn't worked out regularly since his 20s, when he got married and had children. He also hasn't run much since his early 20s and has a history of nagging shoulder problems ranging from soreness to occasional lack of mobility and strength.

Needs Analysis

Needs analysis is just like it sounds and like what we outlined previously in the chapter: we start by analyzing the firefighter's job, specifically the movements and tasks he or she needs to perform. This also relates to specificity of training, which we discussed earlier. Keep your goal in mind as you ask yourself this list of questions to kickstart the process. You can get a handle on your needs by asking the questions in figure 2–41.

This needs analysis, as you can see, gets to the very heart of the distinction between fitness and *performance.*

WHAT ARE YOUR JOB TASKS?

What does your job entail? What are the job-specific physical duties you will be asked to perform?

"I will need to pick up and put down heavy objects (i.e. bunker gear, tools, hoses, ladders, people). Also, climb, walk, hustle, jump, fall (safely), run, and lift."

WHAT IS THE PHYSIOLOGICAL PROFILE OF YOUR JOB TASKS?

In plain English, take the answers from question (1) above and match them with the energy systems and strength systems we learned earlier.

"All of them."

WHAT INJURIES AND ILLNESS ARE COMMON TO YOU & YOUR PROFESSION?

The greatest predictor of future injury is a prior injury, and the best defense against injury is to avoid one in the first place.

"I have shoulder problems. I need to learn which exercises are most appropriate for strengthening them and avoid exercises that aggravate them."

WHAT IS YOUR TRAINING AGE?

How long have you been training for your job specific needs?

"I am 39, haven't run or lifted in over 10 years, but I did play high school football, and track, and spent 4 years in the Navy after school."

WHAT EQUIPMENT IS AVAILABLE FOR YOU TO TRAIN WITH?

Do you have your own workout equipment? Do you belong to a gym? Do you have access to a gym at your department?

"I can workout at the fire house gym, and I belong to a private gym that is a short drive from my home."

Figure 2–41. Needs analysis

Exercise Selection

Your next step should be selecting your exercises based on your needs analysis. What exercises do you want to use to bring about the changes that you are looking for? Additionally, it is critical that you consider what equipment you will have available during your training sessions. You will need to modify the types of exercises and resistance used based on your equipment. Figure 2–42 presents a sample list of exercises to consider.

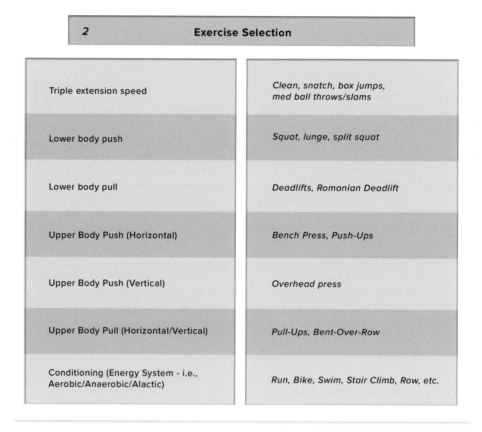

2	Exercise Selection
Triple extension speed	Clean, snatch, box jumps, med ball throws/slams
Lower body push	Squat, lunge, split squat
Lower body pull	Deadlifts, Romanian Deadlift
Upper Body Push (Horizontal)	Bench Press, Push-Ups
Upper Body Push (Vertical)	Overhead press
Upper Body Pull (Horizontal/Vertical)	Pull-Ups, Bent-Over-Row
Conditioning (Energy System - i.e., Aerobic/Anaerobic/Alactic)	Run, Bike, Swim, Stair Climb, Row, etc.

Figure 2–42. Exercise selection

Training Frequency

The next step is to think about your training frequency. That is, how much time can you commit to your training? Figure 2–43 lists a few questions that you should have answers for when thinking of your frequency.

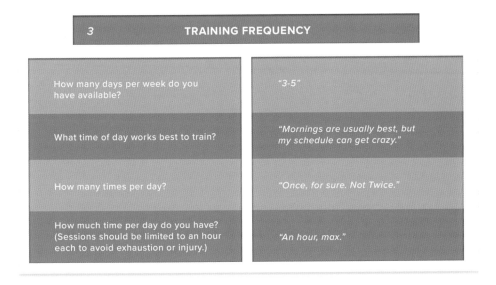

Figure 2–43. Training frequency

Exercise Order

Next you should create a logical sequence of exercises so that you will get the most bang for your buck. In other words, exercise causes fatigue at the neurological level and the energy system level. For this reason, as a general rule, you should complete complex and speed/power exercises early in your daily program. Lower-body exercises should follow, then upper-body exercises. Aerobic conditioning exercises (running, swimming, rowing, etc.) should be done last. The list in figure 2–44 will give you a starting point for designing your own sequence of exercises.

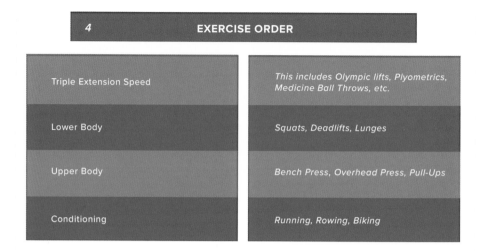

4	EXERCISE ORDER
Triple Extension Speed	This includes Olympic lifts, Plyometrics, Medicine Ball Throws, etc.
Lower Body	Squats, Deadlifts, Lunges
Upper Body	Bench Press, Overhead Press, Pull-Ups
Conditioning	Running, Rowing, Biking

Figure 2–44. Exercise order

Training Load, Reps, Volume, and Rest Periods

The final step in your program development pipeline is to put all the pieces together and map out each training day, week, month, and year for the rest of your life. Armed with the fundamentals above and the practical example in figure 2–45, you can do it.

To begin, let's review the relevant principles. First, based on what you learned about adaptation, you know that your body will adapt and grow in response to training stimulus. You also learned about the various energy and strength systems in your body, and you learned how long development gains last (residual training effects) for each system. This leads, naturally, into arranging the training blocks of these systems into a periodized plan. Finally, we know that formal program design for *performance* (versus general fitness) begins with four important, personalized steps. First, needs analysis: "What do I need to train to be better at my job?" Second, exercise selection: "What exercise will help me train for that?" Third, training frequency: "How often do I need to train to achieve my goals?" Fourth, exercise order: "How do I best structure my workouts for maximum benefit?" And finally, job-specific needs: "I am naturally inclined to be an endurance athlete; however, I need to gain strength and muscle mass for my job."

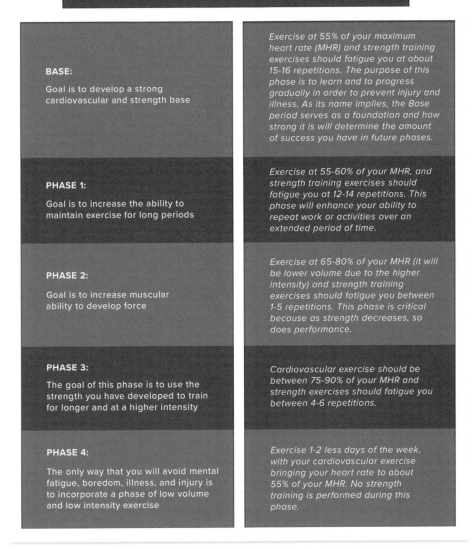

BASE:

Goal is to develop a strong cardiovascular and strength base

Exercise at 55% of your maximum heart rate (MHR) and strength training exercises should fatigue you at about 15-16 repetitions. The purpose of this phase is to learn and to progress gradually in order to prevent injury and illness. As its name implies, the Base period serves as a foundation and how strong it is will determine the amount of success you have in future phases.

PHASE 1:

Goal is to increase the ability to maintain exercise for long periods

Exercise at 55-60% of your MHR, and strength training exercises should fatigue you at 12-14 repetitions. This phase will enhance your ability to repeat work or activities over an extended period of time.

PHASE 2:

Goal is to increase muscular ability to develop force

Exercise at 65-80% of your MHR (it will be lower volume due to the higher intensity) and strength training exercises should fatigue you between 1-5 repetitions. This phase is critical because as strength decreases, so does performance.

PHASE 3:

The goal of this phase is to use the strength you have developed to train for longer and at a higher intensity

Cardiovascular exercise should be between 75-90% of your MHR and strength exercises should fatigue you between 4-6 repetitions.

PHASE 4:

The only way that you will avoid mental fatigue, boredom, illness, and injury is to incorporate a phase of low volume and low intensity exercise

Exercise 1-2 less days of the week, with your cardiovascular exercise bringing your heart rate to about 55% of your MHR. No strength training is performed during this phase.

Figure 2–45. An example of load, reps, volume, and rest

If you could plug all of these answers into a piece of software, and then press Enter to receive a finely tuned program, that would be terrific. But as you have likely noticed, program design is both a science *and an art*. It is a fluid, evolving process that is, and should be, constantly shifting to meet your gains, losses, personal circumstances, and external environmental factors. If that were the final answer, you would be in a tough spot. However, we have developed highly specific tactical athlete plans for you in the appendix. Let's look at a 7-day sample (fig. 2–46) and walk through our design logic together.

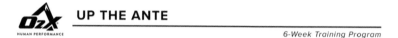

UP THE ANTE

6-Week Training Program

WEEK 1							
Day	1	2	3	4	5	6	7
Notes:	Step 1 - Prepare (8-10m)	Step 1 - Prepare (8-10m)	Step 1 - Prepare (8-10m)	Step 1 - Prepare (8-10m)	Step 1 - Prepare (8-10m)	Step 1 - Prepare (8-10m)	Step 1 - Prepare (8-10m)
	Step 2 - Sweat:	Step 2 - Sweat:	Step 2 - Sweat:	Step 2 - Sweat:	Step 2 - Sweat:	Step 2 - Sweat:	Step 2 - Sweat:
	Clean : 4 sets x 4 reps	Single Arm DB Snatch: 4 sets x 4 reps each arm	Snatch: 4 sets x 4 reps	Rest	Barbell Bent Over Row: 4 sets x 10 reps	Jog or bike 90 min Conversational Pace	Recovery Day
	Squat: 4 sets x 8 reps	Pull-Ups: 4 sets x 10 reps	Single Arm DB Jerk: 3 sets x 4 reps each arm		DB Plank Row: 4 sets x 10 reps each	Or	
	Run: 1.5 miles for time	Rope Climb: 4 sets x 1 climb	Deadlift: 4 sets x 8 reps		MB Chest Press: 4 sets x 10 reps	Ruck 10 mi w/ 25#	
		Run Intervals: 6 sets x 2 min work / 2 min off	DB Split Squat: 3 sets x 10 reps each leg		Run: 3 miles for time		
			Row/Assault Bike: 10 sets x 30 seconds on / 90 seconds rest				
	Step 3 - Recover (10-15m)	Step 3 - Recover (10-15m)	Step 3 - Recover (10-15m)	Step 3 - Recover (10-15m)	Step 3 - Recover (10-15m)	Step 3 - Recover (10-15m)	Step 3 - Recover (10-15m)

Figure 2–46. Up the ante

In the example, the training variables and energy systems are synchronized to produce desired adaptations without overtraining. Each training day takes residual training effects into consideration so that the various energy systems can be conditioned in a properly synchronized cycle (i.e., periodization). This, as we have discussed quite a bit above, allows tactical athletes to train multiple energy systems simultaneously, thereby helping them stay in a continual state of balanced readiness. For example, in the brief example above, the program calls for BB back squat (strength), intervals (anaerobic capacity), BB clean (power), and running or rowing (aerobic), and that is only the first 7 days of an 8-week program. Secondly, the volume (reps) and intensity (load) are designed for specific adaptation goals, and they work together to make gains in strength, power, and endurance.

CONCLUSION

As we stated at the beginning on this chapter, the foundational elements of a successful conditioning plan are:

1. setting a specific goal,
2. planning toward your occupational and personal needs,
3. conducting personal screenings and analyses to identify weaknesses,
4. optimally calibrating stress and training levels to minimize injury, and
5. following the proven O2X PREPARE SWEAT RECOVER methodology.

We also highlighted the extremely important distinction between *fitness* and *performance*. *Fitness* is overall, general physical ability attained through nonspecifically structured fitness programs. We do not mean it as a criticism—someone following a fitness program will improve their general health and well-being. *However, we are focused on tactical athletes and want to do more for you.* Tactical athletes must *perform* with specific goals in mind. Job-specific training will reduce injury rates, improve productivity, and improve efficiency and morale.

Finally, let's be mindful that tactical athletes must maintain perpetual physical readiness, for their entire careers. The careers of firefighters, law enforcement officers, and military personnel last for *decades*. This raises unique questions around sustainability, burnout, periodicity, injury prevention, and longevity. The training programs we provide at the back of this book are designed specifically to meet these unique and important objectives.

CHAPTER QUESTIONS

1. What is the difference between training for fitness and training for performance?
2. What are three benefits of developing a proper conditioning routine?
3. What are the foundational elements of a successful conditioning plan?
4. What is the difference between eustress and distress?
5. How does this relate to conditioning, energy and strength system development, and maximizing performance?
6. What is periodization?
7. What is a needs analysis?
8. What is specificity of training?
9. What is the role of pain in protection and performance?

CHAPTER NOTES

What are three takeaways from this chapter that you can implement in your everyday life?

1. _____
   _____
   _____
   _____
   _____
   _____

2. _____
   _____
   _____
   _____
   _____
   _____

3. _____
   _____
   _____
   _____
   _____
   _____

ADDENDUM

12-WEEK PERIODIZED PROGRAM TEMPLATE

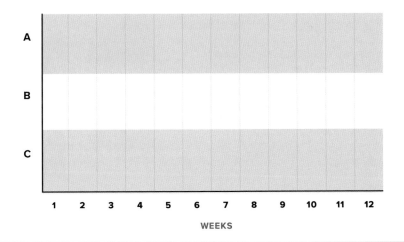

A = Aerobic (Oxidative) and Max Strength
    Residual = 30 days +/- 5

B = Anaerobic (Fast/Slow Glycolysis)
    and Strength Endurance *Residual= 15 days +/- 3*

C = Immediate Energy System (Phosphagen)
    and Power/Speed *Residual = 5 days +/- 3*

9-WEEK PERIODIZED PROGRAM TEMPLATE

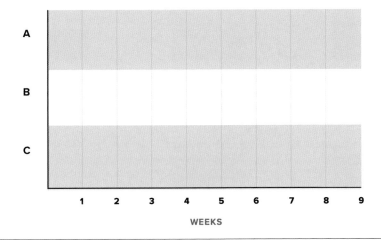

A = Aerobic (Oxidative) and Max Strength
    Residual = 30 days +/- 5

B = Anaerobic (Fast/Slow Glycolysis)
    and Strength Endurance *Residual = 15 days +/- 3*

C = Immediate Energy System (Phosphagen)
    and Power/Speed *Residual = 5 days +/- 3*

HOW TO DEADLIFT

DIRECTIONS:

1. Feet should be shoulder width apart and flat on floor
- Hands placed with pronated or alternating grip outside of your stance
- Hinge down (bar should be in line with shoulders)
- Head in line with spine, looking forward or slightly in front about 8 feet
- Shoulder blades in your back pockets (Lats locked, core tight)
- Deep breath, hold breath, brace vertebral column
- Think about pulling backwards / push the floor with middle to back of feet
- Shoulders lead the hips

1.

2.

3.

2. Keeping bar close to body begin to push hips forward, raising bar off the ground

3. Breathe out
- Squeeze glutes at top of movement

4. Lower bar back to ground in the reverse motion

Alternate Exercises:
SUMO DEADLIFT

CUES:

1. Butt Back   *2. Stand Up*   *3. Squeeze Glutes at the Top*

WATCH OUT FOR:

 Feet Too Close

 Elevated Neck

Incomplete ▲ Extension

 Bar Too Far

 Hunch Back

 Head Down

 Hips Too Far Back

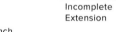

HOW TO OVERHEAD PRESS

DIRECTIONS:

1. Feet should be shoulder width apart
- Head in line with spine, looking forward
- Lats locked, core tight
- Hands at just outside shoulder width
- Elbows tucked
- Deep breath, hold breath, brace vertebral column

2. Drive bar up overhead in as straight of line as possible
- Move your head out of the way
- Arms should be in line with ears in overhead position

3. Squeeze glutes at top of movement
- Do not compromise back position for more range in lift

4. Lower in reverse motion

1.
2.
3.
4.

Alternate Exercises:

SHOULDER PRESS WITH DUMBBELL
SHOULDER PRESS WITH KETTLEBELL
SHOULDER PRESS WITH RESISTANCE BANDS

CUES:

1. Shoulder width grip

2. Push your elbows through your fists

3. Push head through when bar is raised

WATCH OUT FOR:

 Hands Too Close

 Arched Back

 Too Far Back

 Hands Too Wide

 Too Far Forward

HOW TO PUSH PRESS

DIRECTIONS:

1. Hold a barbell with a grip that is a little less than shoulder width apart

2. Pull barbell just above shoulders with elbows close to your body

3. Bend your knees and lower your body into a two inch squat position

4. Press the weight over your head as you press through the heels to explosively stand up

5. Make sure you finish the top of the press by locking out the elbows. Pause and slowly lower the bar back down to the starting position

1.

2.

3.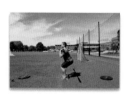

Alternate Exercises:
SHOULDER PRESS WITH DUMBBELL

CUES:

1. Dip   *2. Press*

WATCH OUT FOR:

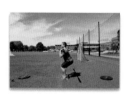

Too deep of a squat.
Only dip two inches.

HOW TO ROCKET JUMP

DIRECTIONS:

1. Feet shoulder-width apart, arms flexed at side of body

2. Pull self down to half-squat position

3. Explosively jump and reach for sky

4. Land by pulling self back to half-squat position

Alternate Exercises:
ALTERNATING PUSH OFF
BOX JUMP
KETTLEBELL SWING

CUES:

1. Pull self down to half-squat position

2. Explosively jump and reach for sky

3. Land by pulling self back to half-squat position

WATCH OUT FOR:

Collapsed
Knees

Too High
Landing

Uneven
Landing

HOW TO SQUAT

DIRECTIONS:

1. Feet should be shoulder width apart and flat on floor
- Toes pointing slightly out
- Head in line with spine
- Look forward or slightly in front about 8 feet
- Deep breath, hold breath, brace vertebral column

2. Descend by sitting back and down
- Femurs should be in line with feet
- Squat to a depth where knee joint is even or lower than hip joint

3. Drive out of hole pushing energy into the ground
- Breathe out on way up

4. Squeeze glutes at the top of the movement

1.

2.

3.

4.

Alternate Exercises:

SUMO SQUAT HOLD   *FORWARD LUNGE*
GOBLET SQUAT   *LATERAL SQUAT/*
REVERSE LUNGE   *LATERAL LUNGE*

CUES:

1. Big chest   *2. Weight back, knees out*   *3. Pull yourself into the hole*

WATCH OUT FOR:

 Bar Too High

 Feet Too Wide

 Knees Too Forward

 Bar Too Low

 Bent at the Waist

 Weight Too Far

 Feet Too Close

 Collapsed Knees

 Not Deep Enough

Plank Hold (max time)

Men	20s	30s	40s	50s	60s
Outstanding	3:48 +	2:17 +	1:58 +	1:34 +	1:25 +
Tactical Athlete	2:08 - 3:47	1:34 - 2:!6	1:17 - 1:57	1:09 - 1:33	1:07 - 1:24
Good	1:30 - 2:07	1:17 - 1:33	1:03 - 1:16	0:53 - 1:08	0:50 - 1:06
Fair	1:06 - 1:29	0:54 - 1:16	0:45 - 1:02	0:36 - 0:52	0:30 - 0:49
Poor	0:35 - 1:05	0:27 - 0:53	0:21 - 0:44	0:15 - 0:35	0:09 - 0:29
Very Poor	0:00 - 0:34	0:00 - 0:26	0:00 - 0:20	0:00 - 0:14	0:00 - 0:08

Women	20s	30s	40s	50s	60s
Outstanding	2:33 +	1:31 +	1:19 +	1:03 +	0:57 +
Tactical Athlete	1:24 - 2:32	1:22 - 1:30	1:08 - 1:18	0:57 - 1:02	0:52 - 0:56
Good	1:06 - 1:23	1:03 - 1:21	0:53 - 1:07	0:43 - 0:56	0:40 - 0:51
Fair	0:49 - 1:05	0:43 - 1:02	0:37 - 0:52	0:31 - 0:42	0:25 - 0:39
Poor	0:24 - 0:48	0:15 - 0:42	0:12 - 0:36	0:09 - 0:30	0:06 - 0:24
Very Poor	0:00 - 0:23	0:00 - 0:14	0:00 - 0:11	0:00 - 0:08	0:00 - 0:05

Push-Ups (max repetitions in 1 minute)

Men	20s	30s	40s	50s	60s
Outstanding	54 +	50 +	42 +	35 +	28 +
Tactical Athlete	39 - 53	33 - 49	27 - 41	24 - 34	23 - 27
Good	26 - 38	22 - 32	18 - 26	15 - 23	14 - 22
Fair	22 - 25	18 - 21	15 - 17	12 - 14	10 - 13
Poor	12 - 24	9 - 17	7 - 14	5 - 11	3 - 9
Very Poor	0 - 11	0 - 8	0 - 6	0 - 4	0 - 2

Women	20s	30s	40s	50s	60s
Outstanding	31 +	27 +	18 +	12 +	7 +
Tactical Athlete	23 - 30	15 - 26	10 - 17	8 - 11	5 - 6
Good	15 - 22	13 - 14	7 - 9	6 - 7	4
Fair	11 - 14	9 - 12	5 - 6	4 -5	3
Poor	8 - 10	6 - 8	4	3	2
Very Poor	0 - 7	0 - 5	0 - 3	0 - 2	0 - 1

Pull Up (max repetitions without dropping)

Men	20s	30s	40s	50s	60s
Outstanding	25 +	20 +	18 +	13 +	8 +
Tactical Athlete	17 - 24	16 - 19	13 - 17	10 - 12	5 - 7
Good	10 - 16	9 - 15	8 - 12	7 - 9	4
Fair	7 - 9	6 - 8	5 - 7	5 - 6	3
Poor	5 - 6	4 - 5	3 - 4	3 - 4	1-2
Very Poor	0 - 4	0 - 3	0 - 2	0 - 2	0

Women	20s	30s	40s	50s	60s
Outstanding	12 +	10 +	7 +	4 +	2 +
Tactical Athlete	6 - 11	5 - 9	4 - 6	2 - 3	1
Good	3 - 5	3 - 4	2 - 3	1	1
Fair	2	2	1	1	1
Poor	1	1	0	0	0
Very Poor	0	0	0	0	0

Bodyweight Squat (max repetitions in 1 minute)

Men	20s	30s	40s	50s	60s
Outstanding	58 +	55 +	48 +	41 +	39 +
Tactical Athlete	44 - 57	42 - 54	35 - 47	29 - 40	25 - 38
Good	39 - 43	35 - 41	30 - 34	25 - 28	21 - 24
Fair	35 - 38	31 - 34	27 - 29	22 - 24	17 - 20
Poor	31 - 34	29 - 30	23 - 26	18 - 21	13 - 16
Very Poor	0 - 30	0 - 28	0 - 22	0 - 17	0 - 12

Women	20s	30s	40s	50s	60s
Outstanding	48 +	43 +	37 +	32 +	28 +
Tactical Athlete	37 - 47	33 - 42	27 - 36	22 - 31	18 - 27
Good	33 - 36	29 - 32	23 - 26	18 - 21	13 - 17
Fair	29 - 32	25 - 28	19 - 22	14 - 17	10 - 12
Poor	25 - 28	21 - 24	15 - 18	10 - 13	7 - 9
Very Poor	0 - 24	0 - 20	0 - 14	0 - 9	0 - 6

Aerobic - 300m Shuttle Run (average of two attempts with a 30 second rest period in between)

Men	20s	30s	40s	50s	60s
Outstanding	0:00 - 0:45	0:00 - 0:48	0:00 - 0:53	0:00 - 1:00	0:00 - 1:08
Tactical Athlete	0:46 - 0:50	0:49 - 0:51	0:54 - 0:57	1:01 - 1:06	1:09 - 1:15
Good	0:51 - 0:54	0:52 - 0:55	0:58 - 1:04	1:07 - 1:14	1:16 - 1:25
Fair	0:55 - 0:58	0:56 - 1:00	1:05 - 1:12	1:15 - 1:23	1:26 - 1:38
Poor	0:59 - 1:05	1:01 - 1:08	1:13 - 1:23	1:24 - 1:34	1:39 - 1:50
Very Poor	1:06 +	1:09 +	1:24 +	1:35 +	1:51 +

Women	20s	30s	40s	50s	60s
Outstanding	0:00 - 0:55	0:00 - 0:59	0:00 - 1:06	0:00 - 1:11	0:00 - 1:28
Tactical Athlete	0:56 - 0:58	1:00 - 1:06	1:07 - 1:12	1:12 - 1:19	1:29 - 1:35
Good	0:59 - 1:02	1:07 - 1:12	1:13 - 1:19	1:20 - 1:35	1:36 - 1:50
Fair	1:03 - 1:11	1:13 - 1:20	1:20 - 1:34	1:36 - 1:50	1:51 - 2:05
Poor	1:12 - 1:18	1:21 - 1:26	1:35 - 1:50	1:51 - 2:05	2:06 - 2:20
Very Poor	1:19 +	1:27 +	1:51 +	2:06 +	2:21 +

Aerobic - 1.5 Mile Run (fastest time)

Men	20s	30s	40s	50s	60s
Outstanding	0:00 - 9:08	0:00 - 9:31	0:00 - 9:47	0:00 - 10:27	0:00 - 11:20
Tactical Athlete	9:09 - 10:08	9:32 - 10:38	9:48 - 11:09	10:28 - 12:08	11:21 - 13:25
Good	10:09 - 11:27	10:39 - 11:49	11:10 - 12:25	12:09 - 13:53	13:26 - 15:20
Fair	11:28 - 12:29	11:50 - 12:53	12:26 - 13:50	13:54 - 15:14	15:21 - 17:19
Poor	12:30 - 13:58	12:54 - 14:33	13:51 - 15:32	15:15 - 17:30	17:20 - 20:13
Very Poor	13:59 +	14:34 +	15:33 +	17:31 +	20:14 +

Women	20s	30s	40s	50s	60s
Outstanding	0:00 - 10:20	0:00 - 11:08	0:00 - 11:35	0;00 - 13:16	0:00 - 14:28
Tactical Athlete	10:21 - 11:56	11:09 - 12:53	11:36 - 13:38	13:17 - 15:14	14:29 - 16:46
Good	11:57 - 13:25	12:54 - 14:33	13:39 - 15:17	15:15 - 17:19	16:47 - 18:52
Fair	13:26 - 15:05	14:34 - 15:56	15:18 - 17:11	17:20 - 19:10	18:53 - 20:55
Poor	15:06 - 17:11	15:57 - 18:18	17:12 - 19:43	19:11 - 21:57	20:56 - 23:55
Very Poor	17:12 +	18:19 +	19:44 +	21:58 +	23:56 +

Aerobic - 1000m Row (fastest time)

Men	20s	30s	40s	50s	60s
Outstanding	0:00 - 2:55	0:00 - 3:04	0:00 - 3:16	0:00 - 3:32	0:00 - 3:56
Tactical Athlete	2:56 - 3:15	3:05 - 3:24	3:17 - 3:34	3:33 - 3:53	3:57 - 4:18
Good	3:16 - 3:40	3:25 - 3:47	3:35 - 3:58	3:54 - 4:26	4:19 - 4:54
Fair	3:41 - 4:20	3:48 - 4:28	3:59 - 4:48	4:27 - 5:17	4:55 - 6:00
Poor	4:21 - 4:58	4:29 - 5:10	4:49 - 5:31	5:18 - 6:13	6:01 - 7:11
Very Poor	4:59 +	5:11 +	5:32 +	6:14 +	7:12 +

Women	20s	30s	40s	50s	60s
Outstanding	0:00 - 3:21	0:00 - 3:48	0:00 - 4:00	0:00 - 4:37	0:00 - 5:03
Tactical Athlete	3:22 - 3:49	3:49 - 4:07	4:01 - 4:22	4:38 - 4:53	5:04 - 5:22
Good	3:50 - 4:17	4:08 - 4:39	4:23 - 4:53	4:54 - 5:32	5:23 - 6:02
Fair	4:18 - 5:14	4:40 - 5:31	4:54 - 5:57	5:33 - 6:39	6:03 - 7:15
Poor	5:15 - 6:07	5:32 - 6:31	5:58 - 7:01	6:40 - 7:48	7:16 - 8:31
Very Poor	6:08 +	6:32 +	7:02 +	7:49 +	8:32 +

Evaluation of Results

Identify your strengths
What areas did you excel in?

Identify your weaknesses
What areas did you struggle in?

What can you do to make adjustments in your program?
Refer back to your Needs Analysis and make sure you covered everything. If you have one, ask your Human Performance coordinator for guidance.

Did you experience any pain during the test?
If yes, incorporate corrective exercises for those areas or see your doctor.

Set goals and prioritize training.
By knowing your current fitness level at the beginning of this program, you are now able to set goals and start working towards them.

Remember to write down your resting heart rate and maximum heart rate. This will be a great way to track your progress.

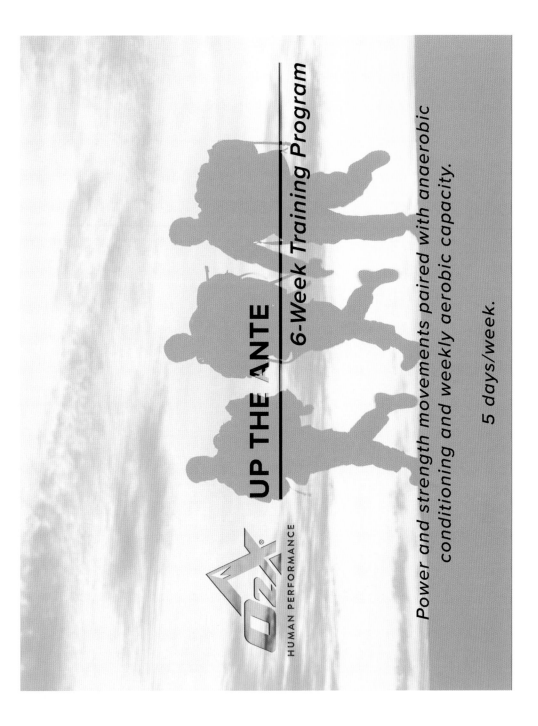

UP THE ANTE

6-Week Training Program

Power and strength movements paired with anaerobic conditioning and weekly aerobic capacity.

5 days/week.

STRENGTH AND CONDITIONING PROGRAMS

O2X HUMAN PERFORMANCE

PREPARE SWEAT RECOVER | The O2X Methodology

Tactical athletes meet physical demands as a job requirement. This includes enduring extended time on their feet, operating on unpredictable terrain, and moving in asymmetrical positions - often while wearing, or carrying heavy gear. As a result, it is crucial for tactical athletes to account for these known factors by targeting potential areas of weakness. Doing so requires proper preparation for workouts, as well as regular prehabilitation routines aimed to prevent injuries and mitigate job-related risks.

So, how do you incorporate injury prevention into your training plan? The PREPARE SWEAT RECOVER methodology: start your workout with 5 minutes of movement (Run/Bike/Row) that will get your blood flowing. Then, focus on warming up individual body parts by moving through the dynamic exercises listed below (Prepare). Finally, after your workout, complete a proper cool down (Recover) to maximize the benefits of your training and enhance your body's ability to recover.

If you miss or skip a workout day, don't stress. Continue with the plan on your next available day, starting from where you left off. Always aim for 3-5 workouts per week, but never more than 3 workout days in a row without a rest day.

Complete the training sessions in this program as efficiently as possible and limit your rest in between sets and exercises. Follow prescribed rest intervals if specified.

Unless otherwise specified, loading for all resistance exercises should be challenging, but you should be able to complete all sets. Fewer repetitions per set require higher intensity loads (heavier) to produce the desired adaptation. For example, a protocol that calls for 3 sets of 5 repetitions (3x5) is meant to be completed with more intense loading than 3 sets of 8 (3x8), but less than for 3 sets of 2 (3x2).

Base your loading on your ability, not your ego and note that some days you'll feel stronger than others. There are a lot of variables that can affect tactical athletes day to day and your training should adjust to account for them.

Before attempting this plan, or any exercise program, please consult with and get approval from your personal health care provider. Significant illness or injury can come from attempting an exercise, or workout program, without proper approval from your personal health care provider. The information contained in this plan is intended to be general and educational in nature, and not meant to replace or supplant the advice of your personal health care professionals.

LEGEND

KB = Kettlebell | DB = Dumbbell | BB = Barbell
RB =Resistance Band | MB = Medicine Ball

PREPARE
(complete each exercise for the provided time/distance)

1. Run/Bike/Row (5 mins)
2. Forearm Plank (20 secs)
3. Straight Arm Side Plank (20 secs)
4. Hip Bridge (20 secs)
5. Mini Band Walk (Lateral) (10 yards/2 sets)
6. Mini Band Walk (For/Back) (10 yards/2 sets)
7. Walking Knee Grab (10 yards)
8. Walking Heel Grab (10 yards)
9. Traveling Butt Kicks (10 yards)
10. High Knees (10 yards)
11. Lateral Lunge (Right/Left) (10 yards)
12. Push Up w/ Inchworm (10 yards)

RECOVER
(complete each exercise for 20-30 seconds)

1. Quad Foam Roll
2. IT Foam Roll
3. Glute Foam Roll
4. Back Foam Roll
5. Shoulder Foam Roll
6. Forward Fold
7. Downward Dog
8. Hip Stretch
9. Quad Stretch
10. Knee to Chest Stretch
11. Hamstring Stretch
12. Spinal Twist Stretch
13. Prone Glute Stretch
14. Bent Arm Chest Stretch
15. Tricep Stretch

For more information on how to complete all exercises, please visit o2x.com/exercise-gallery

WWW.O2X.COM

INFO@O2X.COM

UP THE ANTE

O2X HUMAN PERFORMANCE

6-Week Training Program

WEEK 1

Day	1	2	3	4	5	6	7
Notes:	*Step 1 - Prepare (8-10m)*	*Step 1 - Prepare (8-10m)*	*Step 1 - Prepare (8-10m)*	*Step 1 - Prepare (8-10m)*	*Step 1 - Prepare (8-10m)*	*Step 1 - Prepare (8-10m)*	*Step 1 - Prepare (8-10m)*
	Step 2 - Sweat:	*Step 2 - Sweat:*	*Step 2 - Sweat:*	*Step 2 - Sweat:*	*Step 2 - Sweat:*	*Step 2 - Sweat:*	*Step 2 - Sweat:*
	Clean : 4 sets x 4 reps	Single Arm DB Snatch: 4 sets x 4 reps each arm	Snatch: 4 sets x 4 reps	Rest	Barbell Bent Over Row: 4 sets x 10 reps	Jog or bike 90 min Conversational Pace	Recovery Day
	Squat: 4 sets x 8 reps	Pull-Ups: 4 sets x 10 reps	Single Arm DB Jerk: 3 sets x 4 reps each arm		DB Plank Row: 4 sets x 10 reps each	Or	
	Run: 1.5 miles for time	Rope Climb: 4 sets x 1 climb	Deadlift: 4 sets x 8 reps		MB Chest Press: 4 sets x 10 reps	Ruck 10 mi w/ 25#	
		Run Intervals: 6 sets x 2 min work / 2 min off	DB Split Squat: 3 sets x 10 reps each leg		Run: 3 miles for time		
			Row/Assault Bike: 10 sets x 30 seconds on / 90 seconds rest				
	Step 3 - Recover (10-15m)	*Step 3 - Recover (10-15m)*	*Step 3 - Recover (10-15m)*	*Step 3 - Recover (10-15m)*	*Step 3 - Recover (10-15m)*	*Step 3 - Recover (10-15m)*	*Step 3 - Recover (10-15m)*

UP THE ANTE

6-Week Training Program

O2X HUMAN PERFORMANCE

WEEK 2

Day	1	2	3	4	5	6	7
Notes:	Step 1 - Prepare (8-10m)	Step 1 - Prepare (8-10m)	Step 1 - Prepare (8-10m)	Step 1 - Prepare (8-10m)	Step 1 - Prepare (8-10m)	Step 1 - Prepare (8-10m)	Step 1 - Prepare (8-10m)
	Step 2 - Sweat:	Step 2 - Sweat:	Step 2 - Sweat:	Step 2 - Sweat:	Step 2 - Sweat:	Step 2 - Sweat:	Step 2 - Sweat:
	Clean: 4 sets x 3 reps Squat: 4 sets x 5 reps Run: 1.5 miles for time	Single Arm DB Snatch: 4 sets x 3 reps each arm Pull-Ups: 4 sets x 10 reps Rope Climb: 4 sets x 1 climb Run Intervals: 6 sets x 3 min work / 2 min off	Snatch - floor: 4 sets x 3 reps Single Arm DB Jerk: 3 sets x 3 reps each arm Deadlift: 4 sets x 5 reps DB Split Squat: 3 sets x 10 reps each leg Row/Assault Bike: 10 sets x 30 seconds on / 90 seconds rest	Recovery Day	Barbell Bent Over Row: 4 sets x 10 reps DB Plank Row: 4 sets x 10 reps each MB Chest Press: 4 sets x 10 reps Run: 4 miles for time	Jog or bike 90 min Conversational Pace Or Ruck 10 mi w/ 25#	Recovery Day
	Step 3 - Recover (10-15m)	Step 3 - Recover (10-15m)	Step 3 - Recover (10-15m)	Step 3 - Recover (10-15m)	Step 3 - Recover (10-15m)	Step 3 - Recover (10-15m)	Step 3 - Recover (10-15m)

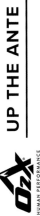

UP THE ANTE

6-Week Training Program

WEEK 3

Day	1	2	3	4	5	6	7
Notes:	*Step 1 - Prepare (8-10m)*	*Step 1 - Prepare (8-10m)*	*Step 1 - Prepare (8-10m)*	*Step 1 - Prepare (8-10m)*	*Step 1 - Prepare (8-10m)*	*Step 1 - Prepare (8-10m)*	*Step 1 - Prepare (8-10m)*
	Step 2 - Sweat:	*Step 2 - Sweat:*	*Step 2 - Sweat:*	*Step 2 - Sweat:*	*Step 2 - Sweat:*	*Step 2 - Sweat:*	*Step 2 - Sweat:*
	Clean : 4 sets x 3 reps Squat: 4 sets x 5 reps Run: 2 miles for time	Single Arm DB Snatch: 4 sets x 3 reps each arm Pull-Ups: 4 sets x 8 reps Rope Climb: 4 sets x 1 climb Run Intervals: 4 sets x 4 min work / 2 min off	Snatch - floor: 4 sets x 3 reps Single Arm DB Jerk: 3 sets x 3 reps each arm Deadlift: 4 sets x 5 reps DB Split Squat: 3 sets x 8 reps each leg Row/Assault Bike: 8 sets x 40 seconds on / 90 seconds rest	Recovery Day	Barbell Bent Over Row: 4 sets x 8 reps DB Plank Row: 4 sets x 8 reps each MB Chest Press: 4 sets x 8 reps Run: 5 miles for time	Jog or bike 120 min Conversational Pace Or Ruck 12 mi w/ 35#	Recovery Day
	Step 3 - Recover (10-15m)	*Step 3 - Recover (10-15m)*	*Step 3 - Recover (10-15m)*	*Step 3 - Recover (10-15m)*	*Step 3 - Recover (10-15m)*	*Step 3 - Recover (10-15m)*	*Step 3 - Recover (10-15m)*

UP THE ANTE

O2X HUMAN PERFORMANCE

6-Week Training Program

WEEK 4

Day	1	2	3	4	5	6	7
Notes:	Step 1 - Prepare (8-10m)	Step 1 - Prepare (8-10m)	Step 1 - Prepare (8-10m)	Step 1 - Prepare (8-10m)	Step 1 - Prepare (8-10m)	Step 1 - Prepare (8-10m)	Step 1 - Prepare (8-10m)
	Step 2 - Sweat: Clean: 4 sets x 2 reps Squat: 4 sets x 3 reps Run: 2 miles for time	Step 2 - Sweat: Single Arm DB Snatch: 4 sets x 2 reps each arm Pull-Ups: 4 sets x 8 reps Rope Climb: 4 sets x 1 climb Run Intervals: 3 sets x 5 min work / 2 min off	Step 2 - Sweat: Snatch - floor: 4 sets x 2 reps Single Arm DB Jerk: 3 sets x 2 reps each arm Deadlift: 4 sets x3 reps DB Split Squat: 3 sets x 8 reps each leg Row/Assault Bike: 4 sets x 60 seconds on / 90	Step 2 - Sweat: Recovery Day	Step 2 - Sweat: Barbell Bent Over Row: 4 sets x 8 reps DB Plank Row: 4 sets x 8 reps each MB Chest Press: 4 sets x 8 reps Run: 5 miles for time	Step 2 - Sweat: Jog or bike 120 min Conversational Pace Or Ruck 12 mi w/ 45#	Step 2 - Sweat: Recovery Day
	Step 3 - Recover (10-15m)	Step 3 - Recover (10-15m)	Step 3 - Recover (10-15m)	Step 3 - Recover (10-15m)	Step 3 - Recover (10-15m)	Step 3 - Recover (10-15m)	Step 3 - Recover (10-15m)

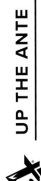

O2X HUMAN PERFORMANCE

UP THE ANTE

6-Week Training Program

WEEK 5

Day	1	2	3	4	5	6	7
Notes:	Step 1 - Prepare (8-10m)	Step 1 - Prepare (8-10m)	Step 1 - Prepare (8-10m)	Step 1 - Prepare (8-10m)	Step 1 - Prepare (8-10m)	Step 1 - Prepare (8-10m)	Step 1 - Prepare (8-10m)
	Step 2 - Sweat:	Step 2 - Sweat:	Step 2 - Sweat:	Step 2 - Sweat:	Step 2 - Sweat:	Step 2 - Sweat:	Step 2 - Sweat:
	Clean: 3 sets x 2 reps Squat: 3 sets x 3 reps Run: 2 miles for time	Single Arm DB Snatch: 3 sets x 2 reps each arm Pull-Ups: 3 sets x 6 reps Rope Climb: 3 sets x 1 climb Run Intervals: 2 sets x 8 minutes / 2 minutes rest	Snatch - floor: 3 sets x 2 reps Single Arm DB Jerk: 3 sets x 2 reps each arm Deadlift: 3 sets x 3 reps DB Split Squat: 3 sets x 6 reps each leg Row/Assault Bike: 4 sets x 90 seconds on / 90 seconds rest	Recovery Day	Barbell Bent Over Row: 3 sets x 6 reps DB Plank Row: 3 sets x 6 reps each MB Chest Press: 3 sets x 6 reps Run: 3 miles for time	Jog or bike 90 min Conversational Pace Or Ruck 10 mi w/ 25#	Recovery Day
	Step 3 - Recover (10-15m)	Step 3 - Recover (10-15m)	Step 3 - Recover (10-15m)	Step 3 - Recover (10-15m)	Step 3 - Recover (10-15m)	Step 3 - Recover (10-15m)	Step 3 - Recover (10-15m)

UP THE ANTE

6-Week Training Program

WEEK 6

Day	1	2	3	4	5	6	7
Notes:	Step 1 - Prepare (8-10m)	Step 1 - Prepare (8-10m)	Step 1 - Prepare (8-10m)	Step 1 - Prepare (8-10m)	Step 1 - Prepare (8-10m)	Step 1 - Prepare (8-10m)	Step 1 - Prepare (8-10m)
	Step 2 - Sweat:	Step 2 - Sweat:	Step 2 - Sweat:	Step 2 - Sweat:	Step 2 - Sweat:	Step 2 - Sweat:	Step 2 - Sweat:
	Clean: 3 sets x 3 reps Squat: 3 sets x 3 reps Run: 1.5 miles for time	Single Arm DB Snatch: 3 sets x 2 reps each arm Pull-Ups: 3 sets x 6 reps Rope Climb: 3 sets x 1 climb Run Intervals: 1 sets x 10 minutes	Snatch - floor: 3 sets x 2 reps Single Arm DB Jerk: 3 sets x 2 reps each arm Deadlift: 3 sets x 3 reps DB Split Squat: 3 sets x 6 reps each leg Row: 3 sets x 90 seconds on / 90 seconds rest	Recovery Day	Barbell Bent Over Row: 3 sets x 6 reps DB Plank Row: 3 sets x 6 reps each MB Chest Press: 3 sets x 6 reps Run: 2 miles for time	Jog or bike 60 min Conversational Pace Or Ruck 8 mi w/ 25#	Recovery Day
	Step 3 - Recover (10-15m)	Step 3 - Recover (10-15m)	Step 3 - Recover (10-15m)	Step 3 - Recover (10-15m)	Step 3 - Recover (10-15m)	Step 3 - Recover (10-15m)	Step 3 - Recover (10-15m)

EQUIPMENT FREE WORKOUTS

Remember to do your prepare work and pre-hab/movement prep prior to each workout as well as recovery exercises post workout.

Strict form... strict form... strict form...

WORKOUT 1

Alternate back and forth for 15 minutes

5 Burpees

5 Push-Ups

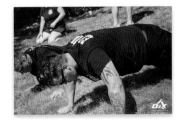

WORKOUT 2

Alternate back and forth for 15 minutes

5 Inchworm Push-Ups

5 Body Weight Thrusters

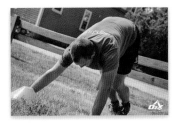

WORKOUT 3

5 Rounds:

15 second Wall Sit with Leg Raise each side

15 Push-Ups

20-30 Supine Glute Bridge with Single Leg Raise

8 Rounds:

40m Sprint / 20 second rest

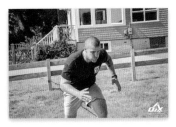

Remember to do your prepare work and pre-hab/movement prep prior to each workout as well as recovery exercises post workout.

Strict form... strict form... strict form...

WORKOUT 4

3 Rounds:

10 Split Squat each leg

30 Lying Hip Abduction

20 - 30 sec Supine Grip Chin Up Hold

1 Round:

1 mile Run

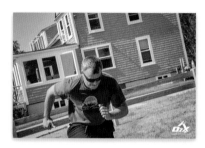

WORKOUT 5

Squat Jumps: 4 sets x 5 reps

Push Up Pyramid: 1 rep - 10 reps, 10 reps - 1 rep (i.e. add one rep to each set. Work your way up to 10, then back down to 1)

Sit Up Pyramid: 1 rep - 10 reps, 10 reps - 1 rep (i.e. add one rep to each set. Work your way up to 10, then back down to 1)

Sprint: 10 sets x 20 seconds / 30 seconds rest

WORKOUT 6

Step Ups: 5 sets x 8 reps each leg

Bird Dogs: 5 sets x 8 reps each leg

Crunches: 3 sets x 10 reps

1 Leg Glute Bridge: 3 sets x 20 reps each leg

Squat Jumps: 3 sets x 10 reps

Jog: 30 minutes

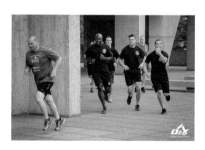

≤ 15 MINUTE WORKOUTS

Remember to do your prepare work and pre-hab/movement prep prior to each workout as well as recovery exercises post workout.

Strict form...form...form...

WORKOUT 1

Complete this workout as fast as possible (AFAP). Complete the first column of each exercise before moving to the second (i.e. 5 squat jumps then 10 push ups)

Equipment Needed: None

Squat Jump	5 - 10 - 15 - 20
Push-Up	10 - 15 - 20 - 5
Squat Thrust	15 - 20 -5 - 10
Lunges	20 - 5 - 10 -15 (each leg)

WORKOUT 2

Complete this workout as fast as possible (AFAP). Complete the first column of each exercise before moving to the second (i.e. 2 pull-ups then 4 thrusters)

Equipment Needed: TRX or Resistance Bands / Barbell or Dumbbell

Pull-Up	2 - 4 - 6 - 8 - 10
Thruster	4 - 8 - 12 - 16 - 20 (BB 75lbs/DB 35lbs/Res Bands)
Row	6 - 12 - 18 - 24 - 30
Push-Up	8 - 16 - 24 - 32 - 40
BW Squat	10 - 20 - 30 - 40 - 50 (Body Weight)

WORKOUT 3

Complete as many rounds as possible in 15 minutes (AMRAP).

Equipment Needed: Barbell, Dumbbell, or Resistance Bands / Box / Pull Up Bar

5 Box Jumps (step down, don't jump)

5 Barbell Press (BB 75lbs or DB 35lbs)

5 Box Jumps

5 Pull-Ups ⎯ 1 Round

5 Box Jumps

5 Burpees

Remember to do your prepare work and pre-hab/movement prep prior to each workout as well as recovery exercises post workout.
Strict form...form...form...

WORKOUT 4

Complete as many rounds as possible in 15 minutes (AMRAP).

Equipment Needed: Barbell, Dumbbell, or Resistance Bands / Pull Up Bar

3 Pull Ups

6 Renegade Rows

9 Burpees — 1 Round

12 Lunges

15 Thrusters

WORKOUT 5

TABATA = 20 seconds of work / 10 seconds rest x 8 sets. 1 set = both exercises in each TABATA

Equipment Needed: Barbell, Dumbbell, or Resistance Bands

TABATA 1 = Tuck Jumps
Renegade Row with Dumbbell

TABATA 2 = Jumping Pull Ups
Barbell, Dumbbell, or Resistance Band Shoulder Press

TABATA 3 = Body Weight Squat
1 Flight of Stairs

WORKOUT 6

Every minute on the minute, begin a new round for 15 minutes.

Equipment Needed: Pull Up Bar (if no pull up bar, replace the 3 pull ups with 10 push ups)

3 Pull Ups

5 Lunges per leg

8 Burpees

TEAM/GROUP WORKOUTS

Remember to do your prepare work and pre-hab/movement prep prior to each workout as well as recovery exercises post workout.

Strict form...form...form...

WORKOUT 1: Head to Head Race

Complete 5 rounds of the circuit. Create 2 lanes and race head to head. Each completing the distances and reps specified. This can be done as a relay with multiple people on a team.

20 Meter Sprint (both people start lying face down)

12 Step Ups (total) to Box (20" recommended)

20 Meter Sprint

15 Kettlebell Swings

20 Meter Sprint

WINNER = FIRST TO FINISH 5 ROUNDS

WORKOUT 2: Teams of Two

Break into teams of two. Split up the reps as needed. Each team gets through the exercises and specified reps as quickly as possible. The team to finish first wins.

If you want to do the workout on your own or only have two people, cut the exercise totals in half and complete the circuit as quickly as possible.

1200M Farmers Carry	40 Push Ups
60 Kettlebell Clean & Press	40 Goblet Squats
60 Pull Ups	20 Pull Ups
60 Goblet Squats	200M Sprint
800M Sandbag Run	

WORKOUT 3: Deck of Cards

Assign each suit an exercise and as you flip through the cards, complete the number of reps shown on the face of the card.

Break into groups or pairs and the first team to get through their deck wins.

 Push Ups   Sit Ups   Air Squats   Lunges

Remember to do your prepare work and pre-hab/movement prep prior to each workout as well as recovery exercises post workout.
Strict form...form...form...

WORKOUT 4: Counter-Timer

Set stations up in a circle. The Counter and Timer exercises should be next to each other.

The group rotates when the Timer completes the reps specified. The Counter counts reps and passes that number on to the next person. The Burpee count is continuous for the group.

The workout ends when the Burpee count totals 200.

COUNTER: Burpees
Accumulate reps as a group. Each person continues the count from where the person before them left off. Rotate when the timer finishes.

TIMER: 10 Lunges Per Leg
This is the timer for the group. When you finish the reps the whole group rotates clockwise to the next station.

STATIONS
Push Ups
Deadlift
Plank Shoulder Taps
Shoulder Press (dumbbells or band)
Mountain Climbers
Flutter Kicks

WORKOUT 5: Partner Circuit

Partner 1 and 2 go back and forth between exercises at each station. The goal is to get through as many rounds between the 2 exercises as possible at each station.

Each station is 2 minutes of work, with 30 seconds off to rotate to the next station.

Station 1:   Partner 1: 20 Squats   Partner 2: High Plank

Station 2:   Partner 1: 20 Push-Ups   Partner 2: Lateral Skaters

Station 3:   Partner 1: 10 Shoulder Press   Partner 2: V-Ups

Station 4:   Partner 1: 10 Bent Over Row   Partner 2: Alternating Single Leg Glute Bridge

WORKOUT 6: O2X Circuit Workout

You can do this circuit individually or as a group. Do each exercise for 1 minute on / 30 seconds off. Use the 30 second rest to transition to the next exercise in the circuit. Do as many reps as possible in the working intervals. Do 1 to 3 rounds of the circuit depending on the amount of time you have available for your workout.

• Bench Press	• Battle Ropes	• Pull Ups	• Band Chest Fly
• Rocket Jump	• High Plank - Knees to Elbows	• Goblet Squat	• Band Reverse Fly

COMPLETE PROGRAM DESIGN EXAMPLE

PROGRAM DESIGN

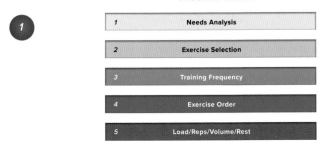

1	**Needs Analysis**
2	**Exercise Selection**
3	**Training Frequency**
4	**Exercise Order**
5	**Load/Reps/Volume/Rest**

PERIODIZATION

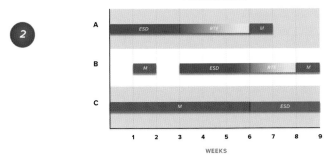

DAILY WORKOUTS

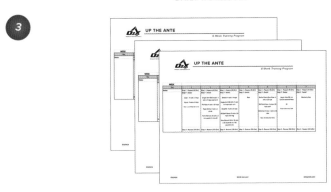

ACTION PLAN

GOALS

NEEEDS ANALYSIS

TRAINING FREQUENCY

EQUIPMENT AVAILABLE

EXERCISE SELECTION (Anything off limits? Restrictions? Regression exercises needed?)

TRAINING LOAD / REPS / VOLUME / REST PERIOD

TRAINING GOALS

What does success look like to you? What's important to you in your training?
What do you want to accomplish? How do you want to feel?

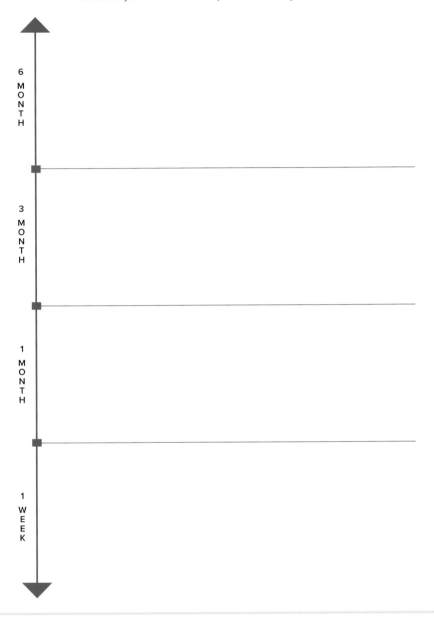

6
M
O
N
T
H

3
M
O
N
T
H

1
M
O
N
T
H

1
W
E
E
K

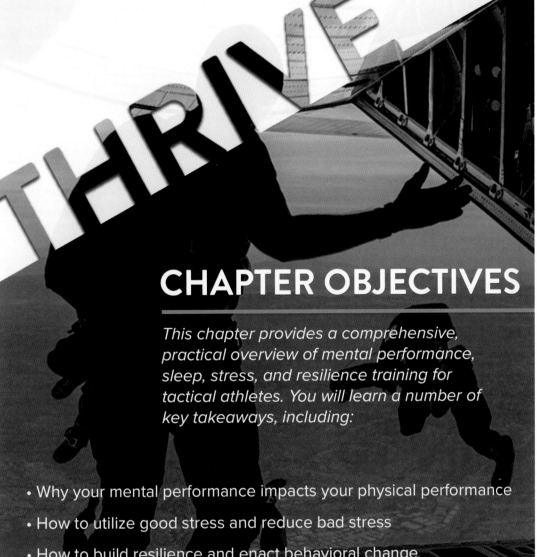

CHAPTER OBJECTIVES

This chapter provides a comprehensive, practical overview of mental performance, sleep, stress, and resilience training for tactical athletes. You will learn a number of key takeaways, including:

- Why your mental performance impacts your physical performance

- How to utilize good stress and reduce bad stress

- How to build resilience and enact behavioral change

- Why sleep is vital and how to improve your rest

- How mindfulness can impact your physical and mental

  performance and how to add these exercises to your day to day

- How mental and physical recovery enhances job performance

WELCOME TO THRIVE

THRIVE. The very word conjures up positive energy! Better than "okay" and better than "fine," *thrive* suggests something beyond "good." Taking it one step further, thrive implies not a momentary feeling or experience, but something that has staying power. One doesn't thrive for a moment; rather, one finds a way of going, perhaps a way of being, that allows him or her to thrive.

Welcome to the THRIVE chapter, the third concept of living that is at the heart of O2X thinking: EAT SWEAT THRIVE. My life's work has been dedicated to helping children, families, schools, and communities respond to some of life's most stressful events: natural disasters, terrorism, life-changing events. I have had the privilege of taking my research outside the walls of academia in order to help adults, children, schools, communities, and unique populations when bad things happen. How do some people face life's stressors and actually become stronger in the aftermath? Can we learn from them? Can we develop and even master the coping skills and habits that define resilience? I believe we can.

Resilience is not the absence of stress; it is, in fact, much more. At the core of resilience is the belief that in the very nature of crisis lies an opportunity for growth. Think about it!

Researchers at Carnegie Mellon University found that from 1983 to 2009 there was a 10%–30% increase in stress levels across all demographic categories. Higher levels of stress can lead to more instances of diabetes, heart disease, and obesity. According to the Centers for Disease Control and Prevention, three-quarters of American healthcare spending goes toward treating such chronic conditions. The Benson-Henry Institute for Mind Body Medicine at Massachusetts General Hospital estimates that 60%–90% of doctor visits are to treat stress-related conditions.[1]

There are evidence-based strategies that indicate we *can* live our lives differently—ways that will make an immediate and long-term difference in our health and happiness.

We know that over time tactical athletes *accumulate* the effects of chronic stress. How important is it to reflect on current stresses and habits and consider new strategies to incorporate as habits into daily living that counter the negative outcomes from living with stress?

The big idea behind this chapter is that your insights lead to action—daily practices and tools that cost nothing and can be done in your chair, your car, at the beach, or wherever.

What's more is the opportunity to reconnect with ourselves. When we work, we tend to leave our lives, important matters, and even our beliefs behind, as though we can pick them up at the end of a shift when we drive into our driveway. We can choose to reconnect to our loved ones (if not now, then when?) and our community. Just think about the possibilities if we were all committed to living the way we believe. So open your minds and your hearts to self-reflection and discovery, and choose to *thrive*!

—*Maria Trozzi, MEd, O2X Mental*
Performance and Resilience Specialist

INTRODUCTION

Until now, we have focused mainly on the physical demands placed on tactical athletes. In this chapter—THRIVE—we will turn our attention to the unique *mental* demands you face. Day in and day out, you are asked to put yourself in potentially dangerous situations to help others, and unfortunately this means dealing with and experiencing traumatic events. Therefore, in order to truly ensure that you finish your career as strong as you started, you must train to develop mental performance skills so you can not only survive, but thrive under these conditions.

Let's start by defining **mental performance** before outlining the tools you can use to develop your skill set. Mental performance is the implementation of psychological and cognitive skills developed to optimize performance, particularly in high-pressure situations. Like going to the gym to get physically stronger, improving your mental performance also requires practice and targeted training of various mental skills.

Mental Performance The systematic implementation of cognitive skills developed to optimize performance, particularly in high-pressure situations.

The mental performance skills we will focus on include mindfulness, breathing, writing, and yoga nidra, to name a few. Developing these skills will help you optimize your mental performance by increasing your readiness to handle unpredictable and relentless stressors, improving your capacity to build resilience through a growth mindset, and enhancing your ability to recover mentally and physically through healthy sleep habits. In contrast, ignoring the mental component of your job and training can lead to corrosive stress accumulation, potential risk of injury, and negative impact on your overall performance and well-being. As a tactical athlete, training to optimize your mental performance is critical to your career longevity and health.

O2X organizes THRIVE into three broad categories: stress, resilience, and sleep (fig. 3–1). You will likely find that practicing skills to develop one category of mental performance also improves the others. One concept you will notice running throughout the discussion of mental performance is mindfulness.

Mindfulness provides the backdrop of many of the mental skills you will learn—from breathing techniques to journaling. Mindfulness is rooted in the idea of being fully present and aware of both yourself and your surroundings. Practiced by elite performers of all backgrounds—from athletes like Michael Jordan and Laird Hamilton to special operations soldiers and Fortune 500 CEOs—mindfulness benefits mental health much like running builds cardiovascular health.

We will explore mindfulness and techniques to practice it in much more detail later in the chapter, but for now, we can ask the question: How does mental performance training help tactical athletes? Skills like mindfulness, breathing, and visualization can help you gain greater self-awareness and situational awareness. This enables you to more effectively make decisions, manage negative reactions, and swiftly respond to high-stress situations. Additionally, improving mental performance allows you to attach *meaning* and *purpose* to your thoughts and actions, which can help you build resilience so that it's there when you need it most.

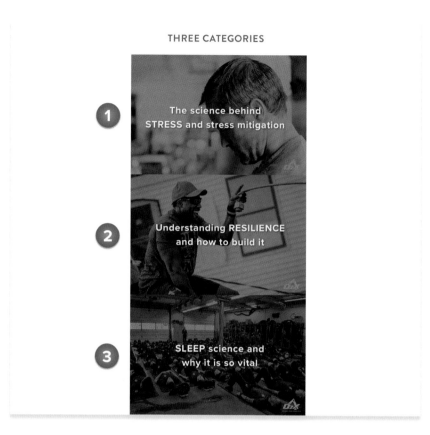

THREE CATEGORIES

1. The science behind STRESS and stress mitigation

2. Understanding RESILIENCE and how to build it

3. SLEEP science and why it is so vital

Figure 3–1. Three categories

KEY TAKEAWAYS

Introduction

⋄ Training to maximize mental performance is as important as physical conditioning and maintaining a healthy diet.

⋄ Mental performance requires developing skills and techniques that allow tactical athletes to face unpredictable situations and meet daily stressors with resilience.

⋄ Self-awareness is a fundamental part of being able to improve mental performance. The remainder of the chapter will outline tools and skills like mindfulness to help you continually improve your self-awareness.

MENTAL PERFORMANCE

One defining factor of being a tactical athlete is enduring daily job-related mental and physical stressors. As a result, a comprehensive human performance program for tactical athletes would be incomplete without training that specifically targets mental performance. As discussed in the introduction of this chapter, mental performance includes a variety of cognitive skills to use in high-pressure situations.

A well-rounded mental performance program develops the plethora of skills highlighted in the accompanying diagram, including anything from attention control to team coordination (fig. 3–2). And like physical conditioning, mental skills training is critical to maximizing human performance. Mental performance is not a new concept (fig. 3–3), and almost every elite organization and team has utilized mental performance concepts to optimize outcomes, including C-suite executives, professional sports teams, and special operations military units.

For corporate professionals, job stress is very real, and many executives feel the pressure of an entire company's success weighing on their ability to make high-stakes decisions. For Olympic and professional athletes, a single point or play can be the defining moment of their lives and the culmination of years of physical training and sacrifice on which their careers depend.

The regularity with which tactical athletes face stressful situations is much higher than that of the average population. This makes mental performance training a necessity for their health and career longevity.

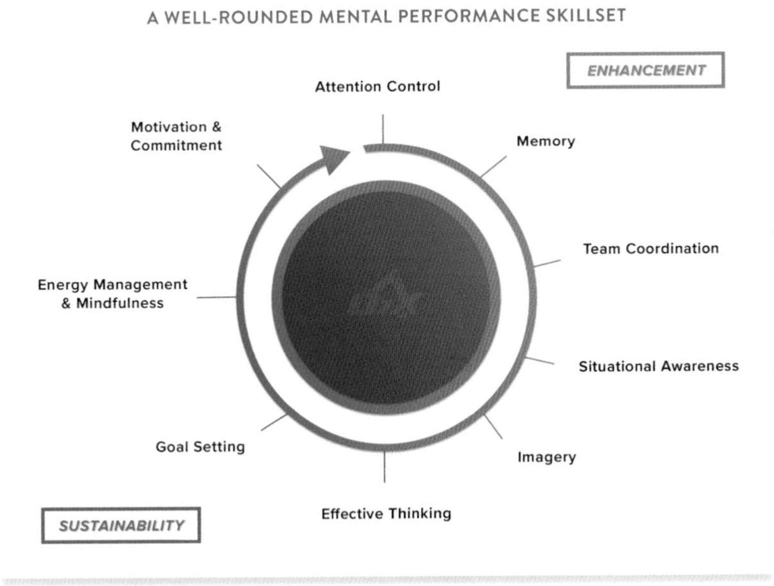

A WELL-ROUNDED MENTAL PERFORMANCE SKILLSET

Figure 3–2. Well-rounded approach to performance

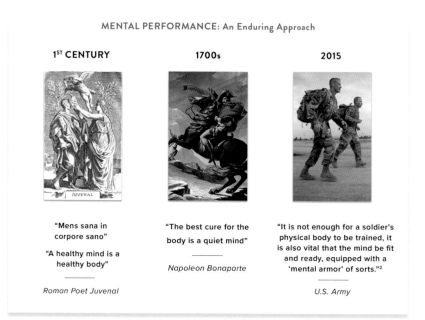

MENTAL PERFORMANCE: An Enduring Approach

1ST CENTURY	1700s	2015

"Mens sana in corpore sano"

"A healthy mind is a healthy body"

———

Roman Poet Juvenal

"The best cure for the body is a quiet mind"

———

Napoleon Bonaparte

"It is not enough for a soldier's physical body to be trained, it is also vital that the mind be fit and ready, equipped with a 'mental armor' of sorts."[2]

———

U.S. Army

Figure 3–3. Mental performance, an enduring approach

For tactical athletes, responding to a call can be nothing short of a life-and-death situation where decisions must be made quickly and under extreme duress. Another component of stress that cannot be overlooked when thinking about tactical athletes' mental performance is the residual stress of constantly responding to high-pressure scenarios. While an Olympic athlete knows when the race will be and a corporate executive typically has ample time to prepare for a high-stakes meeting, tactical athletes show up to work each day not knowing what to expect. This constant need to be mentally ready for anything can be very taxing. By practicing mental skills, tactical athletes can optimize mental readiness in advance of high-pressure situations and refine the tools required to process traumatic events. Practicing your mental skills will help you maintain optimal performance in stressful situations just as it helps a professional athlete get into the zone on game day (fig. 3–4).

For an athlete, getting into **the zone** means she feels that her skill level is high enough to meet the challenge she faces and that her energy level is ideal for performance.[2]

Athletes can use mental skills to find the zone even in extreme situations. For example, if an athlete has to perform at the Olympics but is battling an illness, she can use mental skills to help elevate her energy levels and put herself closer to the zone of optimal performance. Similarly, if a rookie goalie is in the net and has one chance to stop a shootout goal for a championship win, he can use mental skills to mitigate stress and anxiety so he can be fully present and able to react in a split-second. Like professional athletes, tactical athletes can use mental performance training to help get in the zone when the bell rings.

The remaining pages of this chapter will provide you with various skills you can use to manage energy levels and stress. Learning how and when to use these techniques will help you get in the zone more frequently so you can maximize your overall performance.

The Zone
Also known as the individual zones of optimal functioning model or inverted U curve, the zone refers to the idea that some level of anxiety is beneficial to achieving maximum performance. The amount of anxiety varies individually, and one person's zone of optimal functioning may be at a different level of stress as another's

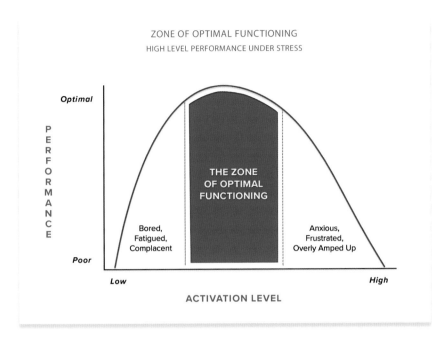

Figure 3–4. Zone of optimal functioning diagram[3]

KEY TAKEAWAYS

Mental Performance

⬧ Mental readiness refers to building a strong and resilient mind so you are ready to face any potential challenges or adversity. Like the body, the mind can be trained and strengthened prior to experiencing stressors.

⬧ Athletes frequently talk about the desire to be in the zone during training and competition. Qualitatively, this is a state where things just seem to be going right and an athlete is focused on the task at hand. Some call this the zone of optimal functioning, where activation or energy level is ideal for the task at hand.

⬧ The optimal energy level to reach a state of maximum performance varies by individual.

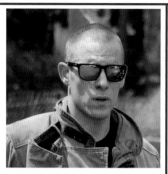

Being the driver/operator of the first arriving engine at working fire is a situation where a lot of things need to happen very quickly and a misstep can cause problems through the rest of the incident. The engine needs to be positioned, water supply established, hoses stretched to the fire, water pumped appropriately, ladders thrown, equipment positioned, radio traffic monitored, and so on. Success here requires finding that zone quickly.

I remember very clearly the times I've had this job at a fire and what it felt like to be in the zone. One time in particular stands out—a fire in a garden apartment building not far from our firehouse. Even several years later, I remember the tones sounding in the kitchen—"engines respond: residential fire"—and our crew jumping up from dinner to run to the bay. I remember taking five slow, deep breaths as I sat behind the wheel waiting for everyone to put on their gear and get in the engine. I recall pulling out of the bay and turning right off the pad. The less-than-a-mile response felt like an eternity as I continued to closely monitor my breathing and listened to instructions from the officer.

As we turned the corner into the apartment complex, the thick smoke rolling across the road made it clear that this would be a working fire. As I set the parking brake and completed the sequence of lever pulls and button presses required to place the engine in "pump," my body entered the zone. I felt as though I was moving in slow motion, dismounting the engine and setting about my tasks. The guys in the back were stretching a long hose line from the rear and I assisted them in getting it from the engine to the stairs of the building. I returned to the engine to charge it with water before attaching a supply hose to the rear intake so the next engine could send us water. I remember stretching a second line to the front of the building, leaving it in the front yard and returning to the engine to grab and place our two ladders.

The second engine crew passed me in the yard and in not-so-patient terms told me to put water in their line, which required a quick trip back to the pump panel to do a recheck of the pressure in the first line. I then returned to the ladders, placing the extension ladder to a balcony above the fire unit and the straight ladder to a window in the rear. A third engine crew arrived, stretched a third line that required my attention, and then I set about laying out all of the tools my company may have needed as the incident unfolded. Hooks, axes, extinguishers, extra air cylinders, and a cooler of water bottles all made their way to a tarp on the front lawn.

I returned to the engine's pump panel, having accomplished all that I needed for the moment, to recheck the pressures and water supply. I remember the second chief that had arrived at the fire walking by and telling me "good job," with a pat on the shoulder. With that I took a breath to relax. My heart rate slowed, my breath returned to normal, and then my hands began to shake.

What had felt like an hour of constant work had actually been closer to seven minutes. I can still picture the slow, deliberate actions—accomplished in the exact sequence—at what felt like a snail's pace. I remember hearing the radio traffic but not the sirens of the other incoming fire trucks. I remember very clearly the apartment building, the smoke, and the fire conditions but not the buildings down the street. I don't recall feeling stressed or overwhelmed but rather prepared and driven.

At that fire, on that day, everything was clicking for me. A culmination of preparation and awareness had produced the desired outcome. I found my way into the zone of optimal performance and am grateful that I did.

—*Brice Long, former firefighter, O2X Director of HP Experience, CSCS*

STRESS MANAGEMENT

Planning ahead is critical to managing stress and staying focused on what's important. With just a little bit of preparation, I can better focus my energy on what matters most, my family and my work.

—*Paul McCullough, O2X cofounder*

Being a tactical athlete is inherently stressful, mentally and physically; however, as we talked about with physical conditioning, not all stress is detrimental. If you practice specific skills that strengthen your mental performance, you can not only survive adversity but come back stronger from it—a process often referred to as *post-traumatic growth*. As with conditioning, we must experience stress and put ourselves in the position of overcoming challenges to become stronger and more resilient.

Much like physical conditioning, there is a level of stress that is productive and can incite growth (eustress), and there is a point at which stress becomes too burdensome (distress) and can lead to burnout or, in the case of physical conditioning, overtraining. Like physical stress, the severity of the psychological stress you can encounter as a tactical athlete on any given day is unpredictable. In addition to potentially acute instances of stress that may come with responding to a traumatic call, you must learn to handle more chronic, low levels of stress you encounter every day or every shift.

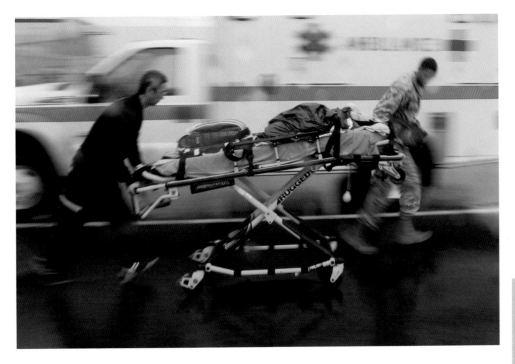

PTSD
Post-traumatic Stress Disorder can be the result of experiencing a traumatic event such as combat, natural disaster, or response to an emergency situation. Not all people who experience a traumatic event develop PTSD. Multiple factors influence whether someone will show symptoms of PTSD.

Both acute and chronic stress can not only impede performance over time but also cause long-term damage to your mental and physical health. Post-traumatic stress (PTS) and **post-traumatic stress disorder (PTSD)** are another category of stress, which we will address in greater detail later in the chapter. Signs of stress impacting your daily life can include irritability, difficulty focusing, and changes in sleep patterns; and after prolonged exposure to stress, you may experience problems with memory, mood swings, and changes in motivation level.[4] This is why it is critical to develop not only the skills to respond to mental stressors, but also more basic skills to increase your self-awareness of when and how you are affected by the daily stressors of your job.

In order to better understand how mental-skills training can improve your performance and your well-being, let's first take a look at the physiology behind how your mind and body react and adapt to stress.

Autonomic Nervous System

Think back to the example of being cold in the SWEAT chapter—the physical stress of being exposed to freezing temperatures triggers our bodies to shiver in order to generate warmth. Our bodies do this without our conscious control, attempting to adapt to a situation and return to a normal baseline state or **homeostasis**. The physiological response that occurs within our bodies when we experience any type of stressor comes from our **autonomic nervous system** (ANS; fig. 3–6).

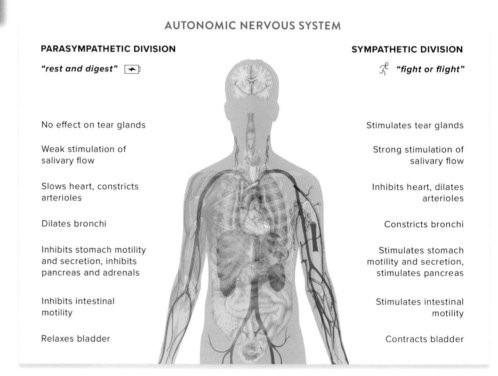

Figure 3–6. The autonomic nervous system

For tactical athletes, the stress response—a function of the ANS—can often be more than a shiver. For example, consider the dynamic environment a special operations team faces when assaulting an enemy compound. These units often operate deep inside hostile areas, supported only by themselves, and acting on uncertain intelligence, so they rely on each other, their training, and their instincts to be successful. One of those key instincts is the body's stress response. Let's look at a snapshot of one of these operators as he and his team advance into an unknown structure.

Making movement toward the compound door, the team is carefully scanning threats. Upon reaching their target building, they stop to make entry into the structure. The lead assaulter checks the door—it's open. A single barrel nod initiates the entry and the first man in the stack moves swiftly through the opening. As he enters the first room, he's laser focused on clearing his sector as the remainder of his team makes movement right behind. He scans his corner through night vision and the outline of a familiar and ominous shape comes into focus. Before his mind has time to fully register the homemade bomb sunken into the dirt floor, his body is already taking action to escape the threat. His pulse quickens, respiration rate increases, and his brain signals the release of hormones and redirects blood to the areas that need it most to make an escape. Fueled by the physiological changes in body chemistry, this operator reverses his momentum and drives his heavily loaded frame back toward the door while alerting his team.

As they move from the structure, their cardiovascular systems are working in hyperdrive to provide their legs with the fuel required to run out of the building to escape the potential blast radius. Less essential functions, like hearing and dexterity, are dialed back to provide more energy for the escape. Time appears to slow down as the way their eyes and brains process information changes to allow for clearer decisions. The team covers ground quickly, distancing themselves from the danger to regroup.

In this example, the special operations team's stress response activated providing the physiological changes needed for survival. We'll now dive a bit deeper into how these systems work, the outcomes, and ways to maximize our body's stress response.

The ANS comprises two parts—our sympathetic nervous system (SNS) and parasympathetic nervous system (PNS). These two branches of the nervous system are responsible for triggering our automatic response to various stressors—like shivering when we are cold or increasing our heart rate, activating digestion, and controlling the release of hormones (like adrenaline), among other things. Let's take a closer look at what the SNS and PNS each do and how they help us respond to stress.

Parasympathetic Nervous System

Have you ever finished a meal and felt totally relaxed and at ease? The most likely example of this is Thanksgiving, and there is something to it—not just the turkey. It is your body's natural tendency to conserve energy and focus its attention on internal processes like digestion. This state of calm and relaxation is often called "rest and digest." It is our body's attempt to reset and replenish resources during nonthreatening situations.[5] When our PNS is activated, our heart rate decreases, blood pressure drops, and breathing slows as we reset. It is during this process that our bodies focus energy on systems that facilitate a quick return to homeostasis, like digestion. This process of returning to normal prepares the body to respond to future stressors.

While our bodies have adapted to naturally reset through activation of the PNS, as a tactical athlete you may not always have a significant amount of time to let your body rest and digest between stressful situations. So it is critical for not only your performance but also your long-term health that you learn how to proactively turn on your PNS through a variety of techniques. Before diving into the mental performance techniques that can help you reset, we will talk about the role of the SNS in stress response. And we will finish this section of our discussion on the physiological response to stress by highlighting heart rate variability and its role in measuring your ability to recover, mentally and physically.

Sympathetic Nervous System

You have likely heard the phrase "fight or flight." Your SNS is the physiological response that enables you to fight or flee when your mind signals that you may be in danger. This is the branch of your ANS responsible for triggering you to meet a threat or outrun it. Unlike the PNS that initiates internal processes like digestion, the SNS activates to respond to external stressors and threats.[6]

It may sound cliché, but think back to the days when humans were truly hunters and gatherers. If you were sitting around a fire and a predator came running toward you with the intention of eating you for dinner, you would think one of two things: (1) I will react and do everything I can to fight off this predator and stand my ground, or (2) I will run as fast and as far as I can to escape the threat of being attacked. This is fight or flight at its most basic, primal level. The SNS triggers a stress response and gets your body ready to deal with the imposing danger the moment you see the threat coming toward you.

This is an extreme example, and the types of danger and stress that tactical athletes face today vary drastically, including sitting in traffic, public speaking, responding to fires and barricaded suspects, and patrolling a combat zone. Whether the potential "danger" comes in the form of an emergency situation, high-pressure athletic performance, or an exam, the SNS prepares our bodies to respond to the impending threat. Specifically, the heart rate increases, blood pressure rises, breathing rate quickens, muscles tighten, and our focus sharpens. These physiological responses are adaptive and necessary to react and respond to danger. But you may also experience stress-induced performance impairment, such as auditory exclusion, tunnel vision, and decreased dexterity. These reactions are the product of the body's redirection of blood flow to the areas that are most vital to a fight or flight response. Large muscle groups and the cardiovascular system are the priorities, while smaller vasculatures, like inner ear canals and fingertips, are not. We will discuss further how mental performance training can help us control our reactions to stress so that we can maximize performance under pressure and recover from stressful situations, while continuously building resilience through encountering adversity.

Heart Rate Variability: Measuring the ANS

Now that you know the basics of the ANS, particularly the roles of the parasympathetic and sympathetic branches, we can dig in to optimizing your body's natural responses to stress. This is where heart rate variability comes into play. **Heart rate variability** (HRV) is a measurement that tracks the physiological manifestation of stress and its impact on the ANS.[7] Here is how it works and why it is a useful measurement for maximizing performance and remaining healthy.

Different from your heart rate, which measures the number of times your heart beats in a given time period, HRV is a more nuanced measurement that requires use of **biofeedback** technology. For tactical athletes, learning how to increase HRV and improve recovery are necessary preparations to handle daily stressors. When looking at a readout from an EKG, you see peaks and valleys like figure 3–7 shows.

Heart Rate Variability
A measurement that tracks the amount of time between heart beats, it is a metric that helps identify the physiological manifestation of stress and its impact on the ANS.

Biofeedback
The use of instruments or technology designed to measure physiological processes. Biofeedback creates awareness of stress responses and enables you to see the impact and effectiveness of using various mental performance tools on your stress response tendencies.

HEART RATE VARIABILITY

LOW VARIABILITY (RR Interval / Interbeat Interval)

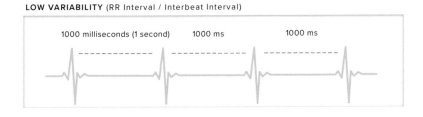

1000 milliseconds (1 second)   1000 ms   1000 ms

HIGH VARIABILITY (RR Interval / Interbeat Interval)

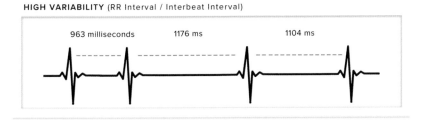

963 milliseconds   1176 ms   1104 ms

Figure 3–7. Heart rate variability

Your heartbeat is identifiable as the peaks in the image, which are used to find your heart rate, typically measured in beats per minute (BPM). It may be intuitive to think that if your pulse is 60 BPM, it is beating exactly one time per second; however, this is not, or should not, be the case for someone who is healthy and well rested. Instead, the interval between each heartbeat varies slightly, and studies have shown that higher variability between beats is indicative of how well you are recovered and ready to respond to potential stressors.[8]

Your HRV measures the push and pull of your SNS and PNS. When you encounter a stressor, your SNS shifts into gear, activating a fight or flight response. In our car analogy, this is like stepping on the gas pedal. On the other hand, when your PNS is activated you slow down as you shift into rest and digest so your body can conserve resources and rebalance. This is like stepping on the brakes. In other words, your SNS is used for short bursts when you need to jump into action for immediate response to a stressor, while your PNS is necessary for long-term sustainment and durability. Higher HRV indicates a more balanced interplay between SNS and PNS, while lower HRV signifies a more active SNS leading to a reduction in your ability to slow down, recover, and rebalance before encountering your next stressor. This imbalance can lead to a variety of negative mental and physical health outcomes from risk of disease to higher stress levels.[9]

Think of it this way: a high heart rate variability means that your SNS and PNS are playing a game of tug of war—and you are in a relatively balanced state, ready to respond to any stressor you encounter. In this state, if a call comes in, your SNS is activated and, using our car analogy, you step on the gas to go from 0 to 60 miles an hour easily in order to respond. When you return from the call, it is important to pump the brakes to activate your PNS so you can rebalance and recover so you are ready to jump into action when you need it next. If you do not take time to reset and are in a constant state of stress or have low HRV, you will put yourself at risk for overreaching and experiencing the negative impacts of chronic stress.

If you are getting the sleep, recovery, and nutrition you need to reset fully from daily stressors, you will likely have a high HRV and be more suited to kick into gear when the light turns green or when you need to jump into action responding to a call. On the other hand, if you encounter stressors, put further stress on your mind and body, or lack the nutrition and sleep you need to recover, you will run on fumes and have limited potential energy at your disposal. It is helpful to track HRV over time to see trends of recovery, particularly if you are on shift work or have schedule demands. Monitoring trends over time can help you modify your training and recovery to help identify when you should take an hour of extra sleep versus wake up early to crush a hard workout.

When we sit down and speak with firefighters, law enforcement officers, EMS or military members, usually they don't recognize how much stress their day-to-day jobs have placed on them. They have the grit to persevere; however, teaching a few tools to be more self-aware and dial in when needed makes all the difference in sustaining performance and living the fullest life they can.

—Adam La Reau, O2X cofounder

Operating under chronic stress without recovering can lead to burnout, overtraining, and injury. The good news is that when you encounter significant amounts of stress, there are tools and techniques you can use to increase your HRV and come back stronger each day. Using mindfulness techniques and mental performance skills to relax is like stopping at the gas station to refuel and bring your body back to homeostasis.

With biofeedback technology you can monitor not only your heart rate but also your HRV. It is important to note a few things when measuring your HRV. First, HRV levels vary by person and decrease with age,[10] so comparing results across individuals is challenging. Second, to get the most benefit from HRV monitoring, track your results over time to identify performance patterns to inform your fueling, training, recovery, and sleep behaviors. Finally, use caution when choosing the tool to measure your HRV; while there are increasingly more products on the market offering this measurement, some are more reliable than others, so be sure to do some research before using an HRV tracker.

HEART RATE VARIABILITY CONTINUED

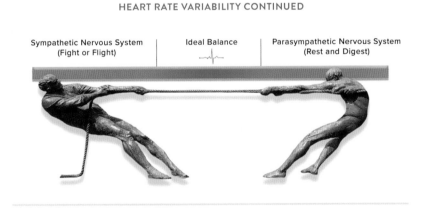

Figure 3–8. Heart rate variability (continued)

When used properly, reliable biofeedback technology can help you track the positive impact of low and slow breathing, mindfulness, and other stress management tools on your HRV levels. A key to this is developing self-awareness so that you know when to tap into your reservoir of mental performance skills and resources. Later in the chapter you will learn these different techniques to help improve your HRV by resetting and activating your PNS.

Biofeedback

How can you learn to reset your system and keep your mind and body in balance? Biofeedback. As mentioned in relation to measuring HRV, biofeedback refers to the technology one can use to measure and quantify the effects of stress on the body and mind (fig. 3–9). This includes monitoring functions that are typically involuntary, like perspiration, heart rate, respiration rate, and temperature regulation, to make necessary adjustments to control those natural processes.

There are signs and symptoms like dry mouth, increased heart rate, stomach discomfort, and dilated pupils that can be indicators of when your body is under stress. Having self-awareness of these signals is the first step toward improving performance. Biofeedback helps show these symptoms as quantifiable measurements, enabling you to address these signs by getting your body back to a state of relaxation. When you monitor your body with biofeedback tools, you can track how different techniques impact your physiology and then actively work toward turning off unnecessary sympathetic arousal to resume functioning at your baseline, or homeostatic, state.

For some people, stress and arousal may constantly impact their functioning over months to years, and it's possible that they may not know how it feels to be in a totally relaxed, parasympathetic state. This is common in all professions that routinely face extremely stressful situations, where stress begins to feel like the norm. While this adjustment can be problematic for people from all walks of life, it is particularly dangerous in tactical athlete populations that operate in environments with razor-thin margins for error, where any misstep can have serious, even deadly, consequences. For this reason, it is imperative that tactical athletes adopt healthy routines and skills to manage stress. Mental performance techniques will help you become more in tune with how you are functioning—emotionally and physically.

EFFECTS OF CHRONIC STRESS ON THE BODY

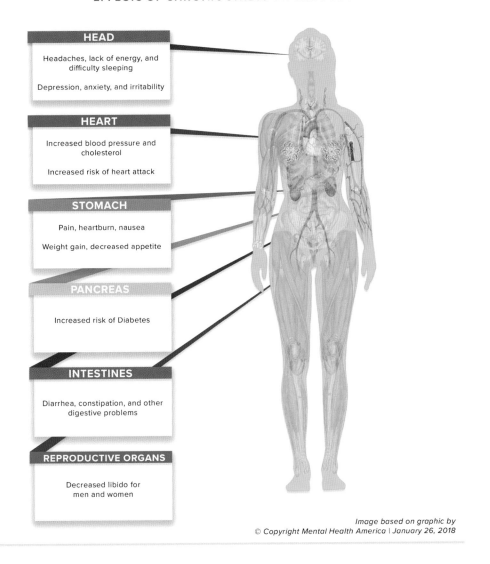

HEAD

Headaches, lack of energy, and difficulty sleeping

Depression, anxiety, and irritability

HEART

Increased blood pressure and cholesterol

Increased risk of heart attack

STOMACH

Pain, heartburn, nausea

Weight gain, decreased appetite

PANCREAS

Increased risk of Diabetes

INTESTINES

Diarrhea, constipation, and other digestive problems

REPRODUCTIVE ORGANS

Decreased libido for men and women

Image based on graphic by
© Copyright Mental Health America | January 26, 2018

Figure 3–9. Effects of stress on the body

SELF-CARE—LEWYN POAGE

From my earliest memories, military service was an understood expectation in our family. My grandfathers were both WWII vets. One was a marine who fought at Iwo Jima, and the 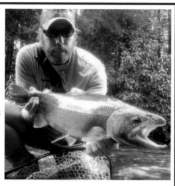 other served in the Air Force. I followed suit and enlisted at 17 years old, retiring 24 years later as a chief warrant officer. I had 20 years in Naval Special Operations and spent the last 12 years at the Naval Special Warfare Development Group. I am honored to have walked those halls with some of the nation's greatest heroes. I participated in countless operations and deployments overseas, and with only a few exceptions, I'd gladly live it all over again. However, that experience comes at a heavy cost.

My service in Naval Special Operations was wrought with both significant accomplishments and devastating tragedies. Decades of exposure to this environment results in compounding mental and physical injury, almost without exception. Like all others at that level, I was programmed to carry an intense burden, complete the operation with a no-fail mentality, and suppress human responses for the greater good of the mission. All of this could not happen successfully without each of my teammates' utmost adherence to this unwritten rule. From 2008 to 2011 in particular, I experienced the great loss of many brothers dear to me. Their deaths reinforced that operating at this level of intense stress, performance expectation, loss, and grief was creating a mental and emotional state that demanded my attention. I was broken. Depressed. At one point, I saw no way out.

Even at my lowest, I excelled at my job, no question about that; it eventually became the one thing I had left that seemed to be going well. Naturally, I thought that spending more time doing what I do best would be my key to coping. But as the intensity with which I pursued work increased, everything else in my life continued to crumble—my relationships, my health, and my mental well-being paid the toll. For the next five years, I would spend days at a time in the team room grinding out work until I couldn't any longer, sleeping there, and then waking up to do it all over again. Desperately seeking a "healthy" outlet, I turned to endurance athletics. I would spend what little time I had off riding my bike hundreds of miles per day and competing in swims of 10-plus miles. I thought that it was a good way to deal with my problems; in reality I was just running, biking, and swimming away from them. This rock-bottom period in my life taught me that the human psyche, by its very design, is created to overcome adversity and trauma. Even without healthy coping mechanisms, the mind does a fantastic job of going into survival mode on its own. Without adaptive, intentional coping strategies, however, the psyche can resort to unhealthy ones: distraction, compartmentalization, denial, numbing, addiction, isolation, and more.

In hindsight, I wish I had known earlier in my career the importance of self-care focused on reflection, resiliency, mindfulness, and a whole-person approach to well-being. Early into my retirement, I was fortunate enough to slowly discover a few modalities that I could incorporate into my own physical and emotional triage: individual therapy, trauma resolution, outdoor rehab (fly fishing), sleep hygiene, mindfulness, breathing, and nutrition. I firmly believe that had I been able to unload and process occupational and personal demons throughout my military career with less stigma, the benefits would have been remarkable and deep reaching. Like most, I was a shooting star on a mission, programmed to believe that I was untouchable, invincible, and bulletproof, never thinking that what I did and saw would catch up with me or, even less, be the undoing of me. There was nothing that could faze me—until something did.

There is zero down side to comprehensive self-care for tactical athletes, organizations, individuals, and families. My goal for those I work with is to help them avoid the mistakes I made on my journey, teaching them not to ignore the mental resiliency and self-care required of tactical athletes in demanding professions.

Similarly, tactical athletes from all backgrounds should lean on solid routines in order to maximize performance. Building a repeatable procedure reduces mistakes, boosts confidence, and helps ensure smooth execution of even the toughest tasks.

—*Lewyn Poage, O2X Operations, Chief Warrant Officer, US Navy (Ret.)*

MENTAL PERFORMANCE SKILLS

Now that you have some background knowledge about how your body and mind react and adapt to stress, we can take a closer look at the tools you can use to manage stress and optimize performance under pressure. Going back to our car analogy, practicing mental skills is like getting your car detailed to make sure it is in top condition. Mental performance training ensures that your windshield wipers work in case of rain and that your tires will not skid if the road gets wet. As a tactical athlete, this type of training will differentiate those who simply survive the job from those who thrive well into their retirement years.

Self-awareness creates the bedrock of mental performance. In order to find what techniques and tools will help you manage stressful situations, you must be aware of how stress impacts you. The good news is that practicing mental performance skills will help you gain self-awareness, so by strengthening those skills you will become more aware of what you need to get in the zone, thrive in high-pressure situations, and build resilience in the face of adversity.

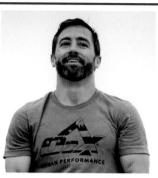

It's just after 0100 when the rear aircraft door opens at 25,000 feet. It's so dark that it's hard to see where the ramp ends and the sky begins. This is the beginning of a nighttime freefall insertion, a complex process refined through hundreds of hours of training. As with many military operations, this one has a razor thin margin for error and our team relied on a precisely choreographed routine to ensure each jump went as planned.

A lot can go wrong on a freefall parachuting operation and there are a nearly infinite number of variables to consider. To counter this, each team member and our unit as a whole had established routines that lead to consistency of performance. Individually and collectively, everyone knew what they needed to do in order to be successful and had a mental and/or physical checklist to ensure compliance.

The jump master and leaders ran through a detailed brief that covered each phase and various contingencies. Each jumper donned equipment at the same time, performed equipment checks, and walked on the aircraft in specific order. One process was for the jump master, who rolled through his own procedure to let the team know when specific benchmarks were reached. He told us when to attach equipment and when to detach from aircraft oxygen onto our own O_2 bottles. He made announcements at various time intervals 10 minutes out, at 5 minutes out, when to stand and perform final equipment checks, 1 minute out, 30 seconds, and until we finally received the green light and as a team we exited into darkness. There was always a range of jumping experience in the team, so utilizing the same script for each jump built a comforting routine that mitigated numerous missteps and set the team up for success.

Additionally, each team member went through a routine and mental process as we zeroed in on the time to jump. There are a lot of things to think through—updates on the radio on what's happening on the ground, aircraft procedures, jump procedures, wind speed and direction, having a strong exit from the aircraft, pulling on the right count, oxygen procedures, contingencies, jump profile, and the rest of the standard operating procedures. Everyone had their own internal procedure and methods that, when paired with SOPs, ensured the jump would go as planned, or that they would be ready if it did not.

For me, my process began with visualizing the environment in exact detail and mentally walking through the aircraft and jump procedures. The key was to feel prepared for the task I was about to perform. In my mind, as in most, thinking through the contingencies and reviewing emergency procedures was critical to feel ready for the jump. The time to think through them and all the possibly ugly scenarios was not while in a high-speed malfunction or entangled with another jumper at 20,000 feet. Visualizing the situation helped me practice and prepare even for the contingencies that can arise. What if I have a parachute malfunction, and it takes me 3,000 feet to clear it? Will I make the drop zone? What alternatives do I have? What radio calls do I need to make? My routine was to rehearse each possible scenario, good and bad, in my mind as I readied my gear to exit the plane.

When it came time to jump, a strong exit was critical. I utilized a mental cue in my head to help. "Wide arms and legs, Dive Down." This was my reminder to be symmetrical and aggressive going off the ramp. Having a great exit put me in a good place for the rest of the jump. I also put great focus into my breathing. Remembering to breathe sounds funny, but the the act of being conscious of my breath and heart rate, being self-aware, and controlling the controllables was reassuring. Although I wasn't the most experienced jumper on the team, the mental preparation helped me perform to the high standards that were required. Through being aware of my level of activation, visualizing and focusing on my mental cue in the same way every time, I built a repeatable routine that I used with success on each jump.

—*Adam La Reau, O2X cofounder, Former Lt. Cdr. US Navy (SEAL)*

Skill: Mindfulness

It's like putting a box in your brain and putting nothing into it.

—*Maria Trozzi, MEd, O2X Mental Performance and Resilience Specialist*

Although it is an ancient philosophy, the concept of **mindfulness** is relatively simple when boiled down to its basic definition: "Mindfulness means paying attention in a particular way: on purpose, in the present moment, and nonjudgmentally."[11] If it were easy, everyone would be fully present all the time without the distractions of phones, screens, music, or any other shiny object that grabs our attention from the here and now. In other words, we would not be dwelling on past mistakes or worrying about what might happen in the future; instead, we would be focused solely on doing what we need to do to optimize our experience in the present moment, wherever we are (fig. 3–10). Although the concept of mindfulness is simple at its core, it is not easy to achieve.

Mindfulness
This is "paying attention in a particular way: on purpose, in the present moment, and nonjudgmentally."[48]

MINDFULNESS

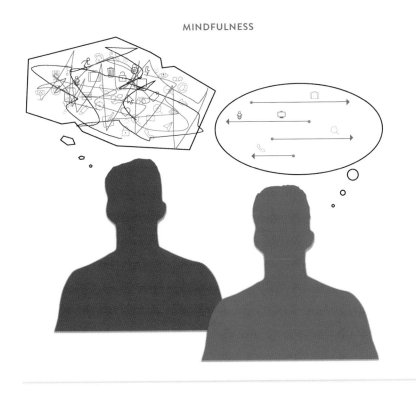

Figure 3–10. Mindfulness

Practicing mindfulness is not as easy as it sounds, but it is a skill that can be trained and improved with extremely positive results. Adding mindfulness into your daily routine allows you to widen your focus, add meaning and purpose to all your actions, gain self-awareness, and effectively manage stressors. Becoming more mindful as a tactical athlete can increase your situational awareness and improve your decision-making in high-pressure scenarios.[12] Additionally, practicing mindfulness can help you manage and mitigate unproductive stress so that your mind is clear of distractions and can process negative emotions.

Here is how mindfulness works—it is actually slightly counterintuitive. Despite the name, the goal of mindfulness is to empty your mind of anything detracting from you being fully present. Mindfulness is not about being relaxed; it is about being fully connected and immersed in your experience from one moment to the next. As you practice mindfulness through different techniques, you will be able to notice bodily sensations like muscle tension, breathing rate, and energy levels.

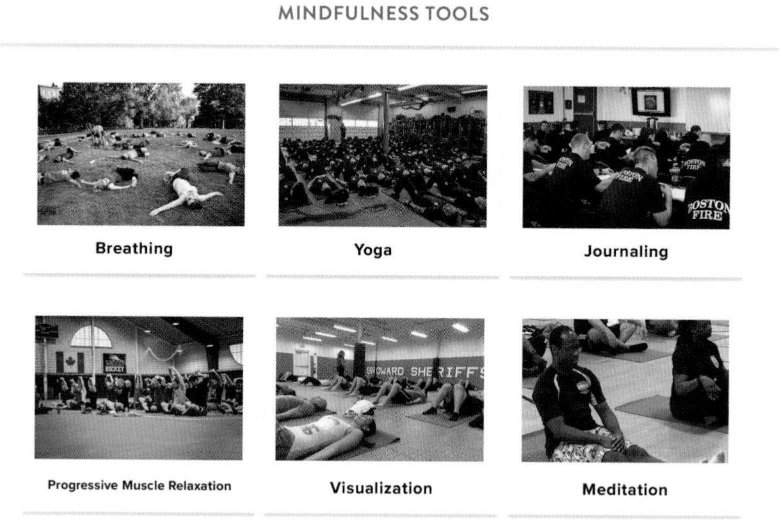

MINDFULNESS TOOLS

Breathing Yoga Journaling

Progressive Muscle Relaxation Visualization Meditation

Figure 3–11. Mindfulness tools

When you are overloaded by stressors, you may have a tendency to lose perspective and make snap judgments. Unfortunately, snap judgments are often biased and inaccurate, and as a consequence, your decisions and actions can be inappropriate. Practicing mindfulness allows you to recognize the moments when the potential for flawed decision-making is high. It also gives you the tools to observe your thoughts and calmly react amid even the most chaotic surroundings.[13]

This ability to remain present and focused among distractions will allow you to thrive in the dynamic situations in which you work. Listening to radio traffic in a firefight, sizing up a building fire, or observing the environment when serving a search warrant can be daunting tasks, but they are of the utmost importance to an operation's success. A mindfulness practice can refine the skills necessary to block out the noise and focus on what matters most.

The question then becomes, "How do you practice mindfulness so the skill is there when you need it?" There are countless ways to practice mindfulness; the key is to find the one that works best for you and that you will actually work to incorporate into your daily routine. A great way to start incorporating mindfulness is to choose a time each day when distractions are minimal, perhaps early in the morning when you first wake up or at night just before you fall asleep. You can even practice mindfulness while you are making your morning coffee or walking from your car to work. Here are three ways to practice mindfulness—one through something you do every day, one through internal reflection, and one through visual focus on an external image.

Tool: Everyday mindfulness

Think of something you do every day that has become so habitual you barely remember doing it (fig. 3–12). Let's use the example of eating your lunch. With a busy schedule, you may rush through lunch without thinking twice, either grabbing a meal on the go or eating so quickly you barely remember it. Adding an element of mindfulness can be simple, although that does not mean it is easy. You can find a more detailed script and description of how to practice mindfulness during daily routines in the addendum, but here is a quick version:

- Pick an activity that you do every day but seldom give much thought. Eating lunch, commuting, walking to work from the parking lot, or brushing your teeth are all good places to start.
- When you complete that activity, say walking into work, tune in and become aware of your body and surroundings. Pay attention to what you see and hear. Notice the scenery, the smells, and each step. Focus only on the present—what you're experiencing now.
- As other thoughts come into your mind and distract you, let them pass, each time gently bringing your attention back to the present moment.

This simple drill can begin to build a practice that will help reduce stress and increase your mindfulness over time.

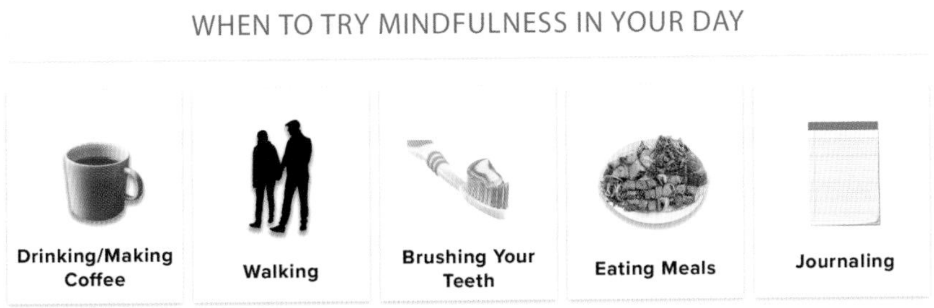

WHEN TO TRY MINDFULNESS IN YOUR DAY

| Drinking/Making Coffee | Walking | Brushing Your Teeth | Eating Meals | Journaling |

Figure 3–12. When to try mindfulness in your day-to-day life

Tool: Find your drive

The next way to practice mindfulness is through internal reflection, which is a tool that you can practice daily and call upon in stressful situations. You might call this "finding your inner resource" or "going to your happy place." By bringing your attention inward and imagining a place that you can associate with strength and calmness, you can quiet your mind and pull your attention away from distracting thoughts so you are better equipped to make decisions with clarity.

To find your drive, bring to mind places, people, activities, and objects that elicit feelings of security, calmness, happiness, fulfillment, and purpose (fig 3–13). Write these down and continue to add to the list as new places and experiences come to mind. Close your eyes, keeping in mind one place from your list. Imagine it in as much detail as possible. Add in sounds and smells you might encounter in that space—birds in the mountains or waves crashing at the ocean. Fill the space with other things like people who would be there or activities you would be doing. Take five minutes a day, or more, to practice recalling your inner resource. As it becomes easier, you will be able to call on the tool in stressful situations and use it as a way to reset and refocus when you feel overwhelmed by too many thoughts.

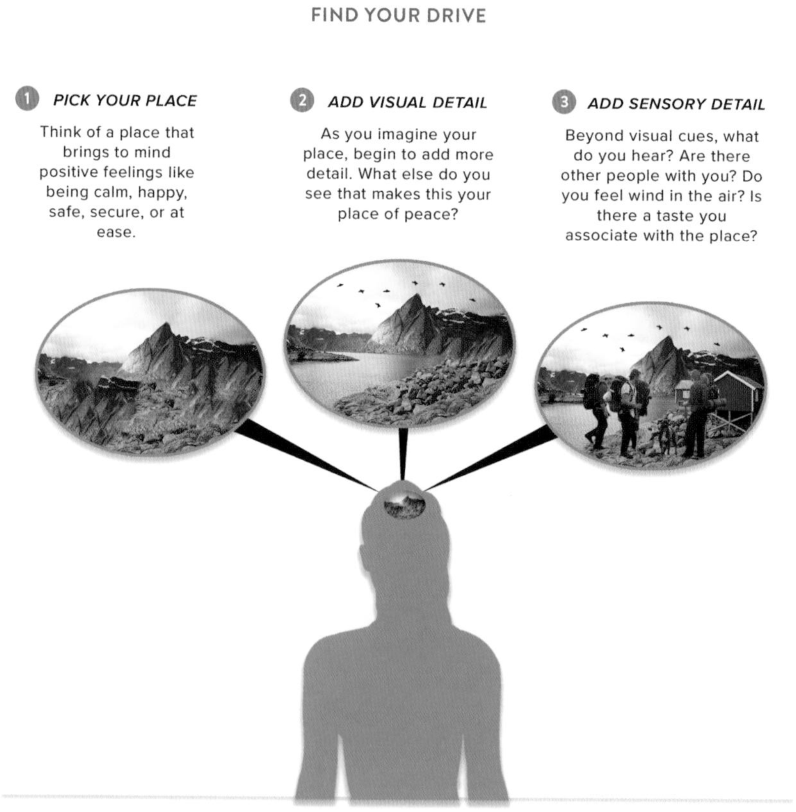

FIND YOUR DRIVE

1 PICK YOUR PLACE

Think of a place that brings to mind positive feelings like being calm, happy, safe, secure, or at ease.

2 ADD VISUAL DETAIL

As you imagine your place, begin to add more detail. What else do you see that makes this your place of peace?

3 ADD SENSORY DETAIL

Beyond visual cues, what do you hear? Are there other people with you? Do you feel wind in the air? Is there a taste you associate with the place?

Figure 3–13. Inner resource

Tool: Focus on an image

The third way to practice mindfulness is to focus on an image for a set amount of time (fig. 3–24); we recommend starting with at least a few uninterrupted minutes, adding time as you improve. Find a photograph or painting, or even a view out your window, and pay attention to it. Do this deliberately. Notice the small details and pay attention only to the image. If your mind or eyes wander or if thoughts start distracting you, bring your focus back to the image. As you practice this you may begin to feel that your mind wanders less and less each time. Much like basic strength exercises, this can seem simple at first, but increasing the length of time and number of sessions you practice will allow you to continue to progress and improve your mindfulness practice.

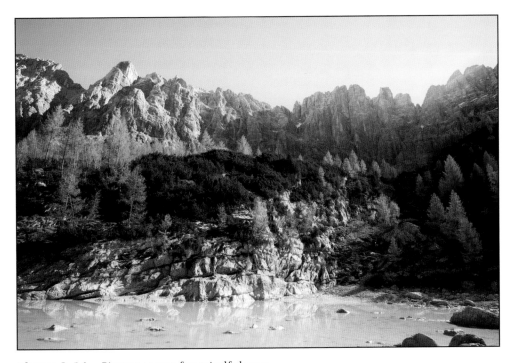

Figure 3–14. Picture to use for mindfulness

Skill: Breathing

Although breathing is a most basic human need, it is rarely something we focus on as a skill to train and improve. Yet the benefits of practicing breathing are vast, for not only mental performance but also physical conditioning and overall health. While there are various styles and different breathing rates you can practice, becoming aware of your breathing and learning how to use it to your advantage is paramount.

Diaphragmatic Breathing

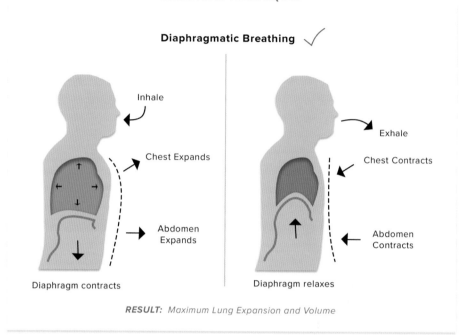

Inhale

Chest Expands

Abdomen Expands

Diaphragm contracts

Exhale

Chest Contracts

Abdomen Contracts

Diaphragm relaxes

RESULT: *Maximum Lung Expansion and Volume*

Chest Breathing

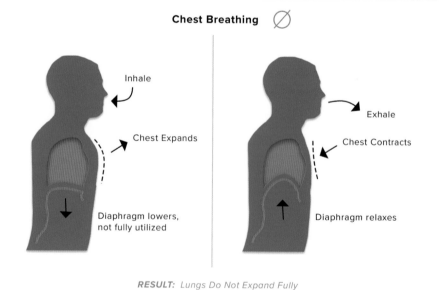

Inhale

Chest Expands

Diaphragm lowers, not fully utilized

Exhale

Chest Contracts

Diaphragm relaxes

RESULT: *Lungs Do Not Expand Fully*

Figure 3–15. Breathing techniques

O2X teaches breath training as "low and slow," although it can also be called differ-ent names like **diaphragmatic breathing**, which references the way you use your dia-phragm to consciously, purposefully breathe (fig. 3–15). If you recall our discussion of heart rate variability and the back and forth between your parasympathetic and sympa-thetic nervous systems, you will remember that your body naturally strives for balance. Our bodies are typically happiest and relaxed when our respiration rate is between four and seven breaths per minute,[14] so we teach using a five-count inhale and seven-count exhale to maximize the benefits. Breathing is a tool that you can use to find balance and manage energy levels in any situation.

Maintaining a slow breathing pace resets your autonomic nervous system by helping rebalance your sympathetic and parasympathetic nervous systems. This elevates your HRV so that you are prepared for your next challenge. For example, if you are too amped up or anxious going into a stressful situation, you can take slow diaphragmatic breaths to calm yourself down. On the other hand, if you are feeling slow and lethargic but need to gear up for a big event or call, then taking deep breaths will help energize you so you are ready to respond swiftly. Low and slow breathing helps bring you back to homeostasis so you can have the right energy level you need for any situation.

How do you train yourself to use low and slow breathing as a technique for mental performance and energy management?

As we mentioned before, breathing is something we do all day, every day without pay-ing much attention. To help you train breathing as a skill, we have broken the practice of low and slow breathing into three key steps, which we will explain below.

Diaphragmatic Breathing Also referred to as low and slow breathing, it is a breathing tech-nique utilizing the contraction of your dia-phragm (the mus-cle between your thoracic and ab-dominal cavity). During this type of breathing, you will feel your belly expand as your lungs fill with air while your chest stays relatively still.

Tool: Low and Slow Breathing
Step 1: Position your body for relaxation
When you begin your low and slow breathing practice, start by lying down or sitting com-fortably in a chair. Comfort is key so that you can focus your attention on your breath rather than be distracted by your posture. However you choose to sit or recline, position yourself so your muscles are as relaxed as possible. Once you find your comfortable posi-tion, bring your attention to your body. Starting at your toes, take note of your muscles and joints. Where do you feel tension? When you notice those areas, consciously try to let go of the tension and relax all your muscles so you feel your weight sink completely into the floor or chair.

Step 2: Check your breathing
This is when you start to bring your attention to your breathing. First notice how you breathe without making any adjustments. Does your chest or abdomen rise and fall as you breathe? Place one hand on your chest and one on your stomach to feel the move-ment. Are you inhaling or exhaling through your nose or your mouth, or both? Are your inhales shorter than your exhales or vice versa? If you're still having trouble, ask a friend to watch as you lie on your back and take deep breaths. Does he or she see your chest rise or abdomen expand?

Simply taking stock of your natural breath patterns will help you identify moments when you are under stress and your breathing changes. Stressful situations cause most people to take short, shallow breaths coming from the chest at an increased rate, as we discussed when considering your body's response to stress.

Step 3: Focus on your breathing, only on your breathing

By practicing low and slow breathing regularly, you will be more relaxed and better equipped to use it as a tool for stress management in challenging situations.

Now that you are in a relaxed position and have taken note of your current breathing rate, here's how you can practice low and slow breathing:

1. Place one hand on your chest and one on your stomach.
2. As you breathe, the hand on your stomach should be moving up and down while the hand on your chest remains relatively still. Imagine a balloon in your stomach inflating and deflating, or imagine that your pants are too big and you need to push your stomach out to hold them up.
3. Breathe in through your nose slowly, pause, and then exhale slowly through your mouth with your lips pursed.

A typical rate is 4 to 7 breaths per minute. To reach this, try inhaling for a count of five and then exhaling for a count of seven, with a pause until you need your next breath.

To start, practice low and slow breathing for a few minutes without interruption. Similar to the earlier mindfulness exercises, if you notice your mind wandering, then bring your attention back to your breath. This is not easy, but remember that like learning any new skill, the more you train, the more relaxed you will be during your practice. As you get comfortable with 5 minutes of breathing, add another minute and continue to add a minute until you are up to 20 minutes of uninterrupted practice. If you do not feel like you have time for 20 minutes in one sitting, include short breaks in your daily schedule and accumulate 20 minutes of breath training over the course of the day. The more you practice, the better you will become and the more you will feel the benefits.

Another way to enhance your breathing practice is to add a **mantra** to your low and slow pattern. You can attach one word to your inhale and another to your exhale. Some people may find it helpful to associate strong words with the inhale and exhale. For example, inhale with the word "strength" and exhale with "power." For each person, a mantra can be extremely personal; what is important is that it helps you focus on your breathing and makes you feel strength and peace as you breathe. This will help you release physical tension and manage psychological stress.

Mantra
A word or sound repeated to aid concentration in meditation.

Tool: Avoid Overbreathing

Overbreathing

As you become more familiar with your breathing patterns, something to be aware of is the risk of **overbreathing** when you encounter actual or perceived stress. Overbreathing occurs when you take several fast, deep breaths in and then breathe out a large amount of carbon dioxide when you exhale. This lowers the amount of carbon dioxide in your blood and signals to your body that its metabolic needs are lower—also known as hypocapnia.

Overbreathing
Also known as hyperventilation and occurs when you take several fast, deep breaths and breathe out a large amount of carbon dioxide. This lowers the amount of carbon dioxide in your blood and signals your body that its metabolic needs are lower.

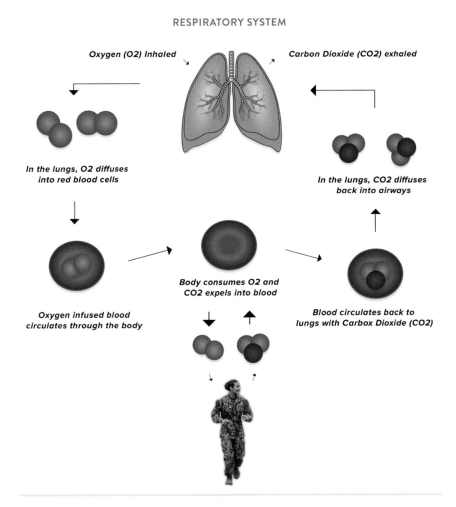

RESPIRATORY SYSTEM

Oxygen (O2) Inhaled

Carbon Dioxide (CO2) exhaled

In the lungs, O2 diffuses into red blood cells

In the lungs, CO2 diffuses back into airways

Body consumes O2 and CO2 expels into blood

Oxygen infused blood circulates through the body

Blood circulates back to lungs with Carbox Dioxide (CO2)

Figure 3–16. Respiratory system

The acute symptoms associated with hypocapnia include shortness of breath, chest tightness, airway constriction, muscle tension, trembling, tingling limbs, sweating, blurred vision, difficulty concentrating, and nausea. Furthermore, chronic overbreathing can contribute to panic disorders, hypertension, migraines, sleep apnea, chronic pain, asthma, and anxiety. Using low and slow breathing can help diminish the tendency to overbreathe and mitigate the negative effects associated with it.[15]

Tool: Pairing breathing with lifestyle

As you continue to practice low and slow breathing, you will begin to notice how it impacts your physiological response to stress and helps your body return to homeostasis. In the context of HRV and our earlier car analogy, breathing helps you slow down and idle at a stoplight so that when you need to react to a situation, you can do so quickly and efficiently.

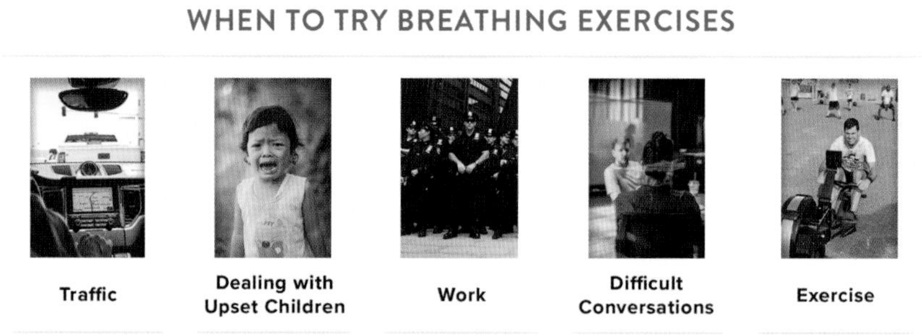

WHEN TO TRY BREATHING EXERCISES

| Traffic | Dealing with Upset Children | Work | Difficult Conversations | Exercise |

Figure 3–17. When to try breathing exercises

Tactical Pause
A strategic moment taken to regain situational awareness and intentionally refocus on the task in front of you.

In addition to a deliberate practice of low and slow breathing during uninterrupted sessions, taking a brief moment for a few low and slow breaths throughout your day can have major benefits. We call this in-the-moment use of breathing a **tactical pause**. You can use low and slow breathing before making a big decision or when you encounter stressful situations. Next time you are dispatched to a house fire, hear "shots fired" on the radio, or just feel your stress level rising, take a tactical pause for a few low and slow deep breaths.

Skill: Progressive Muscle Relaxation

Similar to breathing, progressive muscle relaxation (PMR) is another useful tool that links physical practice to mental performance training. PMR is the systematic tensing and relaxing of muscles, and it can help you become more self-aware of where you hold tension by highlighting the difference between tensed and relaxed states. Along with increased awareness of where and how you hold tension, the practice of progressive muscle relaxation offers a practical tool you can use to release stress.

BENEFITS OF REGULATING THE MIND-BODY CONNECTION

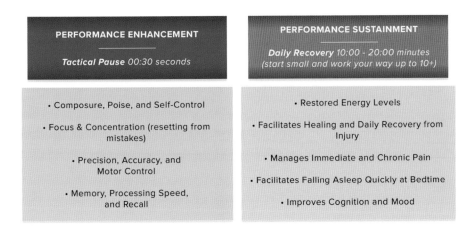

Figure 3–18. Benefits of regulating the mind-body connection

As you become more comfortable with the practice, your body will begin to automatically recognize and release unnecessary tension. This heightened sense of awareness and body control connects your body and mind in a real, profound way. It also gives you a tool to consciously control and train your response to stressors while managing tension.

Like breathing exercises, PMR can be done both as an uninterrupted deliberate practice and as a quick way to manage energy and stress in the moment. While there are different methods, here are two styles of PMR training you can try.

Tool: Full-body progression

1. Lying down or sitting comfortably, take several deep breaths and start to relax your muscles.
2. Beginning with your toes and gradually moving up your body, tense each muscle group until your whole body is tensed and rigid.
3. Starting with your head and moving back down your body, slowly release the tension in each muscle group until your whole body is relaxed.

Tool: Targeted progression

Follow similar steps to the full-body progression, but break it up into targeted areas of the body.[16]

1. Starting with your arms, make a tight fist with each hand.
2. Gradually continue to tense the rest of your arms moving up from your hands.

3. Hold the tension for 8–10 seconds before releasing and stay relaxed for about a minute before repeating the cycle with the next area (i.e., legs, core, and head, neck, and shoulders).

Practicing PMR (fig. 3–19) through systematic routines like those shared above can help strengthen your mind and body connection. It can also be a practical tool for stress mitigation and energy management. Like breathing, PMR can relax you when you are stressed and can energize you when you are feeling slow and fatigued. And just as you can integrate breathing into your daily life, you can do things like clenching your fist and letting it go before you step off a fire truck or out of a patrol car. It could be just the tool you need to reset or refocus your present situation.

PROGRESSIVE MUSCLE RELAXATION

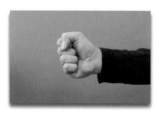

1. Tense a muscle group (arm, fist, etc.), hold for 5-10 seconds.

2. Pay attention to what the tension feels like.

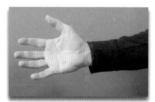

3. Let go of tension.

4. Pay attention to what it feels like to let go.

5. Notice the difference between tense and relaxed state.

Example of muscle group progression:

forehead, nose/cheeks, eyes, jaw/lower cheeks, neck, shoulders, right arm, left arm, back/shoulders/stomach, right leg, left leg

Figure 3–19. Progressive muscle relaxation

Visualization Sometimes called mental rehearsal or imagery, this "practice refers to the cognitive rehearsal of a task in the absence of overt physical movement."[49]

Skill: Visualization

Visualization, or mental imagery, is another tactic you can use to create a mind and body connection that positively impacts your performance (fig. 3–20). It can help you rehearse new skills, build confidence, and increase resilience. The very process of imagining, in full detail, a successful response to any situation will help you carry out that same response when it happens in real life. This is true of all types of scenarios, including visualizing how you would react to adversity or overcome potential obstacles. Here are a few examples of how you can use visualization as a mental performance tool.

TYPES OF VISUALIZATION

INTERNAL	EXTERNAL	**BIG PICTURE**

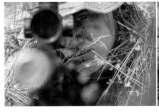 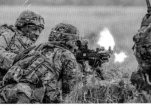 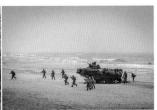

First person visualization allows you to see a situation from your own view point. To develop this skill, complete a task you know how to do well then close your eyes and replay it in your mind.	External visualization is like watching yourself from the lens of a camera. It allows you to visualize your surroundings. To practice, imagine seeing yourself complete a task as though you are watching a recording of yourself.	Many people shift view points from internal to external and to the big picture in a single visualization routine. Practicing to improve clarity and include multiple senses in visualization wil enhance performance.

Figure 3–20. Types of visualization

Tool: Review of a past experience

Bring to mind a situation you have experienced before. This could be responding to a call at work, completing a tough training session, having an open and honest conversation following a bad operation, or playing in a game as an athlete. Close your eyes and begin to bring that scene to life in your head.

1. Start by imagining the scene itself. What did you see? What was around you? Who was with you? Create a vivid picture of the scene.
2. Now you can reflect back on the situation. How did you feel, physically and mentally? What emotions did you feel? What physical sensations did you experience?
3. Next, consider how you reacted. What was your response? Did you rush to respond? Did you react emotionally? How did your response feel? Did you

respond the way you wanted to? If not, imagine what your ideal response would have been and rehearse that in your mind.

As you continue to visualize this scenario, imagine that ideal response. Think not of how it went, but of how you would want it to go if you found yourself in the same situation in the future. By rehearsing your ideal response rather than a past reaction that did not go as planned, you will build confidence and be more likely to achieve your ideal outcome next time.

Tool: Visualization for adversity

It is not easy or enjoyable to think of the worst-case scenarios we might face, but mental rehearsal of adverse situations can help ensure that we will be prepared to respond when the time comes. Similar to the review of a past experience, visualizing a response to adversity provides benefits from imagining your ideal response to the situation. Instead of telling yourself what you would not want to do, frame any visualization by thinking of exactly what you would want to do in your ideal response. Start by thinking of what you want your reaction to be in high-pressure situations or in challenging moments, then imagine yourself responding in that way.

An example of using imagery to plan for adversity is thinking of low-frequency, high-risk scenarios. For law enforcement this may be something like responding to serve a high-risk warrant or being engaged in a foot pursuit. This may not be not something you encounter regularly, but it is something you have to train for physically and be prepared for mentally. By using imagery as a mental readiness tool, you are getting your mind and body ready to respond effectively in high-stakes situations that you do not encounter on a daily basis.

Get detailed in your visualization. Think about the scenario and your response, and dedicate time to imagining what you would see, feel, think, and do. Think about what your tone of voice would be, what words you would use to communicate, and what your ideal outcome would be. Rehearse attaining that goal.

Think of this as building a catalog of worst-case scenarios in your mind—situations that could be difficult to recreate in training and are rare occurrences in the field but are likely enough to require a plan. For firefighters this may be becoming lost and trapped after a structural collapse. Pick actual structures and see yourself experiencing the event. Think through what your next actions would be: How would you radio for help? What tools would you want to have with you? What would your actions be to rescue yourself? Visualize, in detail, yourself successfully escaping. Then do it again. And again. Perhaps change some variables each time, but the end result should always be the same: you get out. This practice will help refine the skills you may need in the actual event and ensure that you have a plan waiting in the hopper when you need it.

VISUALIZATION—ALI LEVY

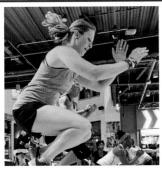

While most Olympic-level skiers grow up skiing every day, I was what they call a weekend warrior. I was lucky enough to have a brother and parents who loved the sport, and we would pack the car and drive to the mountains every weekend to ski two days a week. When I made the jump from skiing recreationally to competing in freestyle skiing, I knew that making the most of my limited time on the ski hill would be critical.

I was determined that only skiing two days a week would not be an excuse to give up on my dream of being on the US Ski Team. Instead, it fueled my work ethic and gave me the feeling of being the underdog bound to break the mold of being a weekend warrior. It allowed me to find ways to practice when I couldn't get repetition after repetition of ski-training runs. This is why I turned to visualization to sharpen my skills off the hill, so I could maximize every moment of ski training.

As a young skier, I thought visualization was just a fancy word for daydreaming—and I was good at daydreaming. I constantly thought about ski competitions before going to sleep, dreamed about wearing a US Ski Team uniform, and imagined competing alongside my skiing idols. That was easy.

But turning my daydreaming into a skill took hard work and practice. It wasn't just dreaming; it was challenging myself to break down technique and recognize what it would take to build up my weaknesses. With the help of my coaches, I developed a script to guide my visualization that got progressively more detailed—from the view of the course below my feet to what I heard my coaches say, all the way down to how my hands felt in my (imaginary) ski gloves.

The images became so vivid that I would have a physical reaction—my heart was beating faster and I could feel my energy rise simply from imagining a ski run. I saw the race from a first-person perspective as though I was looking down the course, but my vision would also shift back and forth as though I was watching a video of myself skiing down from every angle. I could even slow things down, zone in on specific skills, or redo a section of a run if I didn't imagine it exactly as I wanted to execute it. I built imagery into my daily off-season routine.

The real power of visualization didn't hit me until I was on the snow for the first time during the winter after starting off-season visualization. I got on my skis and it was as though no time had passed since the last winter. I had spent so much time imagining exactly what it felt like to click into my skis, to stand at the top of a race course, and to have the snow under my feet that I knew visualization would be the key to progressing with limited training time.

Just like improving physical skills takes practice, so too does learning effective visualization techniques. It is mentally exhausting to clear your mind of distractions and focus on the smallest details of your skiing technique. However, the sense of confidence it gave me while I couldn't be on the ski hill was invaluable to my ability to set an intention for every practice run I skied. While my teammates skied every day and felt like they didn't need to focus as much on using visualization, they sometimes weren't as deliberate about every training run. Bringing intention to my practice enabled me to accomplish more in a single training session than others got done in a week.

Through visualization, I was building confidence and self-efficacy without stepping foot on the ski hill. I imagined tackling the most difficult race courses without making any mistakes, and I saw myself overcoming every bobble, mistake, or bad weather scenario possible. I used imagery to work through any situation—something you don't always have the luxury of doing if you ski all the time.

Visualization gave my physical training meaning and purpose. It allowed me to set specific training goals around what I had worked hard to mentally prepare myself for during time away from skiing. It made me excited to get up the ski hill to test out the new skills I had been thinking about all week.

In freestyle skiing, every second counts, and visualization was a way not only to imagine getting every second right but also to build mindfulness and maintain my composure in high-stress situations. Visualization provided the competitive edge I needed to go from a weekend warrior to being on the US Ski Team. It's something I continue to use in my daily life when I prepare for any high-pressure situation, whether it's getting the most out of a workout session, preparing for a public speaking engagement, or finishing an ultramarathon.

—Ali Levy, MEd Sport Psychology, US Ski Team Member, O2X Marketing Director

Tool: Mental rehearsals

As a tactical athlete, your job requires a specific skill set, and you need to learn new techniques for performance regularly. Visualization can be a great tool for practicing new skills and mastering old ones that you may not practice regularly. To use visualization in this way, think of a technique or skill that you do well as an example of how you can use mental imagery for any skill you are trying to master.

Once you select a skill or activity, break it down movement by movement and imagine yourself fluidly progressing through each step toward your desired outcome. You may find that you see the situation internally from a first-person perspective, or you may be looking at the scene and yourself as though you are watching it on a TV screen. There is no wrong perspective, and over time you may realize that you jump between the different viewpoints.[17] The key is learning what works for you and continuing to practice positive mental imagery to maximize your performance.

Imagining yourself encountering challenging situations allows you to practice your response without facing actual physical or mental stress. You can use visualization to recreate past experiences and imagine yourself doing them differently, or you can place yourself in new scenarios so you can pre-plan your response to potential challenges.[18] Think about the situations in your life that would benefit from positive mental imagery and add dedicated visualization practice to your daily training routine.

Skill: Self-Talk

Self-talk is as simple as it sounds—it is what you tell yourself when nobody else is listening. And it can have a profound impact on your performance. Self-talk can help get you in a positive mindset for performance, direct your attention to an outcome you want to see, or it can be a mantra to help you practice mindfulness. A key to using self-talk to your advantage is to think in terms of things you want to have happen, not things you want to avoid. In other words, if you are in a stressful conversation or high-pressure situation, your first instinct may be to think "do not lose your temper" or "do not fail." However, this often has the reverse effect because what your mind latches on to is not "do not" but rather the action "lose your temper." So you are more inclined to act on that thought. Instead, reframe your self-talk to focus on what you want to have happen. For example, change your thought from "do not lose your temper" to "stay calm."

For tactical athletes, you may find it helpful to remind yourself that you thrive in tense situations and that you do your best work under pressure. Your training has prepared you for your job and you want to be ready in that moment. If not you, then who? This type of positive reframing can improve your focus on the task at hand and increase the belief you have in yourself to achieve the outcomes you desire. As you continue to read, you will learn additional ways that self-talk can help you enhance and maintain attention control.

Skill: Attention Control

Attention control is a foundational element of situational awareness. It is the process of bringing your full *sensory awareness* to the present moment and maintaining that focus. Effective attention control allows you to shift between broad and narrow points of focus in a situation so that you are well equipped to make accurate appraisals and decisions.

When firefighters or law enforcement officers arrive at a vehicle crash, they must very quickly observe what is happening at the scene as a whole. *What are the big hazards? Is traffic still moving? Any risk of fire?* Next, they direct focus to the incident itself. *What happened? Are there people injured or trapped?* Then they develop a plan of action. *What can we do to fix this problem? What is our plan?* Finally, they select a path and execute it. *Time to go to work.*

At its core, attention control is the process of focusing on the present moment, sustaining your attention, shifting focus as conditions change, and resetting focus if you become distracted. There is a clear link between practicing mindfulness and improving your ability to maintain attention control in high-pressure situations. Another helpful tool for training attention control is what we will call the channel approach (fig. 3–21). This can be used for single events or for big-picture planning and to help you make major decisions in your work and personal life.

Tool: Channel approach to attention control

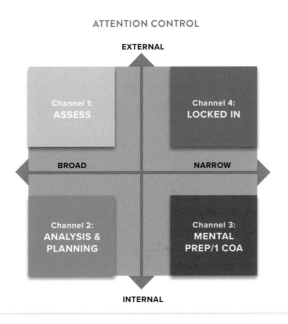

Figure 3–21. Attention control

1. **Assess:** Begin with a basic assessment of your situation—think of this as a broad, external view as though you are looking from an overhead viewpoint of everything around you. Take in your surroundings.
2. **Analysis and Planning:** In this channel, shift your attention inward, so your viewpoint is less broad than your original assessment of the situation. Think of the scenario from an internal perspective and make plans for how you would ideally want to handle the situation. This may sound similar to the visualization exercise explained previously, and it is. These tools can be used together to improve mental performance and attention control.
3. **Mental Prep and Course of Action:** Now narrow your focus to a single course of action. Take the various possibilities you came up with in channel 2, and mentally prepare to execute that plan.
4. **Locked In:** This is the final phase of the channel approach, and it is all about executing your plan and staying focused on your chosen course of action. This is where you want to direct your attention once you set your plan in motion.

You will notice that when you begin the exercise, your focus is extremely broad and external, but with each step, or channel, your focus narrows until your attention is directed toward the exact course of action you need to take. Think of this like flipping back and forth between camera angles. As new challenges or variables come into play during a situation, you may need to reassess by switching channels back to a broad focus and then once again narrowing your attention to address new obstacles. The ability to systematically shift focus and redirect attention control can be critical to maximizing performance and achieving desired outcomes in unpredictable, high-pressure scenarios.

It can be tempting or easy to get stuck on a single channel, particularly if the situation seems overwhelming or overly complex. For example, say that you are considering putting in for a new promotion. That can feel daunting and overwhelming when you are looking at the big picture in the assessment stage. The broad view of seeking a change would include things like promotional opportunities available, location, and the possibility of having to go back to school for a specialty degree. This can seem like so much that you get stuck spinning your wheels without even beginning to analyze and plan next steps.

If you are able to get past the assessment stage, you may get stuck in the planning phase. This could happen if you feel that you have too many options and cannot commit to making a clear plan. On the other hand, just to get moving forward, you may jump straight to a course of action without fully analyzing and planning for it. This would cause you to miss important details and risk missing the mark with your plan. Later in the chapter you will learn the three Rs, which form another technique you can use to get yourself out of a rut. If at any point you feel stuck in a channel or overwhelmed by the situation, you can refocus your attention by taking a tactical pause to reset.

Tool: Listening

One way to practice attention control without being in a high-pressure situation or having the weight of an important decision on your mind is by listening to music deliberately. To do this effectively, pick your favorite song or a song that has several different instruments and that you will not mind hearing multiple times.

Start to play the song and listen as you normally would. Gradually bring your focus to one specific sound or set of instruments within the song. As you focus on that segment of the music, see if you can quiet the other components of the song so that your attention is entirely on that one layer of the music.

As you continue to listen, shift your attention to a new part of the song. Perhaps this time you focus solely on the vocals. Think about what you notice as you attempt to shift your attention. Is it easy or challenging? Does your attention easily shift back and forth between the two parts? Try to maintain focus on multiple parts of the sound at once, then shift back to an individual component of the music. This is not an easy task; however, with practice you will become more aware of how you shift attention, what cues you use to do so, and how to limit distractions when necessary. This exercise is a training tool that will help build your stamina for focus while increasing your self-awareness and improving your mindfulness. Like focusing on breathing, focusing on one part of a song helps clear your mind of distractions so you can reset and intentionally refocus your attention.

Additional tools

Another helpful tool for attention control is called WIN—what's important now. This is a way to direct your attention toward whatever is most critical to your success in a given moment. When you feel overwhelmed or find your thoughts drifting away from the present moment, ask yourself, "What's important now?" WIN is an easy-to-remember acronym to help bring you back to the present situation.

Echoing our discussion of self-talk, verbal and physical cues can also be a tool for attention control. You can use a **mantra**, which is a cue word you say repeatedly to direct your attention toward the goal you want to accomplish. Or you can use task-specific cues to direct yourself to a specific action or physical motion that brings your attention back to the task at hand. "Aim small, miss small" is a popular self-talk phrase among shooters. This simple bit is repeated over and over before a shot to remind the person on the trigger to be as precise as possible when taking aim.

Think about cues or routines that you can use regularly to help focus your attention. This may involve running through a list in your mind of gear you need when you get ready for a shift, or it could be using simple words that bring your attention back to the moment when you feel your mind drifting. Practicing attention control is critical to decision-making and situational awareness during high-pressure circumstances, and the tools listed above will help ensure you can focus on the present when you need to most.

Skill: Writing

Practices like diaphragmatic breathing and progressive muscle relaxation are physical ways to train mindfulness, while writing is a cognitive technique that can be equally useful in optimizing mental performance. Writing is a great way to make sense of and organize your thoughts so you can mentally hit reset and approach your next task with a clear mind. As a mindfulness technique, writing can widen your focus and scope of attention. It can also reduce stress by helping you identify and address any stressors taking up space in your mind.

Preoccupation with unresolved issues or worries can shift our attention and energy away from the present moment. This disrupts our connection to others and distracts us from being focused and productive. There are a number of ways that you can use writing to enhance mental performance, and we will share a few examples that you can incorporate in your daily routine.

Tool: Journaling
Mindful writing

Writing down your thoughts each day is a valuable skill. This can help you clear your mind so that you can focus your attention.[19] Additionally, you can use writing as a tool for debriefing and recollecting thoughts after a stressful or exciting situation, so you can then look back and create a plan to improve performance for the next event. Finally, you can make writing a daily practice by using it to reflect on each day.

The way you choose to write down your thoughts and emotions as a daily practice is extremely individual; some people may write in lists while others may type out a stream of consciousness, jotting down everything that comes to mind. You do not need to be a great writer to use journaling as a tool for mental performance. When you finish your daily writing practice, you can choose to read it and reflect in the moment or come back to it days later. You may even evaluate your journal entries weekly to see if there are patterns or changes over time.

If you have trouble getting started with journaling, then set a timer. Sit in a quiet place with no other distractions available—no phones, screens, or people. Set a timer for 10 minutes and sit with nothing except a pen and paper. Eventually you will become more comfortable with the practice and will not need to set a timer. You may find that you turn to writing in times of stress or when debriefing from events.

Tool: Gratitude

Another way to incorporate writing into your routine is through what is often called gratitude journaling. This can be as simple as writing down (or even making a mental note of) three things you are grateful for at the end of each day. This practice allows you to become more aware of things that are going well and can shift attention to those positive thoughts and away from worry. Practicing gratitude writing can improve your perceived well-being, and it promotes prosocial behavior. In other words, when you practice gratitude you are more likely to feel better and more inclined to help others.[20] Try it now: stop and write down three things that you are grateful for.

Tool: Control what you can

Using writing, like the mindful journaling described previously, not only helps us identify areas of worry but also enables us to create action plans to address those concerns. Being consumed by worries or unproductive thoughts depletes our physical and mental energy and negatively impacts our focus. This diminishes our ability to be fully present and make clear decisions. Writing down your worries can help you let go of things you cannot control, and it can empower you with a sense of influence over your situation and an idea of how you can alleviate stress.

For this writing exercise, find a time you can consistently set aside each day. Then you can follow these steps (fig. 3–22):

1. List out your worries or concerns. You can choose a specific topic like work or something in your family life, or write generally with no topic in mind. Do not censor your list; write down anything that is causing worry or feels unresolved. Even the seemingly small stuff can cause stress.
2. Break the list up and separate the worries into two categories—things you can control and things that you cannot. (You may want to write each worry on a separate flashcard or label each worry on your existing list.)
3. Starting with the list of things you can control, organize the worries by how severe each worry is for you (small, moderate, and big concerns).
4. Beginning with the small worries, outline a solution or something you can do to plan for each stressor and alleviate that worry. Then go through the same process for the medium and big concerns, outlining a plan for encountering the stressor and a solution that will limit that worry. It is often helpful to think about what the worst-case scenario is for a worry and then work backwards to find the solution or an action you can take to eliminate or diminish that worry.
5. Move on to the list of things that are not in your control, starting the same process as outlined above and writing down a plan to put in place if the worst-case scenario happens. You may find small things that you can control within each worry, and even that realization can help diminish the concern.

You can repeatedly reuse the list you make until the worries subside, or you can create a brand new list each day and reflect on patterns or changes in your worries over time. The key to this exercise is to identify areas that are in your control and to create action plans to address and cope with concerns that are not. As you get more comfortable doing this, you will likely notice that the writing exercise helps you see concerns and worries from a more balanced and level-headed perspective.

1 **Set a goal**
Example: I want my kids to be healthy.

2 **List what you can control**
Example: I can control...

... noticing signs of any sickness as quickly as I can.

... giving them the proper medicine and vitamins needed to fight illness.

... their cleanliness while at home.

3 **List what you can't control**
Example: I can't control...

... the health of their friends at school.

... what they touch when I am not around.

... the strength of their immune system.

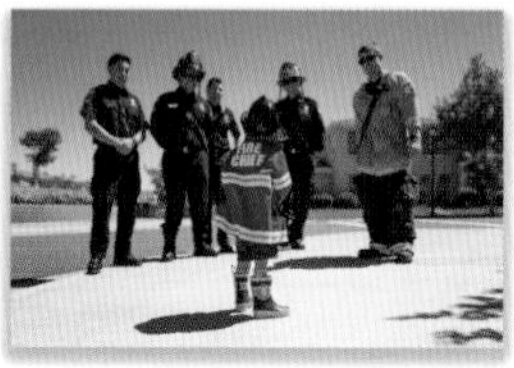

4 **Control the controllables.**
Example: I will...

... schedule a physical for my children.

... make sure they get their annual flu shot.

... encourage them to wash their hands and partake in other cleanliness habits around the house.

Figure 3–22. Control what you can[21]

Tool: Prioritizing (must, should, could)

While to-do lists can be a great tool for time management and organization, they can also become so long that they distract us from being present. Our list of tasks feels so long and daunting that we freeze because we do not know where to begin. Whether it relates to work or your family and home life, organizing your to-do list will help you manage your time and limit the distractions that a long, overwhelming list can cause.

Start by writing down everything you need to get done in a day. Then label each task as either something that must be done, should be done, or could be done. For example, a firefighter's list might include some things like this:

1. Clean the kitchen
2. Wash the fire truck
3. Reorganize the tool room
4. Check gear and SCBA

Next, attach a label to each task (fig. 3–23). A good rule of thumb is to think of things that have deadlines as "must do," things that need to get done but are without time constraints as "should do," and things that you would like to do if you could as "could do." For the list above, the labels would look like this:

1. Clean the kitchen—should do (if you put this off too long, it will become a must do)
2. Wash the fire truck—must do
3. Reorganize the tool room—could do
4. Check gear and SCBA—must do

Beginning with the must-do tasks, start to complete the things on your list. This will help structure your time and give you a sense of accomplishment as you get things done. Prioritizing your to-do lists in this way will help you manage your time and reduce stress.

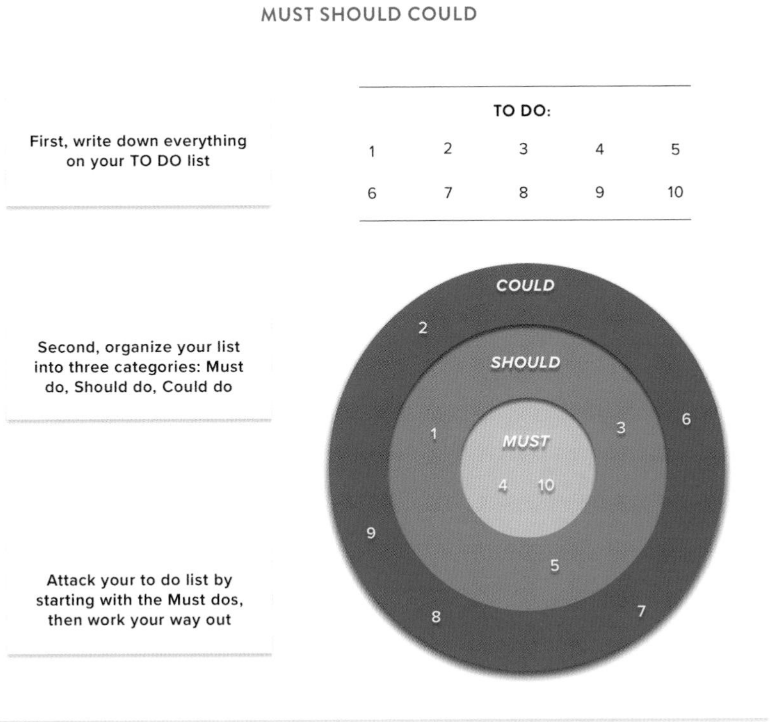

Figure 3–23. Must, should, could

Using writing as a tool to manage time, mitigate stress, and refocus on what is important allows us to find balance in our lives. Strategies like making a "must, should, could" list or writing out worries help us foster a healthy balance between work and life while creating space and time to add more things we want to do. Whether you add more time with friends and family or start a new hobby, being able to prioritize is a key part of finding balance and recentering yourself.

Recentering—Do What You Love

Beyond finding balance, recentering is a simple concept that can also be called self-care. Recentering is about having better balance in your life so that you have time to do what you love and what drives you. We do not have an endless pool of energy and resources to draw on, so it is important that we refill our reservoir whenever we have the chance. Recentering comes from finding the thing that refills your tank and keeps you going. It is about creating the time and space in your daily life for activities and relationships that replenish your energy and feelings of self-worth. For a tactical athlete who devotes a significant amount of time to serving others, self-care and recentering is critical to preventing burnout and ensuring career longevity. Try it now: stop and write down three things that you would never give up (without mentioning family or work). You may find this to be quite a challenge, but prioritizing balance is key to a long career.

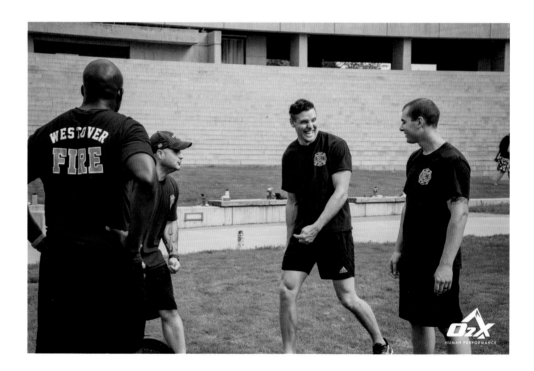

The concept of recentering and finding balance relates directly to our ability to build resilience. By learning how to replenish our mental and physical energy, we can be better equipped to handle new stressors after each challenge we face. Just as proper nutrition and recovery fuel strength gains after physical training sessions, the mindfulness techniques outlined in the chapter allow you to grow and strengthen your resilience after experiencing adversity. The next section will help explain in more detail how you can develop a growth mindset and build resilience.

KEY TAKEAWAYS

Tools and Skills for Mental Performance

◇ Mindfulness: "It's like putting a box in your brain and putting nothing into it."

◇ Diaphragmatic breathing: Maintaining a low and slow breathing pace resets your autonomic nervous system by helping rebalance your sympathetic and parasympathetic nervous systems.

◇ Overbreathing occurs when you take several fast, deep breaths and breathe out a large amount of carbon dioxide when you exhale. This lowers the amount of carbon dioxide in your blood and signals to your body that its metabolic needs are lower—also known as hypocapnia.

◇ Other mental performance tools include progressive muscle relaxation, visualization, self-talk, attention control, and journaling. These tools help manage worries, process stress, maintain focus, and allow you to become fully present and aware of your surroundings.

◇ Recentering is about having better balance in your life so that you have time to do what you love and what drives you.

◇ Finding which tools and skills are most effective for you and embedding them in your daily routine is key to short- and long-term success as a tactical athlete.

RESILIENCE—ANDY HAFFELE

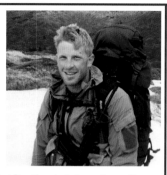

Four months after joining my first SEAL platoon, I was shot in the upper right chest from 15 feet away with an M4 assault rifle. The accident occurred during a training exercise in Hawaii on March 18, 2004. After the shot, I was immediately stabilized by our exceedingly capable team medic and flown to the nearest level one trauma hospital where I was taken straight to the operating room. By the end of the initial surgery, I had lost 50 units of blood, almost died 3 times on the operating table, and was still bleeding internally. At that point, the lead surgeon told my wife of 7 months that they had done all they could do, and it was in God's hands now. By the next morning, I had gone through another 20 units of blood but had miraculously stopped bleeding. The next couple of weeks brought an additional 4 emergent surgeries. In the recovery room after one of these close calls, I was intubated and motioned to my wife for a pencil and paper as that was the only way for me to communicate. I grabbed the pencil and wrote, "I WILL NOT DIE!!!!"

After nearly a month in the hospital, I was released to a very different life from the one I knew prior to the accident. The bullet had pierced my axillary artery and the subsequent shockwave had created a softball-sized hole in my chest that caused severe nerve damage to my entire right arm and shoulder. My arm was completely useless and I didn't know if I would have use of it again. Oddly, this incident was just the first hurdle in my race.

Two months prior to my injury, I had noticed an abnormal lump forming on one of my testicles. Due to our platoon's training schedule, I delayed my check-up until March 19th. I was shot on March 18th and I was not able to get it checked out for another 6 weeks. On the day I went in, I had 3 different urologists tell me I had testicular cancer and they would need to remove the affected testicle the following morning. You have got to be kidding me. Before the surgery my wife wrote on the inside of my thigh in big, black marker, "RIGHT ONE ONLY." We did that for a couple of reasons. First, you always hear those horror stories of a doctor operating on the wrong arm or knee or something else. My wife and I did not want to have anything like that occur given all that we had already been through. Second, we needed to add some levity to the situation. I can still remember the chorus of laughter that echoed off the walls in my operating room when the doctors saw that written on my leg. Fortunately, the operation was a success and further lab results would verify that the cancer was in its earliest stages. I would still need some low-dose radiation treatments to eradicate any lingering cancer cells, but the cancer has been in remission ever since then.

These physical trials were the easiest part when compared to the mental obstacles that lay ahead. My wife and I nearly lived in a hospital for a year post-injury between rehab and follow-up appointments. When we were not at the hospital, the threat of having to return was always just a heart or respiratory issue away. However, the real pain started when confronted with all the unknowns. Will I ever be able to use my arm again? Will I ever be able to return to being an operational SEAL? Will I ever be able to have children? Why did this happen to me? Why me?

To complicate matters, as I recovered from my injury, my platoon completed their work-up and deployed to Afghanistan. That deployment would result in great tragedy and the loss of many SEALs during a single operation and rescue mission in the Hindu Kush Mountains. Members of my platoon were among them. Subsequently, I buried many of my fallen brothers in the weeks to come and was left with very similar questions but in an entirely different context...Why me? Why was I spared this fate? Why am I still here because of this injury? Why can I not trade places with any of my men?

I continued physical therapy and received numerous surgeries to improve the function in my arm for another 3 years. My team of therapists, specialists, and doctors from every section of the hospital worked tirelessly to put humpty dumpty back together. But no matter how much time and effort you may put into something, on occasion your goals are simply not attainable. After a very long battle, my arm had reached its maximum potential near the end of 2007. The injury had resulted in permanent and irreversible nerve damage. I was subsequently medically discharged from the Navy.

Despite what may seem like a loss to many, I would not take back the events of March 18th, 2004, if ever given the opportunity. I gained an insight and perspective on life that never would have happened without the catastrophic events of that day. Conversely, I would gladly take the place of any of those fathers, sons, uncles, and brothers that died in the Hindu Kush of Afghanistan all those years ago. But somewhere along the way of my journey, I realized that that choice is not up to me no matter how much I may disagree. I have been blessed in countless ways throughout my life. I come from two very loving and caring parents and a great little brother. I have a beautiful and loving wife who has stuck by my side through some of my darkest days. We have three dear sons who light up our life and make my world complete. Those are just some of the highlights. Since being given this precious second chance, I try to live a life that honors my men and all the men and women who have sacrificed everything for this incredibly priceless gift. My only resiliency advice is pretty simple...lean on your faith, lean on your family, and lean on your friends. Do that and in that order of priority and everything else will fall into place.

—*Andy Haffele, Lt. (Ret.) US Navy SEAL*

RESILIENCE

Resilience is the ability to withstand stress and adversity and then rebound as strong as you were before. Consider this a form of post-traumatic growth, meaning that challenging experiences can be opportunities to strengthen, adapt, and be better prepared for future adversity. Resilience is not something you are born with; it is something you develop and is a skill that needs to be continually strengthened to help you overcome obstacles and maximize your potential. Our life experiences, and the stress they sometimes produce, lay the foundation for our ability to build resilience. Each experience or challenge we face teaches us how to cope effectively so we can overcome future obstacles. It is the process of dealing with adverse situations that teaches us resilience, not the situations themselves. We only realize how resilient we are after persevering in the face of adversity.

ATTITUDE, MINDSET—GOEFF KRILL

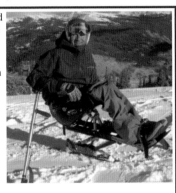

As a disabled athlete, I am often asked how I have been able to achieve such a positive outlook and accomplish so much in my life after being paralyzed. There are consistent questions: *Weren't you depressed? Didn't you want to die, because I don't think I could have lived that way?* When I hear those questions, I can't believe that people actually feel that way. Life is a precious gift, and your charge is to live it in all the ways that it manifests. I think back to the night of my spinal cord injury (SCI), and there were moments of fear for what was to come, what would change, and how my life would play out. But when you really break everything down to the bare bones, I am alive and that is enough. Above all else, being alive is a pretty incredible cornerstone to begin building anything you want for yourself. I know that for many this is easier said than done.

Step one for me was acknowledging my situation and the reality that I would never be able to walk again. Take account of your situation—whatever it is—and don't sugarcoat it, believing that it will just get better. Yes, it may, but you can waste a whole lot of time wishing and dreaming when there is a life of doing out there waiting for you. From the very onset of my SCI, the medical industry has been talking about a cure. If I had spent my life hoping, waiting, and dreaming of that day, I would have missed out on the most epic and fulfilling years of my life. Yes, I can't walk, but it hasn't stopped me from traveling the world through sport and having an amazing family and kids. The doom and gloom is the easy road to take, and it's what people expect from you when you're in the midst of a life-altering situation. Those around you may listen and comfort you for a while, but eventually they do not want to be subjected to misery.

Step two involves your ability to adapt to a situation. I know that the best-laid plans always have their hiccups and alterations from the originally intended path. It is the ability to morph and meet the challenges in the moment that allows us to win, survive, and conquer. Resilience is based on your ability to be flexible in all aspects, not just physically but mentally, changing your mental status to meet the needs of the situation. This is critical to "survive-ability" and success.

The bottom line for me, and the continued outlook that has kept me going in the game of life the past 23 years, is a simple lesson that has been consistent in my life ever since I started playing sports and was a part of a team. You may be sidelined, put on the bench for a while, but in the end you are always a part of that team. This is the same in life: you have to be there for family and friends and most importantly for yourself to be in the game. Injuries and unforeseeable situations in life happen, but life is good, amazing, and simply awesome to live when you continue to just be in it.

—*Geoff Krill, O2X Specialist, Adventure Athlete, and Professional Ski Instructors of America (National Team)*

Special operations forces, professional sports teams, and top corporations focus on resilience and mental-toughness training for performance enhancement. These top-tier organizations understand that resilience can be taught and is a critical component to maximizing the potential for success.

The first, critical step toward building resilience is to acknowledge that we face a challenge or stressor and to then recognize the negative effects and emotions we feel as a result of the situation. Only after acknowledging the adversity can we begin to make sense of it and take steps to move on from the negative experience, becoming more resilient in the process. This requires using mental performance tools to obtain a high level of self-awareness and self-compassion.

Skill: Understanding Post-Traumatic Stress Disorder (PTSD)

Before jumping into the tools and techniques you can use to build resilience, we want to first address and open a discussion on the topic of mental health as it relates to experiencing trauma and subsequently building resilience.

As we have talked about repeatedly, tactical athletes face heightened levels of physical and mental stress daily. The degree of stress can vary from low-level chronic stress to the high-level stress of responding to traumatic calls or life-and-death situations. As a result, it is increasingly important that you recognize how stress and trauma impact you and that you have the tools and resources to address and recover from stressful events.

Traumatic stress can come from a single event or from continued exposure to difficult situations, and it can manifest as post-traumatic stress disorder (PSTD). Most often, PTSD is associated with combat experience, but emergency room personnel, law enforcement officers, firefighters, EMS providers, and investigators are also regularly exposed to traumatic events of varying degrees and must prioritize coping with and handling these stressors.

The risk of experiencing PTSD for first responders and tactical athletes is related to the amount and intensity of exposure to repeated trauma.[22] This can be compounded by personal relationships, sensitivity to specific incidents (calls involving children, for example), and, in the case of many first-responders, the proximity of work to home. Symptoms to look for include the following:[23]

1. **Re-experiencing:** Having repeated memories or thoughts of a past experience. This can include nightmares or flashbacks, and the memories are often accompanied by physical reactions of anxiety. These thoughts and dreams often feel intrusive and out of control.
2. **Avoidance:** The tendency to avoid, ignore, or try to forget past events. This can also include isolation and the physical avoidance of being in crowds, watching movies, or doing activities that remind you of the traumatic event. Participation in these events or situations could elicit agitation or panic.

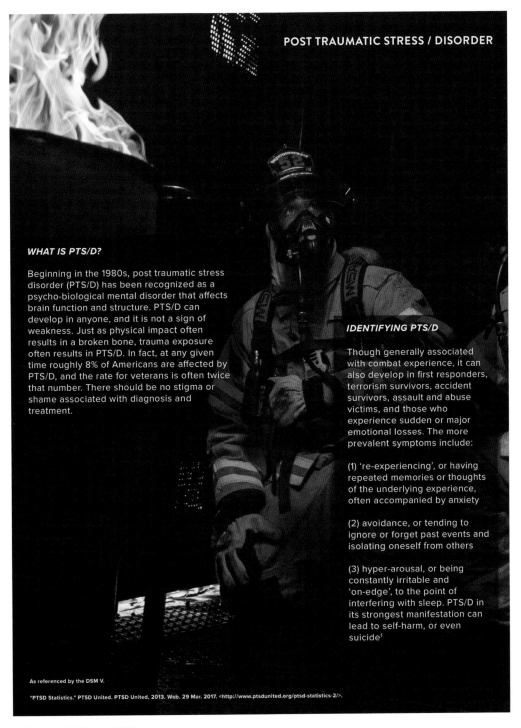

WHAT IS PTS/D?

Beginning in the 1980s, post traumatic stress disorder (PTS/D) has been recognized as a psycho-biological mental disorder that affects brain function and structure. PTS/D can develop in anyone, and it is not a sign of weakness. Just as physical impact often results in a broken bone, trauma exposure often results in PTS/D. In fact, at any given time roughly 8% of Americans are affected by PTS/D, and the rate for veterans is often twice that number. There should be no stigma or shame associated with diagnosis and treatment.

IDENTIFYING PTS/D

Though generally associated with combat experience, it can also develop in first responders, terrorism survivors, accident survivors, assault and abuse victims, and those who experience sudden or major emotional losses. The more prevalent symptoms include:

(1) 're-experiencing', or having repeated memories or thoughts of the underlying experience, often accompanied by anxiety

(2) avoidance, or tending to ignore or forget past events and isolating oneself from others

(3) hyper-arousal, or being constantly irritable and 'on-edge', to the point of interfering with sleep. PTS/D in its strongest manifestation can lead to self-harm, or even suicide[1]

As referenced by the DSM V.

"PTSD Statistics." PTSD United. PTSD United, 2013. Web. 29 Mar. 2017. <http://www.ptsdunited.org/ptsd-statistics-2/>.

Figure 3–24a. PTSD

VERY HIGH RISK SYMPTOMS

- Threatening to hurt or kill oneself
- Looking for ways to kill oneself
- Sharing suicidal ideations
- Talking or writing about death, dying or suicide

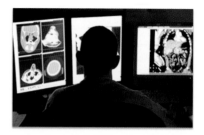

HIGH RISK SYMPTOMS

- Hopelessness
- Rage, anger, seeking revenge
- Acting reckless or engaging in risky activities
- Feeling trapped – like there's no way out
- Increasing alcohol or drug abuse
- Withdrawing from friends, family or society
- Anxiety, agitation, disrupted sleeping patterns
- Dramatic mood changes
- No reason for living, no sense of purpose in life

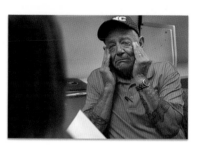

OTHER RISK FACTORS

- Recent losses – physical, financial, personal
- Family history of suicide
- History of abuse (physical, sexual or emotional)
- Co-morbid health problems, especially a newly diagnosed or worsening problem
- Age, gender, race (elderly or young adult, unmarried, white, male, living alone)

What to do if you sense a friend or colleague is symptomatic:

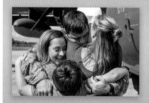

- ☐ *Begin a conversation, be straightforward*
- ☐ *Encourage them to share their thoughts and plans*
- ☐ *Encourage them to seek help*
- ☐ *Do not minimize the problem or cause the person to feel shame*
- ☐ *If you feel the person isn't in immediate danger, acknowledge the pain is legitimate and offer to work together to get help*

RISK MITIGATION TOOLS

- Receiving positive social support
- Seeking spirituality
- Feeling a responsibility to family
- Having children in the home

- Experiencing life satisfaction
- Building positive coping skills
- Building problem-solving skills
- Developing a therapeutic relationship

Figure 3–24b. PTSD (continued)

3. **Hyperarousal:** Being constantly on edge or irritable. This is sometimes referred to as being keyed up, and it is the notion that you are constantly vigilant and looking out for potential signs of danger. It can lead to sleeplessness, difficulty focusing, and being easily startled.

4. **Negative Thoughts:** A shift in your belief about yourself and the world around you. This can manifest as self-harming thoughts and behaviors and even an increased risk of suicide. It can also lead to a negative shift in your interactions toward others, resulting in feelings of isolation.

Additionally, the symptoms listed above can manifest across a wide spectrum of severity and even those who experience them can still function at a high level.

An important note is that not all people who experience stress develop PTSD; if two people experience the same traumatic event, one may develop PTSD while the other may not. Part of being a good teammate is understanding this, and it is not easy. You must empathize with others and be mindful of your own needs—for your whole career. It is critical that you recognize how trauma impacts you as a tactical athlete. It is also important to understand that acknowledging and addressing your symptoms and signs of stress is a courageous and necessary part of fulfilling your job and ensuring a long, healthy life.

Skill: Finding Your Mindset

Throughout this chapter you have learned various techniques that highlight the link between the thought–performance interaction. In other words, what you think is directly connected to how you feel and ultimately how you perform. Now, we will take a closer look at the types of thoughts you may have and how they can help or hinder your performance. This is where your **mindset** comes into play.

Pioneered by psychologist Carol Dweck, mindset is your belief in yourself and your most basic, fundamental qualities.[24] This can include your belief in your intelligence, personality, or general talents. Although having a positive mindset produces better results,[25] that does not always come easily, and building a growth mindset takes work.

Dweck's research differentiates mindset into two categories: a growth mindset or a fixed mindset. Someone with a fixed mindset regards intelligence, talent, and fundamental abilities as inherited, unchangeable traits. With a fixed mindset, you are likely to view a failure as inevitable and see obstacles as insurmountable tasks rather than opportunities for learning and development. On the other hand, someone with a growth mindset views intelligence, talent, and basic abilities as things that can be developed and improved through dedication and effort.

A growth mindset lays the foundation for a healthy attitude of learning from challenges, and it leads to continued growth and progress even in the face of obstacles. In terms of its role in resilience, a growth mindset allows you to use experiences as feedback for growth and to see adversity as an opportunity to build resilience and come back stronger. Developing a growth mindset is vital to building resilience, as it allows you to shift your perspective and see new challenges, feedback, and setbacks as channels for progress.

Mindset
Pioneered by psychologist Carol Dweck, mindset is your belief in yourself and your fundamental abilities, and it is often broken into two categories—growth and fixed mindset.

There are a few key points when it comes to a discussion of mindset. A growth mind-set does not always equate to positivity and only seeing good things. Also, you may exhibit a growth mindset in certain areas of your life and fixed mindset in other areas. And you have the ability to change your mindset from fixed to growth through height-ened self-awareness and purposeful practice.

Next time you meet an obstacle or do not get the outcome you desired, think about your reaction. If you feel yourself jumping to a fixed mindset like the examples shared in the fixed versus growth chart (fig. 3–25), take a tactical pause and refocus on how you might approach the setback with a growth mindset. Consider any debriefs and after action reviews (covered in depth later) that occurred and how you received the feedback. Again, although this difference can be subtle and the concept may seem simple, it is not always easy to make the shift from a fixed to a growth mindset. It is something that takes dedicated practice, like all of the mental performance skills we have discussed, but the outcome can, quite literally, be life changing.

FIXED VS. GROWTH MINDSET

	FIXED	vs.	GROWTH
SKILLS	**Something you are born with** "I am unathletic and cannot finish a road race."		**Comes from hard work** "If I spend time working out, I can definitely improve my endurance."
EFFORT	**Going through the motions** "Even though I show up for work, I will never get promoted."		**A path to mastery, learning** "If I tackle new skills and projects, I will be worthy of a promotion."
CHALLENGES	**Something to avoid** "A marathon would be far too difficult for me."		**An opportunity to grow** "If I am disciplined about the training plan, I could get across the finish line!"
FEEDBACK	**Take input personally** "I can't believe my squad leader criticized my reputation on deployment."		**An opportunity to learn** "If I work on those skills, and communicate better, I will be a valuable team member."
SETBACKS	**Blame others, be discouraged** "That guy has been undermining me from the get-go . . . "		**Use as a wake up call** "If I make a concerted effort to know him, he will understand my approach better."

Figure 3–25. Fixed vs. growth mindset

Skill: Extending the Comfort Zone

The concept of stress as a tool for growth is not a new one in this book. Earlier we discussed the importance of physical stress for strength gains and how the only way to build resilience is to experience some level of stress. The same is true of personal progress toward reaching our goals and continuing to strive for optimal performance. In order to move the needle forward and expand what you are comfortable with, you have to get uncomfortable with added stress.

Many elite athletes and high-performing individuals will talk about learning to be comfortable being uncomfortable. For a race car driver, this may mean pushing the speed just a little faster than normal to test his limits on the track. For a professional who does not present often, this may mean committing to a bigger public speaking engagement than she has ever experienced. For a tactical athlete, this may mean learning a specialty skill that does not come naturally—like learning to conduct confined space rescues when you struggle with claustrophobia. As we put ourselves in new, less-comfortable situations, our confidence grows and our comfort level expands so we can continue pushing ourselves more and more toward higher levels of performance and new learning experiences.

The drive to get outside our comfort zone does not always come naturally, and sometimes we get in our own way and let fear of the unknown or the possibility of failure limit us from maximizing our potential. We get stuck in routines and miss taking the opportunity to learn new skills or take on new challenges (fig. 3–26), particularly when we deal with stress daily. This can be detrimental and make us forget the things that drive us and that allow us to progress and grow so we can improve our performance.

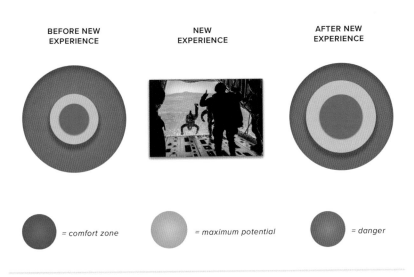

BREAKING OUT OF YOUR COMFORT ZONE

BEFORE NEW EXPERIENCE   NEW EXPERIENCE   AFTER NEW EXPERIENCE

= comfort zone   = maximum potential   = danger

Figure 3–26. Breaking out of your comfort zone

You may know someone with an "I'm up for anything, anytime, anywhere" mentality. Chances are that the person who has this mindset has fostered the belief that personal growth and learning come from pushing outside the comfort zone. If this does not come easily for you, then how do you jump start your personal growth and get out of your comfort zone?

Think of something you have been meaning to do or always wanted to try. This may involve learning a new skill or doing something that you avoid because you know it's tough, like learning to swim in swift water or practicing shooting off-handed. Commit to doing it. Make a plan for how you will try this new activity and set a timeline for yourself. Then you can think about what worries you about the task and use some of the previously outlined mental performance skills to help you get into the proper mindset for completing your goal.

As with any skill, the more you practice, the easier it will be for you to get outside your comfort zone. As you expose yourself to new experiences, you will begin to notice an increase in your confidence. The more opportunities you say yes to, the more chances you have to learn and grow. All it takes is a reason to get started. From a scientific standpoint, allowing your brain to build new connections and your body to build muscle memory by addressing weaknesses through new experiences will improve your motivation.[26]

> *Motivation*
> This is what drives us and what allows us to set goals and continually push ourselves to face new challenges, overcome obstacles, and maximize performance. People can be intrinsically motivated by internal factors or extrinsically motivated by outcome-oriented goals.

Skill: Building Motivation

Motivation is what drives us. It drives us to set goals to continually push ourselves to face new challenges, overcome obstacles, and maximize our human performance. Understanding what motivates you and how to tap into it in hard times is what separates those who are good at what they do from those who are the best. In fact, motivation is the foundation of goal setting—it allows us to answer the question of why we do what we do and why we set certain goals. Paired with a growth mindset and strong mental performance skills, motivation allows us to see a purpose greater than ourselves so that we can rise above any obstacles and achieve our goals.

Motivation varies from person to person and even from task to task. It is important to reflect on and understand what drives you—what you are passionate about and find rewarding—and then set goals to combine your passion with your drive so you can fulfill a purpose greater than yourself. This will enable you to manage fears and self-doubts, creating a positive mental attitude as you work toward your goals.

To start, you will need to think about what type of motivation drives you. The two main categories are intrinsic and extrinsic motivation. Intrinsic motivation is an internal desire to do something because it is inherently enjoyable to you.[27] This would be doing something solely because it is rewarding for you, without regard of an external reward or the need to do it for someone else's benefit. On the other hand, extrinsic motivation is outcome oriented and is your desire to do something based on the results it can yield.[28] It may be the motivation of pleasing someone else or getting recognition for your work.

Motivation is a spectrum, and you may be both intrinsically and extrinsically motivated to some degree—you might really enjoy what you are doing but also have some motivation to do it well to receive accolades for your work. Like mindsets, the two forms of motivation are not mutually exclusive, and you can work toward increasing your intrinsic motivation with deliberate thought and practice. Using motivation to learn from mistakes and failures is what builds resilience and increases your confidence as you approach new challenges. This enables you to come back stronger from setbacks so you can forge a warrior spirit and help others overcome any adversity they face.

MOTIVATION—ARNO ILGNER

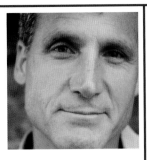

I've been teaching mental fitness to rock climbers for a *few* decades. My many years of teaching have helped me identify core principles that build one's mental power for approaching challenges. I've found that motivation is a critical foundational process to observe. Our motivation determines the decisions we make and the actions that flow from those decisions.

You want to win? Of course you do. But will such a motivation help you win? No, it won't. It's a matter of attention. Focusing on the goal shifts your attention into the future and on what you can't control. All control exists in the present moment. A big shift you need to make, then, is being excited about what happens in the present moment more than winning. This is a seemingly simple shift to make; however, our tendency to overvalue the achievement of goals makes it extremely difficult. Victims remain unconscious to this tendency; warriors don't. Warriors continually observe their attention and redirect it to the current task.

Current tasks happen currently, in the now. Therefore, you must identify what the current task is and focus your attention totally on it. You use your attention in two main ways: to think with the mind and to do—to take action—with the body. Thinking is the process of focusing your attention in the mind, to think about past experiences and future possibilities. You think to prepare, to identify the future goal and a plan for achieving it. Then, when preparation is over, it's time for action. Stop thinking and go in; shift attention out of the mind and into the body.

The starting line of a race is where you shift your attention into the body, to do the actual work required to move toward the goal. Joseph Campbell, who wrote about the hero's journey, said that people are looking for a feeling of being alive. Feeling is not about thinking; it's a process that occurs in the body. The body doesn't exist in the past or future like the thinking mind does. The body exists only in the present, where all action also occurs.

Visualize exerting effort, not achieving the goal. Desire to be in the stress of the experience—yes, the stress—and not at the finish line. We're inundated by information about reducing stress and how bad stress is. Yet it's in stress, not our comfort zones, that we learn. Therefore, lean into it, desire it, focus your attention on it and on processes that occur in the body. Breathe, stay as relaxed as you can, and appropriately use your body for the task, holding it with proper posture and using it efficiently. Tune in to and visualize those qualities.

You'll get tired when you're deep in stress. Your attention will shift out of the body processes and into the thinking mind as you doubt your ability to continue. Notice this shift and then deliberately redirect your attention to the body. Feel how it's processing the stress. Feel how the body is breathing and moving. Monitor how well you're engaging it. This is not a time to distract yourself with music or anything else, so leave your iPod at home. It's time to get in touch with your body, which is doing the work. You'll need to know what's occurring so you can discern between fatigue and injury. If you're fatigued, then stay committed and soldier on; if you feel that you're injuring yourself, then pay attention to it. You may need to stop. Pay attention so you know what to do.

This shift in motivation allows you to focus your attention on what you actually can control. Think about how powerful this shift is. This is what warriors do. Making this shift in motivation will make you feel alive, not in the future but now, in the current stressful event.

—Arno Ilgner, O2X Specialist, Pioneering Rock
Climber, and Founder of The Warrior's Way
(www.warriorsway.com)

Skill: Forging a Warrior Spirit

As we alluded to in our discussion of motivation, being able to call your attention to a bigger purpose and add meaning to what you do is a way to foster resilience and move forward through difficult times. Those who possess the intangible and often overlooked **warrior spirit** embody this and serve a cause greater than themselves. Warriors come in all shapes, sizes, ages, and types. They reveal themselves in the most unexpected moments. They are often unassuming, soft-spoken hard workers who are not looking for the glory of a spotlight.

Those with a warrior spirit are internally driven, filled with grit and perseverance that come from overcoming adversity. Warriors run toward challenges and face fear of the unknown to help others get through difficult situations. People with a warrior spirit use their own scars and experiences to encourage, support, and help others see how to overcome their own obstacles. A warrior's ultimate reward is helping others become resilient in difficult times in order to achieve their goals.

The warrior spirit is one that finds calm in the midst of chaos and that sees adversity as a personal challenge and opportunity for growth. Everyone can have a warrior spirit, but like resilience, it must be developed over time and through experience. To develop or strengthen your warrior spirit, you can use many of the mental performance skills outlined in this chapter to build your ability to handle stressors and create opportunity out of adversity.

Developing a warrior spirit comes one step at a time; it is not immediate. It is about visualizing your goal, finding your passion, and making small, incremental steps in the relentless pursuit of fulfilling your purpose. The ability to see fear as a challenge to overcome, to manage emotions, and to strive for optimal performance is what forms the center of the warrior's soul. The impact you want to have on others is what drives you.

Having a warrior spirit requires that you write the legacy you want to leave. This spirit is what pushes you to serve a purpose greater than yourself. It enables you to find strength in difficult times and allows you to continually build resilience despite any level of adversity. Think about the lessons you want to teach and how you want others to remember you. Then think about the values and traits that you need to embody to leave a legacy you can be proud of. If there were to be a newspaper story about you in 5 years, what would it be about and how would it describe you? Think in terms of not only the outcome, but also the way that the article would describe you achieving your goal. Then go out and live in a way that would make you proud to read that story. This will help you find purpose in times of adversity and will guide you toward developing your warrior spirit.

PUTTING MENTAL SKILLS IN ACTION

Throughout the THRIVE chapter you have been introduced to a number of mental performance skills and learned how to use them to manage stress, build resilience, and forge a warrior spirit. You have learned about the physiological impact of stress on performance and how to use mental performance training to physically improve your recovery by activating your PNS, increasing your HRV, and finding balance. The chapter has outlined how you can practice mindfulness through dedicated focus on internal and external images, create inner resources to promote calmness amidst chaos, and use visualization and breath work to prepare for potential stressors and mitigate their negative effects on performance. Understanding how to use mental performance skills and mindfulness to take tactical pauses and for daily recovery is one step in maximizing performance, and the next is systematically implementing goal setting, refocusing, and after action reviews into your work.

Skill: Goal Setting
Pre-event

Mental Readiness
Building a strong and resilient mind so you are ready to face any potential challenges or adversity.

Mental readiness is a key ingredient to success, not only on the job but also in other areas of our lives. The amount of trust you have in yourself affects your ability to set goals and maximize performance. It is one thing to have skills and abilities but another to trust that those skills and abilities will meet your needs when the stakes are high. This level of self-belief and mental readiness comes from the ability to set appropriate goals and attack them with discipline and persistence.

Effective goal setting is key to establishing action plans and optimizing performance. Goal setting helps you resolve worries, visualize success, and navigate anything you encounter. It applies to all areas of performance including nutrition, conditioning, family life, hobbies, and career advancement. Goal setting allows you to identify short-term steps and a process you can follow as you work toward long-term achievements.

When setting goals, begin with the end in mind. Like visualization, think about what your ideal outcome is and then work backward to list the steps it will take to end up with that result. For example, let's say you want to be selected for an elite unit—rescue company, SWAT team, or special operations unit. You can break that down into more detail including what gates you need to pass along the way, but your end goal is to make the team. With this in mind, your next step would be to create a training plan to follow leading up to the date you plan to try out.

With the long-term goal of making it onto the unit, you can treat each training day as its own event and set small, daily goals. Identify and write down the requisite mental and physical skills, then figure out how to train in those areas. Accomplishing every workout and achieving process-oriented goals can help you maintain motivation even when you feel burnt out or overwhelmed by larger goals. At the outset the big goal may seem unattainable, but taking each step one day, one hour, or even one second at a time can give you the strength to succeed.

One of the most grueling training evolutions in the military is known as "hell week," a rite of passage for all aspiring Navy SEALs. During these long days, trainees are exposed to intense physical challenges and extreme environmental conditions without the luxury of more than a couple hours of sleep the entire week. Success during hell week requires a laser focus on the near term: completing the next evolution, the next 100 m, the next step. Those who look too far into the future can become overwhelmed with the seemingly impossible task and often fail. Those who take the week one moment at a time and accomplish a series of small, manageable goals have a much better chance of advancing beyond hell week.

While physical goals seem to naturally lend themselves to a goal-setting process, it may take more practice to do this with less tangible goals that do not have a clearly defined path. The principles of goal setting (fig. 3–27)[29] will help guide you to set realistic and achievable goals, and to enjoy the process of working towards them.

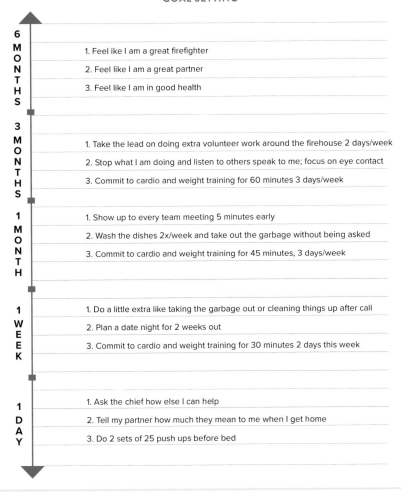

Figure 3–27. SMART goal setting

Tool: Discipline and persistence

If you are setting goals that are slightly out of your comfort zone and truly pushing yourself to improve, it is likely that some steps toward achieving your desired outcome will not come easily. That is okay. In fact, it makes us more resilient, and it makes accomplishing our goals rewarding. This is where discipline and persistence come into play.

Once you have set a goal, you need to build an action plan and follow through with it. Focusing on the process of reaching small, daily milestones can help you maintain focus and commitment on reaching a long-term goal. This also helps you plan for and handle obstacles or unexpected challenges that cross your path. To return to our example, you want to make it on to your agency's elite team. It is likely that balancing training with your normal work schedule and personal life is going to be a challenge. Regular 5 a.m. interval workouts to prepare for the run test before heading to work will get old very quickly. It is inevitable that there will be a day you want to hit snooze on the alarm clock. That is okay. Missteps and sick days are something you should plan for so you are prepared and know how to navigate without derailing your progress.

This is where discipline becomes a factor. Being disciplined about what you need to do to reach your goals does not mean giving up everything that may get in the way. It does mean, however, that you will need to plan ahead to account for potential setbacks and plan frequent reminders of your motivation. If you think you will hit snooze, plan ahead by moving your alarm clock across the room, or think about the motivation behind your goal. What is its greater purpose? Think of the opportunities you'll have when you make it to the unit of your dreams. Planning ahead and focusing on your purpose will help you see something small you can do each day that will help you get to your goal.

Along with discipline comes persistence—continuing on even when it gets difficult and bouncing back if you do get off track. Goals that require persistence will help you grow and become more resilient. As you begin to set goals, remember that there will be times when you fail and are not able to get the outcome you desire. Be compassionate toward yourself in times of failure, and consider that even those who have achieved the greatest success have experienced failure.

Do not give up after a failure; instead use it as fuel toward reaching your next goal. Acknowledge what went wrong, where you fell short, and learn from the experience so you do not make the same mistakes twice. Avoid apprehension to setting new goals for fear of failure to achieve them. Setting goals can be fear inducing and exhilarating, and having a positive mental attitude and growth mindset will help you turn anxiety into excitement so you stay committed to your plan.

In the Moment

Focus and effective self-regulation are required for maximizing performance in any situation, particularly those with high-stakes outcomes. Whether you are a firefighter responding in a truck through a crowded city street or a fighter pilot landing an F-18 on a moving aircraft carrier in limited visibility, maintaining focus is crucial to your success. But focusing solely on the potential outcome of your actions can intensify the pressure you feel and impair your performance. Top performers in high-pressure situations learn not to get distracted by a potential outcome. Instead they shift their focus internally to the aspects of the situation they can control. Rather than being stressed by the environment, they use mental performance skills to mitigate worry and redirect their attention to the process that will lead them to a desired result.

Tool: Self-regulation

As you learned previously, stress can negatively impact your performance in a variety of ways. This is when knowing how you physiologically respond to stress can be your best tool. When it comes to handling stress, **self-regulation** is the process of bringing your body and mind back to homeostasis. The first step to being able to rebalance is recognizing when a situation is eliciting fear, anger, apathy, or any emotion that is negatively impacting your performance. When you acknowledge your detrimental responses to pressure, you must self-regulate to come back to your optimal zone for performance.

Self-Regulation
Your ability to recognize and manage your thoughts, emotions, and behaviors, which is particularly useful in high-pressure situations.

When you get called to action or find yourself in the middle of a hard workout as you progress toward accomplishing a goal, situational awareness and the ability to reset and refocus if you get off track is imperative. What do you do when things are not going the way you planned?

In these moments, taking a tactical pause will help you maintain awareness of your surroundings so you can redirect your focus on the task at hand. Breathing, self talk, and PMR are all examples of techniques you can use to control your emotions and reactions in high-pressure circumstances. Knowing when those tools can help you comes down to using two processes: the three Rs and RSVR.

Tool: The three Rs

The three Rs—Recognize, Reset, Refocus—are a quick and straightforward tool to put into action in the midst of a stressful or high-pressure situation (fig. 3–28). Being able to recognize, reset, and refocus creates a tactical pause, maintaining situational awareness and focus on the present moment.

Tool: RSVR

Similar to the three Rs, RSVR—Recognize, Stabilize, Visualize, Re-engage—is another systematic method to help you maintain physiological stabilization and reset when you are in the midst of chaos (fig 3–29). This is a process designed as a practical guide to use whenever you begin to feel the effects of stress. Thinking back to the beginning of our mental performance discussion, you will recall that when you perceive stress your sympathetic nervous system is triggered, causing increased heart rate, rapid breathing, racing thoughts, and other physiological responses aimed at preparing your body to fight or flee.

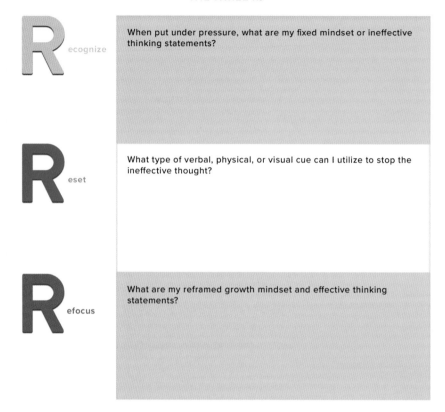

THE THREE Rs

Recognize — When put under pressure, what are my fixed mindset or ineffective thinking statements?

Reset — What type of verbal, physical, or visual cue can I utilize to stop the ineffective thought?

Refocus — What are my reframed growth mindset and effective thinking statements?

Figure 3–28. The Three Rs

If you can teach yourself to take a tactical pause and maintain physiological stabilization in these intense moments, you will be able to remain fully aware of your situation so you can make clear and rational decisions. In our car analogy, this would be the equivalent of downshifting into a lower gear when you are speeding to a curve. RSVR is the process of realizing you are going too fast and taking action to slow down before you swerve out of control.

Over time, you will become familiar with recurring triggers that cause you stress, and you will be able to build RSVR scripts specifically for each of those scenarios and their optimal outcomes. For example, a firefighter might enact RSVR before getting to the scene of a call by running through an internal dialogue like this one.

RSVR

First, make an effort to Recognize when you're overly aroused by your "fight or flight" system. Indicators include muscle tension, increased heart rate, racing thoughts, chest tightness, and amped up anger or fear. Over time, build awareness by noticing patterns in your counterproductive thoughts, and negative emotions. Also, try to notice recurrent triggers – whether they be people, situations, or something else - that cause arousal. You can likely list recurrent triggers as you're reading this. For example, a siren, accident scene, or difficult colleague, could be a recurrent trigger. When you become aware of arousal, this is your cue to initiate step 2, Stabilize.

Second, you should Stabilize your mind and body. As you sense arousal occurring in your body, or you anticipate a trigger, you can physiologically stabilize your mind and body by taking a few diaphragmatic breaths. The old adage "take a deep breath" is actually rooted in physiology. As you learned above, diaphragmatic breathing helps "throttle down" your sympathetic nervous system, and thus helps you get a handle on what is going on around you. It also leads to better decision making, and overall performance under stress. As you're taking deep breaths, begin step 3, Visualize.

Third, you should Visualize what you want to say, how you want to act, and your desired outcome. This is short-term goal setting, and helping your thoughts lead you to a desired (ideally safe and optimal) result. In longer-term contexts as well, visualization is an excellent technique for training your mind to lead your actions toward a successful outcome. Athletes, public speakers, dancers, and many other disciplines use visualization to improve results. Here, for you, anticipating recurrent triggers in your life, and mentally role playing how you could optimally handle these triggers, will build your resilience. Now, it is time to Re-engage.

Finally, you are prepared to optimally Re-engage in the situation. At this point in the RSVR process, you have recognized the triggers, taken a few diaphragmatic breaths to physiologically re-stabilize yourself, and visualized how you would like this situation to play out. So, get back in the moment, get after it. With a calm, quiet mind, move forward in whatever activity you're engaged in, while keeping your antennae tuned for the next recurrent trigger.

Figure 3–29. RSVR—Recognize, Stabilize, Visualize, Re-engage

"Here we go: a working fire." (This may trigger some anxiety or some sort of energy for you). "Take a few deep breaths, stay calm and in control. Focus on listening to the radio traffic and check out my gear. Make sure everything is in its place. No distractions. Mentally run through what will happen when we get on scene and that parking brake sets. I'm well trained and I have a great crew. We know what to do and it's going to happen quick—stay out of our way. Few more deep breaths. Unbuckle my seatbelt and let's get after it."

RSVR provides a clear plan for taking a tactical pause and refocusing on the present during high-stress events. The next step is implementing practices that intentionally promote recovery from these experiences at ideal times—during performance transitions. Some examples of the optimal time to downshift and reset after intense experiences include: on your way home from work, at the halfway point in your day, or before going to bed. You may downshift multiple times during the day, depending on the amount of stressors you encounter. The final piece of putting mental performance into action is not only how you recover from an incident but how you learn from each experience through effective debriefing.

Post-Event Debrief

The final component to maximizing human performance and building resilience is conducting effective debriefing following any experience or training exercise. These after action reviews allow you to reflect on a situation and think critically about how you and your team responded (fig. 3–30). The intention is to create action plans to improve future performances. In order to produce useful results, tactical athletes must use after action reviews as deliberate, purposeful reflections with a focus on continual learning and growth.

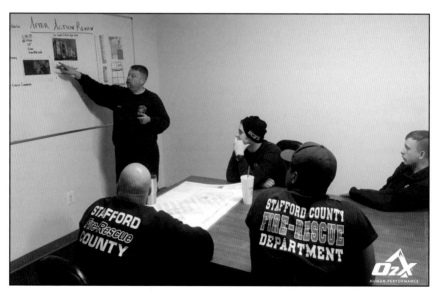

Figure 3–30. After action review

Tool: After action review

Using debriefing as a tool for performance requires that each individual involved develop a growth mindset and acknowledge that the reviews are critical to progress. The sessions should not be considered a casual conversation but should be standardized, methodical recaps of each factor involved in a scenario. A systematic review of any situation—training or real—should include analysis of pre-event, during-event, and post-event elements.

To become comfortable with debriefing and after action reviews (aka "hot washes"), leaders can make them a standard component of any training exercise. Once the training drill is complete, the after action review takes place. The O2X AAR template is offered here (fig. 3–31) as a framework for conducting an effective debrief. Take this example and make it your own. Create an AAR template that matches the values and battle rhythm or your unit or organization and use it to get 1% better every day. Building this guide into standard operating procedures following all training events will allow the team to become comfortable with the practice. It will also facilitate more impactful AARs after high-stakes, real-life events.

KEY TAKEAWAYS

Mental Performance in Action

- Goal setting helps you resolve worries, visualize success, and navigate anything you encounter. It allows you to identify short-term steps and gives you a process to follow as you work toward long-term achievements.

- Discipline and persistence allow you to do anything you need to do to reach your goals without giving up when you face adversity or challenges.

- The three Rs is a systematic method you can use to recognize, reset, and refocus when you are in the midst of a high-pressure situation.

- RSVR is a technique you can use to take a tactical pause to maintain physiological stabilization and reset when you are in a chaotic situation.

- The O2X AAR template is a tool you can use for effective after action reviews to debrief a training event, emergency call, or operation that can help you develop a growth mindset and team culture of continuous learning and progress.

AFTER ACTION REVIEWS

PHASE 0 - PRIOR PREPARATION

• All individuals have required baseline training
• All firefighters current on all SOPs
• New guys know roles and responsibilities – trained up by vets
• All physically able
• Any distractors in team? How to remove them?
• Any new equipment being introduced? New tactics?
• Plan for detailed members?

PHASE 1 - SHIFT TURN OVER

• In Brief from officer / chief
• Everyone clear on Roles and Responsibilities
• Detailed members briefed on roles
• Individual equipment checked – SCBA, PPE
• Team equipment checked – Apparatus, tools, etc
• Any atmospherics need to take into account – Heavy winds, Environment dry, holidays, road closures, traffic
• Mental State of Crew
• Physical State of Crew
• Energy level
• Attitude
• Distractors in group?
• Feeling overall prepared / dialed in?

PHASE 2 - DISPATCH TO ARRIVAL ON SCENE

• Dispatch initial information provided
• Turnout time in acceptable range
• Response time in acceptable range
• Details passed along route regarding situation

PHASE 2 (CONTINUED)

• Route taken – most efficient
• Decisions made along transit
• Pre-deconfliction of other units on ground or enroute
• Positioning of apparatus on scene
• What we expected when arrived on scene? If not, why?

PHASE 3 - ON SITE

• Situational awareness on site
• Communication / De-confliction other ground elements – EMS, Ladder, Engine, Law Enforcement
• Offensive or defensive operations?
   o Entry team details
• Clear, Concise calls made from entry team to leadership
• Leadership calls
• Additional alarms needed?
• Other teams – Roof Team, Support Elements
• Updates passed amongst group
• Everyone have PPE on entire time?
• Overhaul

PHASE 4 - MOVEMENT BACK TO THE HOUSE AND RE-JOCK

• Organization back to apparatus
• Route back
• Team gear reset while prepared for next call
• Individual gear reset – change out bunker gear, hoods, new bottles, etc
• Anything learned during call? Tactics changed? Role changes?
• Paperwork generated up chain by officer / chief

Figure 3–31. After action reviews template

FINAL THOUGHTS—MENTAL PERFORMANCE

As with any skill, using mental performance techniques takes time and practice. Start by learning how your body and mind are impacted by stress and then begin to try different management strategies. You do not need to become an expert in yoga and mindfulness to begin to see and feel the benefits of the practice, just as you do not need to become a bodybuilder to feel the impact of following a conditioning program. The key here is to become familiar with the various mental performance tools available to you and discover which ones work for you. The final piece to the puzzle is learning how and when to use the skills you learn. We hope that this section has given you the information you need to use mental performance to reach your goals.

SLEEP—HABITS, MINDSET, ENVIRONMENT

We will end our discussion of THRIVE with the topic of sleep because it is not only critically important but also something that many of us are lacking. Sleep affects every aspect of your overall health and tactical performance, both mentally and physically. While good sleep can help you optimize health and performance, a sleep deficit and extended wakefulness can have serious consequences on your well-being and lead to significant health risks (fig. 3–32).

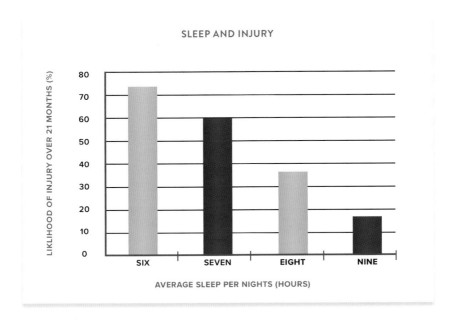

Figure 3–32. Sleep and injury

The benefits of sleep cannot be overstated; they are plentiful and quality sleep can improve every aspect of your health, well-being, and performance. Adequate sleep is linked to processes including memory consolidation, tissue repair and regeneration, immune system functioning, and rebalancing of neurotransmitter and metabolic systems. On the other hand, sleep deprivation results in decreased cognitive functioning, slower reaction times, and deficits in communication, coordination, endurance, and strength. Additionally, poor sleep can lead to mood swings, emotional instability, and an increased likelihood of accident-related injuries.[30]

If sustained over time, inadequate sleep is also associated with a weakened immune system, altered eating habits, weight gain, insulin resistance, diabetes, high blood pressure, and other cardiometabolic diseases.[31] The good news is that there are things that you can do to get the rest you need to mitigate these risks and reap the benefits associated with adequate sleep. The standard recommendation is that adults over the age of 18 get 7 to 9 hours of sleep per night.[32] Like nutrition, focusing on the quality, quantity, and timing of sleep is key to ensuring that you get the sleep you need to perform at your best.

Shift Work, Sleep, and the Impact on Performance and Health

The number one cause of death among firefighters is cardiovascular disease, followed by motor vehicle accidents. Sleep disorders double the risk for both, while also tripling the risk for experiencing mood and anxiety disorders like depression and PTSD.[33] Beyond these major consequences, lack of sleep or extended wakefulness can negatively impact our ability to complete daily tasks, decrease our cognitive functions, and diminish our psychomotor vigilance task performance.[34,35] Tactical athletes who are commonly required to work on shifts that include extended hours and overnights must take these consequences related to sleep into consideration to minimize the potential risks.

Normally, shift work is characterized as a work schedule that divides a 24-hour day into periods that are roughly the same duration and requires three or more teams to fulfill 24-hour coverage.[36] For many tactical athletes, a 24-hour period is *one shift*. Both 12- and 24-hour schedules are commonly found among tactical athletes like firefighters, law enforcement officers, and medical professionals, and these shifts can cause disruptions in circadian rhythms leading to disordered sleep patterns. Long shifts can be even harder for units deployed to disaster areas and military operations abroad. This leads us to look at sleep science and the physiological process of sleep so you have a better understanding of what you can do to mitigate the potential risks of operating under sleep deficit or extended wakefulness.

Physiological Process and Impact of Sleep

Let's discuss at the processes involved in sleep regulation—sleep drive and circadian rhythm—that serve as triggers to signal our bodies that it is time to sleep. While both sleep drive and circadian rhythm have their own role in the sleep process, it is their coordination that allows humans to maintain approximately 16 hours of continued wakefulness and 8 hours of uninterrupted sleep.[37] If and when these processes get out of sync, sleep issues can ensue, and you can use the tools outlined later in the section to reset your sleep schedule.

Sleep drive

Sleep drive—or sleep process—is your body's natural process for maintaining homeostasis and finding balance between rest and wakefulness. If you are fatigued or have been awake for a long period of time, you will have a high sleep drive—your body's need for sleep is heightened.

Sleep Drive
Your body's natural process for maintaining homeostasis and finding balance between rest and wakefulness.

Physiologically, sleep drive is the buildup of sleep-promoting metabolites (the breakdown of energetic processes) in the brain during waking hours. While you sleep, these metabolites are cleaned out and your sleep drive dissipates.[38]

Back to our car analogy, think of your sleep drive (or sleep process) as the fuel gauge. If you get a sufficient amount of quality sleep, your tank will be full and your sleep drive is low. As you sleep, the needle moves and your sleep drive decreases. On the other hand when you become sleep deprived, the gauge signals that you need to refuel and your sleep drive increases.

Circadian rhythm

The second process involved in sleep regulation is **circadian rhythm**, which is our internal clock that helps dictate the timing of our sleep/wake pattern over the course of a 24-hour period.[39] The circadian rhythm uses environmental input—like light—to appropriately coordinate internal biological rhythms with the external day/night cycle.[40] For humans and most animals, bright light exposure from the sun manages this cycle (fig. 3–33).

Circadian Rhythm
Your internal clock, which uses environmental input (like light) to coordinate biological rhythms with your external environment.

More scientifically, a master circadian clock is located in the brain—specifically the suprachiasmatic nucleus (SCN) of the anterior hypothalamus—which is hard-wired to receptors in the retinas of your eyes.[41] Bright light stimulates these receptors and sends a clear message to your master clock that it is daytime and your body should be alert and awake to engage with your surroundings. Getting bright light first thing in the morning is a powerful way to synchronize your internal rhythm with your external environment.

On the other hand, darkness or a lack of bright light signals that it is night and an appropriate time for your body to prepare for rest, relaxation, and sleep. This daily cycle is linked to a variety of physiological processes like brainwave activity patterns, hormone production, energy management, and cell regeneration. Coordinating your circadian rhythm and sleep drive promotes healthy sleep patterns so you can be well-rested and fully alert when you need to be.

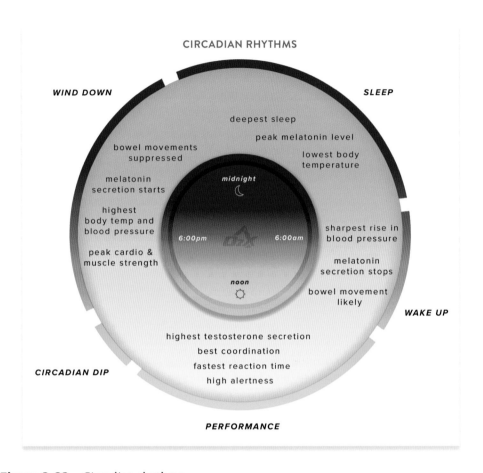

Figure 3–33. Circadian rhythms

Let's take a more in-depth look at how this process works in your body. When it starts to get dark around you and your eyes detect less light, retinal cell receptors transmit a message to your brain's master clock. This prompts the SCN to initiate the process of getting your body ready for sleep. Specifically, the SCN signals to the pineal gland that it is time to start winding down. The pineal gland secretes melatonin, which causes your adrenal glands to slow down and bring your body to a relaxed state as it prepares for sleep.[42]

This process runs smoothly if you are only using light exposure from the sun; however, if you alter your light exposure and begin to see bright, artificial light at night, your master clock can be thrown off its natural schedule. Unfortunately, limiting exposure to only sunlight is difficult to achieve in the modern world where we are surrounded by multiple sources of artificial light that impact our natural sleep/wake cycles and can cause sleep problems.

Exposure to artificial light like phone and computer screens has the same effect as sunlight and tells our body to stay alert and awake even if it is nighttime. Broad spectrum white light, like that from phones and screens, contains many bands of visible light. Research indicates that the short waves of blue light have a more profound effect on your master clock than other bands of light. This is sometimes referred to as "blue light wakefulness." Studies have demonstrated that blue light suppresses melatonin levels and delays the onset of sleep to a greater degree than other bands of light, like orange light, which can actually help promote restfulness.[43]

The prevalence of artificial light in your daily life, particularly at night, can confuse your natural clock and cause a condition—circadian rhythm misalignment. This causes a disconnect between your internal clock and external environment that results in difficulty sleeping. By managing and limiting your exposure to light and creating healthy sleep routines, you can mitigate the possibility of experiencing this disconnect and the related health risks.

As a tactical athlete, you deal with an additional challenge as you do not always have the luxury of a regular schedule where you can sleep all night and work during the daytime. Instead, you may be on a 24-hour shift or working nights. You may sleep all night some nights but not at all on others and there is typically no warning as to when either may occur. As a result, understanding how internal and external processes impact sleep is important and you must use the knowledge to ensure you get adequate rest when you can. The next section will provide tools and tips you can use to incorporate healthy sleep habits into your daily routine so you can maximize the time you have to rest.

Creating Healthy Sleep Habits

Now that you understand how your body signals and prepares itself for sleep, you may have a few questions. How do you know you are getting adequate sleep? How do you create habits to help you improve or maintain healthy sleep patterns?

Here are some signs that you are getting an adequate amount of quality sleep:

1. You fall asleep relatively easily within about 15 minutes of going to bed.
2. Your sleep is uninterrupted or perceived as uninterrupted.
3. Your sleep schedule is "regular," and you fall asleep and wake up at approximately the same time every day (including weekends).
4. Your sleep feels restful and restorative.

If you are not experiencing all of the signs of healthy sleep, there are many different tips and tricks you can use to get your sleep back on track. Figure 3–34 categorizes these tips by mindset, habits, and environmental factors that can help improve your sleep hygiene. Beyond those tips, we will also share information on other strategies—like yoga nidra and napping—that you can incorporate into your routine.

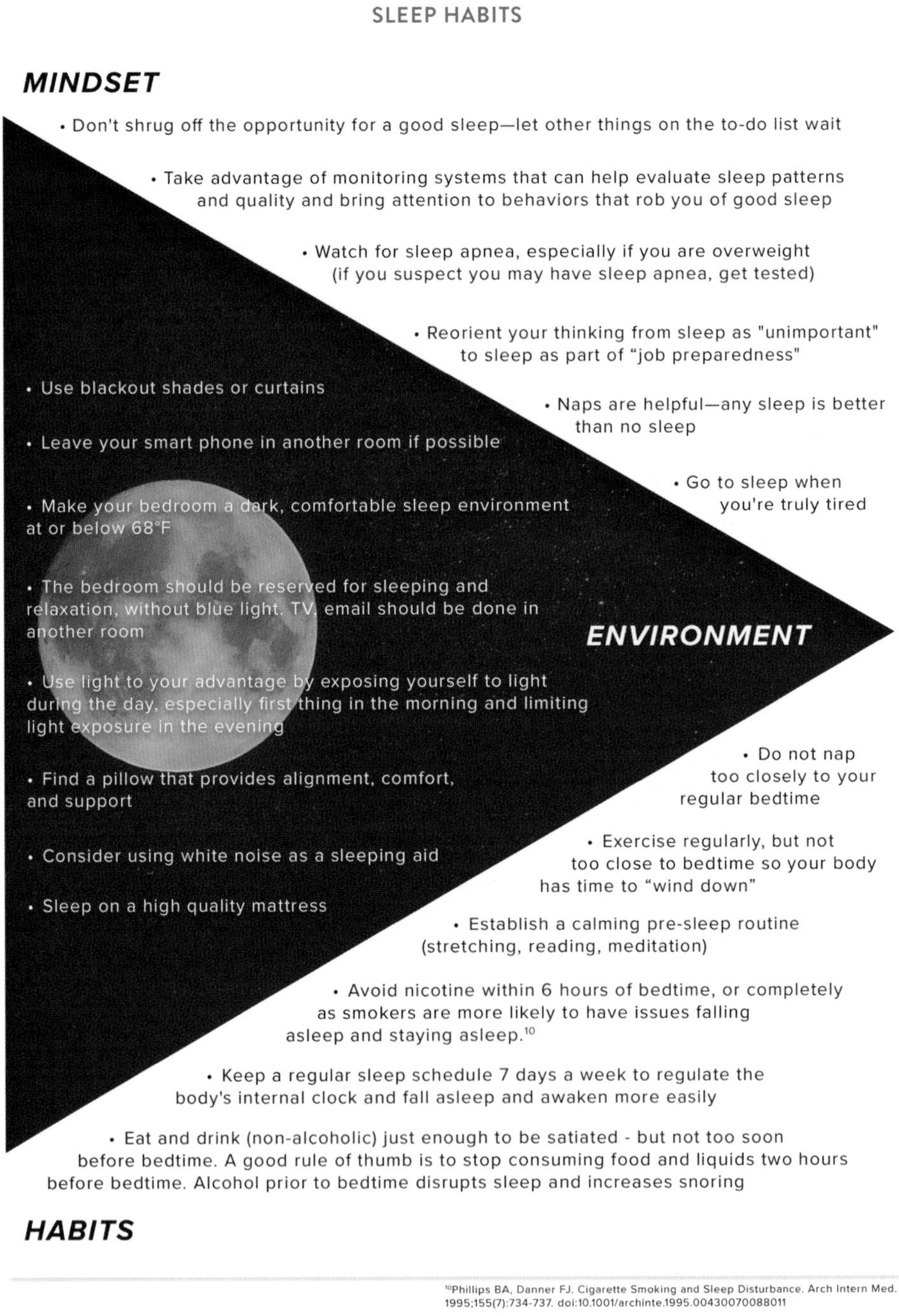

MINDSET

- Don't shrug off the opportunity for a good sleep—let other things on the to-do list wait

- Take advantage of monitoring systems that can help evaluate sleep patterns and quality and bring attention to behaviors that rob you of good sleep

- Watch for sleep apnea, especially if you are overweight (if you suspect you may have sleep apnea, get tested)

- Reorient your thinking from sleep as "unimportant" to sleep as part of "job preparedness"

- Use blackout shades or curtains

- Naps are helpful—any sleep is better than no sleep

- Leave your smart phone in another room if possible

- Go to sleep when you're truly tired

- Make your bedroom a dark, comfortable sleep environment at or below 68°F

- The bedroom should be reserved for sleeping and relaxation, without blue light. TV, email should be done in another room

ENVIRONMENT

- Use light to your advantage by exposing yourself to light during the day, especially first thing in the morning and limiting light exposure in the evening

- Find a pillow that provides alignment, comfort, and support

- Do not nap too closely to your regular bedtime

- Consider using white noise as a sleeping aid

- Exercise regularly, but not too close to bedtime so your body has time to "wind down"

- Sleep on a high quality mattress

- Establish a calming pre-sleep routine (stretching, reading, meditation)

- Avoid nicotine within 6 hours of bedtime, or completely as smokers are more likely to have issues falling asleep and staying asleep.[10]

- Keep a regular sleep schedule 7 days a week to regulate the body's internal clock and fall asleep and awaken more easily

- Eat and drink (non-alcoholic) just enough to be satiated - but not too soon before bedtime. A good rule of thumb is to stop consuming food and liquids two hours before bedtime. Alcohol prior to bedtime disrupts sleep and increases snoring

HABITS

[10]Phillips BA, Danner FJ. Cigarette Smoking and Sleep Disturbance. Arch Intern Med. 1995;155(7):734-737. doi:10.1001/archinte.1995.00430070088011

Figure 3–34. Sleep habits[44]

Yoga nidra

In addition to the tips and tricks shared previously, you may also turn to breathing and mindfulness practices for relaxation. **Yoga nidra** is another tool to use when you need to relax and prepare your body for sleep. Also known as yogic sleep, yoga nidra is a yoga practice specifically designed to elicit complete relaxation. During yoga nidra practice, you are able to focus your attention inward to draw on your inner resources of bodily awareness and breathing. At the same time, you are letting go of distracting thoughts and practicing mindfulness. There are a variety of scripts and meditations for yoga nidra, but what is important is finding the tool that works best for you.

Yoga Nidra Also known as yogic sleep, this is a yoga practice specifically designed to elicit complete relaxation.

YOGA NIDRA—BYRON

I was amazed at how my jaw released. I didn't realize how much I'd tensed it or that I had probably been clenching my jaw for so long, until I came out of the iRest yoga nidra class with Annie Okerlin, an O2X THRIVE specialist. It gave me a really great perspective on how I hold my body and the patterns of movement I have created over time. Aches that I accepted would be with me forever were gone because I finally rested deeply enough to let them go. Instead of my aches making me cranky or irritable, I now feel like I can be kinder to my loved ones because I am no longer uncomfortable or in pain. After years in the Marine Corps, I accepted that pain would be with me for the rest of my life. I'm young with a lot of life to live and now

I know I can do it peacefully. I've been adding 2 to 3 iRests a week and I can really feel the difference. My wife commented that she noticed I don't plop down on the couch anymore and that I seem more gentle in my movements. I can play with my son longer too, although he still tires me out!

I am also starting to see how I am less reactive to daily stressors. Things that used to really send me into flames can still happen, but I feel like I have the choice now to be reactive or responsive. That is teaching me to be a better human, which is something that will help everyone around me.

—*Byron, 29, US Marine Corps (Ret.)*

How to use napping

Napping is another great way to hit the reset button and fill up your tank. Going back to the concept of your sleep drive, taking a nap can help you lower your sleep drive as you replace some of the fuel in your sleep tank. This can be particularly beneficial if you have a night of bad sleep where you were not able to fully refuel your tank. But when you nap, it is important not to sleep too much; otherwise you run the risk of excessively decreasing your sleep drive, which will leave you less tired at night when you want go to sleep.

As a general rule, naps should not be more than 120 minutes and should not take place too late in the day—or too close to your natural bedtime. If you would like to increase alertness and boost creativity, a short nap between 10 and 30 minutes is usually sufficient if you had adequate sleep during the previous night. To replenish your focus, reasoning, and problem solving—or to increase creativity—a longer nap between 30 and 90 minutes can be beneficial. To prepare for a hard workout after work or to cope with a substantial sleep loss from the prior night, a longer nap of 90 minutes can improve your performance. As you try napping, take note of how you feel when you wake up. If you wake up too groggy, try shortening your nap so you do not reach your deeper stages of sleep, or extend your nap to 90 minutes so you complete a full sleep cycle (90 minutes is the average length of a full cycle).[45] To summarize, the ideal length of a nap varies based on the time you have available and the purpose of the nap.

As a tactical athlete, you may be required to work night shifts or rotating shifts that alter your pattern of light exposure and can lead to chronic circadian misalignment. Similarly, traveling frequently can disrupt regular sleep, as can unresolved stressors that cause our minds to race, poor nutrition, and constant stimulation from external light sources. Despite all of these factors that have the potential to interfere with our natural physiology, the greatest thing that can impact sleep is not making it a priority. Sleep is a function of job preparedness and should be viewed as such. Just like being physically fit, hydrated, and tactically proficient, being well rested is a requirement for effective performance. Naps are a helpful tool to use when you want to take control and prioritize sleep so you can maximize your performance.

Overcoming jet lag

As we alluded previously, frequent travel can impact sleep patterns. This is particularly true when you cross multiple time zones and are forced to quickly readjust your internal clock. The internal clock is capable of adjusting to about one time change per day. As the master clock scrambles to adjust and catch up to a new time, our biological processes are disrupted and we experience what is commonly known as "jet lag." Symptoms of jet lag include fatigue, excessive sleepiness, disorientation, lightheadedness, loss of appetite, gastrointestinal disturbances, insomnia, and difficulty concentrating. Being able to create habits and routines to limit these symptoms is helpful for anyone traveling regularly.

Before you even begin handling your jet lag, there are ways to prevent some of the physical stress of traveling. The US Olympic Committee published some helpful guidelines to deal with jet lag.[46] First, make sure to drink enough water—think back to our discussion of hydration in the EAT section and make hydrating a priority when you travel. Second, when you are flying get up and move around or stretch at least every two hours to prevent muscle and joint stiffness. Third, again thinking back to the EAT chapter, making sure you have good, quality foods with you will help you stay on track and keep your blood sugar stabilized during long stretches of travel.

There are some easy ways to deal with light jet lag. First, using earplugs and eye masks can help shut out light and noise so you can sleep or nap when needed, particularly on the plane. Second, once you arrive at your destination, brief napping in the new time zone can help improve your alertness and diminish fatigue brought on by jet lag. However, these naps should remain short so that you allow your body to adjust and sleep in the new time zone. Third, it is important to get light exposure during the day time in the new time zone so that your internal clock can adapt to the environmental light/dark cycle of your new location.

Because light is the single most important factor in establishing healthy circadian rhythms and ensuring quality sleep, getting natural light exposure in a new time zone will help your master clock adjust.[47] If it is still daytime when you arrive at your destination, go for a walk outside to get exposure to natural light and cue your internal clock for the new time zone. A more advanced technique is to start adjusting your light exposure and sleep schedule to a new time zone before you start traveling. This will require that you start going to bed and waking up earlier or later than your normal sleep schedule.

For example, if you are traveling from New York to London, you will need to adjust to London's time zone, which is 5 hours ahead of New York. If you normally go to bed at 11:00 p.m. and wake up at 7:00 a.m., you may want to try shifting your sleep schedule by 2 hours before you leave. This would mean going to bed at 9:00 p.m. and waking up at 5:00 a.m. for a few days leading up to your travel date and making sure you get immediate light exposure when you wake up at 5:00 a.m. By doing this, you will have already started getting used to a new time zone so the 5 hour adjustment will be easier to make once you arrive in London. The bottom line here is understanding how travel and time changes can impact your sleep, and the things you can do to help limit the potential for experiencing jet lag.

Tips on making your own healthy sleep habits

As you have seen throughout this discussion, sleep is critical to our overall well-being and job performance. While there are many different things that can prohibit us from getting adequate amounts of high-quality sleep, it is possible to eliminate many minor sleep problems through creating healthy habits. This includes developing a sleep routine, creating a comfortable sleep environment, and maintaining focus on proper nutrition and exercise in our daily lives. Keeping a regular sleep schedule, even on weekends, allows our body to maintain homeostasis and alignment of our sleep drive and circadian rhythm.

Even when life gets in the way and changes our schedule, there are adjustments we can make that can improve sleep dramatically. By following the sleep habits outlined earlier in this chapter and keeping your sleep schedule as consistent as possible, you will be more well rested and ready to tackle anything that comes your way. Adopting healthy sleep habits will help you stay healthy, focused, and better prepared to meet new challenges each day.

SLEEP KEY TAKEAWAYS

◇ Adequate sleep is linked to processes including memory consolidation, tissue repair and regeneration, immune system functioning, and rebalancing neurotransmitter and metabolic systems.

◇ Like nutrition, focusing on the quality, quantity, and timing of sleep is key to ensuring that you get the sleep you need to perform at your best.

◇ The prevalence of artificial light in your daily life, particularly at night, can confuse your natural clock and cause a condition of circadian rhythm misalignment.

CONCLUSION

Mental preparation bears a striking resemblance to physical conditioning. Like going to the gym to increase strength and fitness, mental performance also requires training and dedicated practice to develop mental fortitude so that it is there when you need it. As a tactical athlete, you face stressors that can range from witnessing and experiencing traumatic events to low levels of chronic stress from the daily unpredictability of your job. Understanding the physiological signs and impact of stress and increasing self-awareness about how you handle stressors is critical to learning what mental skills you can develop to mitigate stress, build resilience, and optimize performance.

Whether you have 5 minutes while you brush your teeth or 20 minutes spread throughout the day, there is always time to practice mindfulness. The benefits are undeniable. Making improvements to your mental performance does not require broad, sweeping changes, but it can lead to major lifestyle improvements. Practicing mindfulness exercises and fostering a growth mindset will improve your ability to respond to stress and help you finish your career as strong as you started.

Throughout this chapter, you were introduced to the science behind stress, practical stress management tools, resources and a framework for building resilience, and a deeper understanding of why sleep is a foundational element of human performance. Just as you learned rules for healthy eating habits and for developing a periodized physical conditioning program, you now have the tools and resources to set goals and create an action plan to enhance your mental performance.

CHAPTER QUESTIONS

1. O2X organizes mental performance into what three categories?
2. What is mindfulness?
3. What is the "the zone of optimal functioning"?
4. What role does the parasympathetic nervous system play in response to stress?
5. What role does the sympathetic nervous system play in response to stress?
6. What does heart rate variability help measure?
7. How can low and slow breathing impact your performance?
8. What are three mental performance tools you can use in your daily life?
9. What is resilience and how does it relate to mindset?
10. What are 4 common symptoms of PTSD?
11. What are the key components of effective goal setting?
12. How does sleep impact risk of injury?
13. What are three healthy sleep habits you can incorporate into your daily routine?

CHAPTER NOTES

What are three takeaways from this chapter that you can implement in your everyday life?

1. _____
   _____
   _____
   _____
   _____
   _____

2. _____
   _____
   _____
   _____
   _____
   _____

3. _____
   _____
   _____
   _____
   _____

ADDENDUM

CONCENTRATION GRID

The concentration grid is a mental performance tool that can be used to develop a number of skills including, but not limited to: focus, attention control, and stress management.

There are 100 numbers randomly scattered on this grid (00-99). Your goal is to find as many numbers in consecutive order during the time limit specified. You must find the numbers in order and cannot jump ahead until you've found each number consecutively.

Follow the instructions below:

• Set a timer for 60 seconds
• Think of a number between 00 and 99 in your head
• When you hit start on the timer, find the number you thought of on the grid and continue to find consecutive numbers until your time runs out.
• Count the amount of numbers you found.
• Each time you try the concentration grid, your goal is to improve the amount of numbers you are able to find within the time limit.

If you choose a high number, work your way down by counting backwards. For example, if you choose 98 you will find 97 - 96 - 95, and so on as far down as you can count within the time limit.

65	8	50	31	6	13	66	49	94	95
58	48	78	98	25	89	68	10	42	70
57	52	74	69	91	41	97	76	85	18
44	60	83	39	40	96	47	32	54	75
00	55	29	37	11	90	27	77	38	99
34	23	61	7	4	15	12	59	45	92
80	28	86	26	2	46	3	71	67	17
43	14	20	84	51	9	19	5	62	79
24	35	53	21	88	72	33	22	63	73
93	64	82	87	81	56	1	30	36	16

MINDSET QUIZ

1. Intelligence is something people are born with that can't be changed.

    ○ Strongly Agree   ○ Agree   ○ Disagree   ○ Strongly Disagree

2. No matter how intelligent you are, you can always be more intelligent.

    ○ Strongly Agree   ○ Agree   ○ Disagree   ○ Strongly Disagree

3. You can always substantially change how intelligent you are.

    ○ Strongly Agree   ○ Agree   ○ Disagree   ○ Strongly Disagree

4. You are a certain kind of person, and there is not much that can be done to really change that.

    ○ Strongly Agree   ○ Agree   ○ Disagree   ○ Strongly Disagree

5. You can always change basic things about the kind of person you are.

    ○ Strongly Agree   ○ Agree   ○ Disagree   ○ Strongly Disagree

6. Musical talent can be learned by anyone.

    ○ Strongly Agree   ○ Agree   ○ Disagree   ○ Strongly Disagree

7. Only a few people will be truly good at sports—you have to be "born with it."

    ○ Strongly Agree   ○ Agree   ○ Disagree   ○ Strongly Disagree

8. Math is much easier to learn if you are male or maybe come from a culture who values math.

    ○ Strongly Agree   ○ Agree   ○ Disagree   ○ Strongly Disagree

O2X
HUMAN PERFORMANCE

MINDSET QUIZ

9. The harder you work at something, the better you will be at it.

○ Strongly Agree   ○ Agree   ○ Disagree   ○ Strongly Disagree

10. No matter what kind of person you are, you can always change substantially.

○ Strongly Agree   ○ Agree   ○ Disagree   ○ Strongly Disagree

11. Trying new things is stressful for me and I avoid it.

○ Strongly Agree   ○ Agree   ○ Disagree   ○ Strongly Disagree

12. Some people are good and kind, and some are not—it's not often that people change.

○ Strongly Agree   ○ Agree   ○ Disagree   ○ Strongly Disagree

13. I appreciate when people give me feedback about my performance.

○ Strongly Agree   ○ Agree   ○ Disagree   ○ Strongly Disagree

14. I often get angry when I get negative feedback about my performance.

○ Strongly Agree   ○ Agree   ○ Disagree   ○ Strongly Disagree

15. All human beings are capable of learning.

○ Strongly Agree   ○ Agree   ○ Disagree   ○ Strongly Disagree

16. You can learn new things, but you can't really change how intelligent you are.

○ Strongly Agree   ○ Agree   ○ Disagree   ○ Strongly Disagree

MINDSET QUIZ

17. You can do things differently, but the important parts of who you are can't really be changed.

   ◯ Strongly Agree   ◯ Agree   ◯ Disagree   ◯ Strongly Disagree

18. Human beings are basically good, but sometimes make terrible decisions.

   ◯ Strongly Agree   ◯ Agree   ◯ Disagree   ◯ Strongly Disagree

19. An important reason why I do my work is that I like to learn new things.

   ◯ Strongly Agree   ◯ Agree   ◯ Disagree   ◯ Strongly Disagree

20. Truly smart people do not need to try hard.

   ◯ Strongly Agree   ◯ Agree   ◯ Disagree   ◯ Strongly Disagree

O2X
HUMAN PERFORMANCE

MINDSET QUIZ SCORING

GROWTH QUESTIONS

Strongly Agree = 3   Agree = 2   Disagree = 1   Strongly Disagree = 0

FIXED QUESTIONS

Strongly Agree = 0   Agree = 1   Disagree = 2   Strongly Disagree = 3

1. Fixed	5. Growth	9. Growth	13. Growth	17. Fixed
2. Growth	6. Growth	10. Growth	14. Fixed	18. Growth
3. Growth	7. Fixed	11. Fixed	15. Growth	19. Growth
4. Fixed	8. Fixed	12. Fixed	16. Fixed	20. Fixed

RESULTS

Strong growth mindset	45-60 points
Growth mindset with some fixed ideas	34-44 points
Fixed mindset with some growth ideas	21-33 points
Strong fixed mindset	0-20 points

Adapted from:

McKenzie, K. (2013). Developing a growth mindset: The secret to improving your grades. [PowerPoint slides]. Academic Success Summit Program. East Stroudsburg University, East Stroudsburg, PA. Retrieved from http://www4.esu.edu/academics/enrichment_learning/documents/pdf/developing_growth_mindset.pdf

WHAT WE VALUE AND WHAT WE DO

Take this time to think about what you value in your life and the things you do on a daily basis. Write 3-5 things down for each category and then consider how what we say we value and what we do either align or are different.

1) *What do you value? How do you DO your life presently? Think about what is important to you.*

_____

_____

_____

_____

_____

2) *What aspects of your life would you not want to give up?*

_____

_____

_____

_____

_____

AFTER ACTION REVIEWS

PHASE 0 - PRIOR PREPARATION

PHASE 1 - SHIFT TURN OVER

PHASE 2 - DISPATCH TO ARRIVAL ON SCENE

PHASE 2 (CONTINUED)

PHASE 3 - ON SITE

PHASE 4 - MOVEMENT BACK TO THE HOUSE AND RE-JOCK

DAILY DEBRIEF

1) *What did you do well today?*

_____

_____

_____

_____

_____

2) *What can you improve upon?*

_____

_____

_____

_____

_____

3) *What can do you do 1% better tomorrow?*

_____

_____

_____

_____

_____

What is your 6 month goal?

To lose 6 pounds

What is motivating you to accomplish your goal?

Having more energy and feeling more confident

How motivated are you to accomplish your goal?
1   2   ③   4   5   6   7   8   9   10
Not at all   *Somewhat*   *Extremely*

Less than 10 on the scale? Ask yourself the next round of questions and try again.

Why is the goal you set important to you?

Really about feeling well, not about the weight loss

What activities do you enjoy? How often do you currently get to do these activities?

Hiking, walking, and running. Not much

How would reaching your goal impact your ability to do the activities you enjoy?

They make me feel well in of themselves, therefore they embody something I value both in the activity of them, and their outcomes, and so I am motivated to re-engage with them

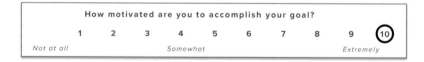

How motivated are you to accomplish your goal?

1   2   3   4   5   6   7   8   9   ⑩

Not at all   *Somewhat*   *Extremely*

What are three things you will do to achieve your goal?

1. Start with "feeling" goals and seeing things as activities that support how I want to feel, not just the outcomes they produce.

2. Dust off my hiking shoes tonight when i get home.

3. Tonight, I will set a time this weekend to go onto my favorite trail.

What is your 6 month goal?

What is motivating you to accomplish your goal?

How motivated are you to accomplish your goal?
1   2   3   4   5   6   7   8   9   10
Not at all   *Somewhat*   *Extremely*

Less than 10 on the scale? Ask yourself the next round of questions and try again.

Why is the goal you set important to you?

What activities do you enjoy? How often do you currently get to do these activities?

How would reaching your goal impact your ability to do the activities you enjoy?

How motivated are you to accomplish your goal?
1   2   3   4   5   6   7   8   9   10
Not at all   *Somewhat*   *Extremely*

What are three things you will do to achieve your goal?

1.

2.

3.

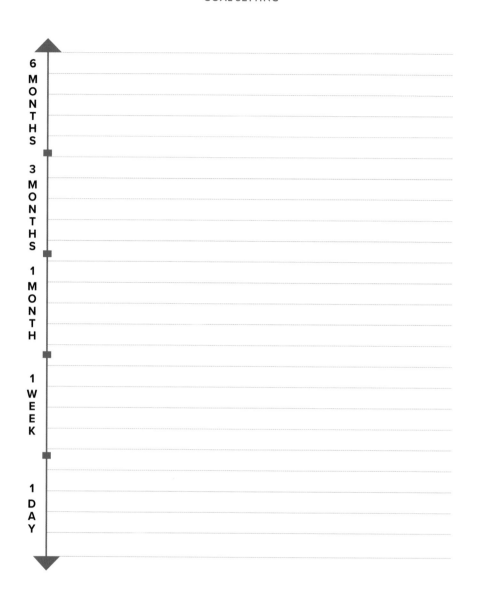

6 MONTHS

3 MONTHS

1 MONTH

1 WEEK

1 DAY

Sleep Rationing

The weight lifting metaphor

- Don't lift more than you can handle
- Start low and build your way up
- Don't increase the level until you have mastered the level you are at
- Once you have mastered your level for 2-3 days, increase by a small amount (30min)

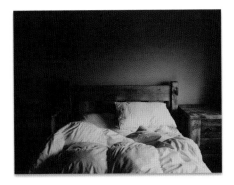

Sleep Efficiency

$$\frac{\text{Time Asleep}}{\text{Time in Bed}} = \text{Sleep Efficiency \%}$$

If you lay in bed for 6 hours, but only get 4.5 hours of steady sleep, what is your sleep efficiency?

If you lay in bed for 8 hours, and get 6 hours of sleep (2 hours at a time, then 40 minutes of tossing and turning), what is your sleep efficiency?

Which scenario is better, and why?

---

* Always consult a medical professional if you are having difficulty sleeping. The recommendations listed here can help you build better sleep routines and habits, but are not a substitute for the guidance of a trained medical professional.

SLEEP PATTERNS

What Dave wants:

- 7 hours of sleep (going to bed at 2300 and waking up at 0600)

What actually happens:

- Dave can't actually fall asleep until 0130. He wakes up feeling very groggy and has even slept through his alarm.

- He takes a 75-minute nap around 1600 because he is very tired.

- He cannot fall asleep until 0130 the following night.

What should Dave do?

Week	In Bed	Asleep	Wake	Total Sleep	New: In Bed	New: Out of Bed	New: Total Sleep Time
1	2300	0130	0600	4.5 hrs	0130	0600	4.5 hrs
2					0100	0600	5 hrs
3					0030	0600	5.5 hrs
4					0030	0600	6 hrs
5					2330	0600	6.5 hrs
6					2300	0600	7 hrs

No Naps!

Phase	Day	In Bed	Out of Bed	Total Sleep Time
1				
2				
3				
4				
5				

HP ON THE ROAD

CHAPTER OBJECTIVES

This chapter provides a comprehensive, practical overview of maximizing your performance while on the road. You will learn a number of key takeaways, including:

- How to utilize the 80:20 rule for ideal nutrition
- How to stay on schedule while travelling
- What to pack and to look for on the road
- What workouts can be completed from anywhere
- How to be a healthier when flying

MAINTENANCE AND ADAPTATION

If you've reached this point in the book, ideally you have mastered a certain pattern that works for you. You may have stocked your pantry with the nutrient-rich foods you need to thrive and have found a few restaurants within walking distance where you can eat out without sacrificing your new commitment to your health. However, as any athlete or special operations soldier will tell you, the whole game changes when you get on the road. This section will teach you how to use the tools that you have mastered at home, in your comfortable environment, to maintain fitness and nutritious eating when on the road—or just out of your element. *One of the most important concepts for sustainable health and fitness is to have a formula that works for your lifestyle. If you do not, it will be extremely difficult to maintain and you will likely experience repeated setbacks.* A workout regimen is no better than a fad diet if it disappears whenever you work overtime or travel for training.

PILLARS OF GOOD HEALTH ON THE ROAD: EAT SWEAT THRIVE

- Nutrition and Hydration
- Exercise
- Sleep
- Stress Management
- Resilience

Above are the five pillars of performance on the road. They mirror the standards we strive to maintain at home, of course, but each deserves extra focus when you are in a new setting. For example, O2X Specialist Maria Urso says, "Eating healthy does not mean you need to eat 'perfectly.' Perfect is not sustainable, at home or on the road. If you aim to make healthy choices 80% of the time, the choices you make during the other 20% of the time should not derail you or your nutrition and fitness program." This may mean packing your own snacks to avoid overly processed airport food and binging at tourist traps. The same rules apply whether you're at a 2-week conference, weekend tactical training, or stringing together back-to-back shifts—consistency is key. Now what does she mean by not needing to be perfect? For that, we refer to the 80:20 rule.

THE 80:20 RULE

Essential to successful travel is becoming comfortable with the 80:20 rule (fig. 4–2). It dictates that you should approach each of the pillars of performance with the mindset that absolute perfection (100%) is difficult to sustain. For this reason, when you approach each pillar, 80% of the time you should aim for optimal performance, and 20% of the time you should allow yourself to do what comes naturally or whatever is dictated by circumstances outside of your control (work, family, travel, etc.). With time (for those who are adopting new healthy behaviors), that which comes naturally will increasingly contribute to your 80% rather than 20%.

One benefit of the 80:20 rule is that a treat or a bad decision does not mean the day is "ruined." By giving yourself a grace period for about one-fifth of your choices, you can stay on track and not slip into the mentality of throwing in the towel over a small indulgence.

THE 80:20 RULE

**80% of the time, aim for optimal performance.
20% of the time, do what comes naturally.**

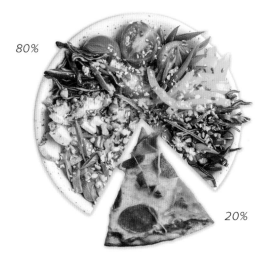

80%

20%

Figure 4–2. The 80:20 rule

Framework of the 80:20 Rule

- Nutrition
  - 80% of the time you should focus on clean eating, while optimizing nutrient intake.
  - 20% of the time you can allow yourself to enjoy the foods and drinks that may not necessarily be classified as nutritious. (Note: "enjoy" does not mean a gluttonous splurge.)
  - 80%: Spinach and grilled chicken salad with sunflower seeds and a vinaigrette.
  - 20%: A large sweet tea.
- Exercise
  - 80% of your exercise should be purposeful and planned, with variation between cardiovascular and strength-focused exercises depending on your personal goals.
  - 20% of your exercise can be unstructured—exercise that may be considered leisurely or play.
  - 80%: Wake up early for 45 minutes of resistance training.
  - 20%: Play an hour of pickup basketball at a local gym or hike to the best view in the area.
- Sleep
  - 80% of the time (or 5–6 nights per week) you should aim for 6–8 hours of uninterrupted sleep. You should aim to go to bed and wake up at the same time 5–6 days per week.
  - 20% of the time (1–2 nights per week), you may have to compromise given the demands of family, work, and travel.
  - 80%: You've set your alarm for a training session, so you turn in by 10:00 p.m.
  - 20%: Stay out past midnight for a birthday dinner and move your workout to the afternoon.
- Stress Management
  - 80% of the time you should follow a pattern of self-care along the lines of your specific needs.
  - 20% of the time feel free to blow off steam in a way that gets your blood pumping.
  - 80%: Track your schedule and set aside time each day for planning and mindfulness.
  - 20%: After a major disappointment, change up plans by canceling a run and throwing in a boxing class.

If you can incorporate the 80:20 rule into your life, you will find that maintaining health and fitness on the road is as simple as you make it.

Once you have the concept, it's time to put it into practice. Use this checklist (fig. 4–3) on the road to keep to the system.

ON THE ROAD CHECKLIST

WEEK BEFORE

☐ Optimize well-being

☐ Make nutrition and exercise accessible

DURING YOUR TRIP

☐ Stick to a plan

☐ Eat clean

☐ Exercise daily

☐ Get at least 6 hours of sleep

☐ Minimize distress and focus on eustress

Figure 4–3. On-the-road checklist

INCORPORATING THE PILLARS

Master your approach to nutrition and exercise on the road by including the following:

1. EAT
   - Stabilize your blood sugar through proper meal planning. Eat breakfast and consume a snack or a meal every 3–4 hours so that you do not feel hungry. Eat until satisfied at every meal or snack.
   - Maintain proper caloric intake. (See nutrition section for what that entails for you and your health and fitness goals.)
   - Consume enough macronutrients to meet your dietary needs. Macronutrients are protein, carbohydrates, and fat. Make sure you are eating complete (animal or complementary plant-based) proteins, complex carbohydrates, and foods that are low in saturated fat and high in omega-3 fatty acids.
   - Adequate hydration will prevent you from feeling hungry, aid digestion, and improve performance. When traveling, you need to be vigilant about staying hydrated since many modes of travel can dehydrate you and water in large quantities may be hard to come by.

2. SWEAT
   - Cardiovascular: On most days of the week, you should aim to complete at least 30 minutes of exercise that increases your heart rate. Your effort should be between a 5 and a 7 on a 1–10 scale (with 1 being "no effort" and 10 being "extremely difficult").
   - Strength: At least 1–2 days per week, you should incorporate resistance training exercises that target each of your major muscle groups (legs, back, chest, abdominals, arms, shoulders). Each exercise should be performed to failure or fatigue.
   - Stretching and Stability: Stretching exercises, whether yoga or range-of-motion exercises, will help you feel more limber. Stability exercises (e.g., planks, balancing, isometric holds) will engage your core and reduce the amount of strain on your lower back. You should aim to spend 5–10 minutes per day stretching and working on your core stability.
   - Unconventional: Although structured exercise is important, learning how to incorporate unstructured exercise (e.g., hiking, walking, playing sports) into your schedule will work wonders when you do not have a gym or structured location nearby. Find activities that you can do anywhere that incorporate various elements of fitness. These can be cardiovascular (e.g., walking, hiking, jumping jacks), strength (e.g., body-weight exercises like wall-sits and burpees), or stretching and stability (e.g., planks, foam rolling).

3. THRIVE
   - Sleep
     ◇ The body needs sleep to repair tissues, restore mental well-being, and manage stress. No human can exist without sleep. Practice good sleep hygiene (more on that later), and aim for 6–8 hours of sleep per night.
   - Stress Management
     ◇ The body and the mind are constantly faced with eustress (good stress) and distress (bad stress), and both of them should be managed for optimal well-being. Eustress is the type of stress that makes the body or the mind adjust to a stimulus and become more resilient. Exercise and brain teasers are examples of things that induce eustress. Deadlines, illness (of yourself or a loved one), or loss will induce variable levels of distress.
     ◇ Learn how to cope with the good and bad stressors in your life. Just like you establish an exercise program, you should establish a stress management program. Identify ways that you can manage your stress. Minimizing distress (or the impact of the distress) will impact the other pillars of your life.

WHY DOES TRAVEL DERAIL US?

- **Nutrition:** You usually prepare your own meals with high-quality foods.
  Travel: There is no kitchen or fridge.
- **Hydration:** You have convenient access to water and are in a routine of staying hydrated.
  Travel: Long flights are dehydrating, and you only get 8 ounces of water the entire flight.
- **Exercise:** You have specific equipment that you use at the gym or at home.
  Travel: You don't have access to your gym or equipment.
- **Exercise:** You run, bike, swim, or walk familiar routes of known distances (that are safe).
  Travel: You have no familiar path to follow.
- **Sleep:** You are used to a certain bedtime and a comfortable room.
  Travel: You sleep at odd hours in different time zones in an unfamiliar room (or plane).
- **Stress:** You have a routine, and most of your life is manageable and predictable
  Travel: Schedules can make or break your day. Missed flights, long lines, delays, traffic, and inconsiderate travelers add stress.

HOW TO PREVENT TRAVEL FROM DERAILING US

- Establish coping skills to reduce the stress that you might encounter and to improve how you respond to the stress that you cannot avoid. For example, take a different mode of transportation to the airport so that you do not have to deal with the additional stress of finding parking or locating your car.
- The thing about traveling is that it does not have to totally derail you. You can choose to be on plan or off plan, but ultimately it is about making a *choice* and making a *plan* (fig. 4–4).
- Depending on whether your trip is for business or leisure, you can decide how you want your trip to look from a health and fitness perspective.
- For each trip you take, you should commit to an approach before you leave. Once you have a mindset for your behavior, you will be much more likely to stick with your plan.

NUTRITION ON THE ROAD

The Necessities

No matter how you approach your trip, it is important that you incorporate the necessities (fig. 4–5). Including these key components will keep your body in a physiological balance, preventing things like dehydration and gastrointestinal issues.

DIFFERENT TYPES OF TRAVEL

	FAMILY/FRIENDS VACATION	WORK TRIP ALONE	WORK TRIP WITH COLLEAGUES	TRAINING TRIP
NUTRITION	Be mindful of the quantities you consume, do not binge because you can.	Best control over your environment. Stick as closely to your nutrition plan as possible.	Less control over restaurant/meal times. Make healthy choices wherever you go. Bring healthy snacks to avoid hunger.	Nutrition is key - what foods MUST you have? Will you purchase at destination or bring? What restaurants/grocers are nearby?
EXERCISE	Exercise when you feel like it; participate in novel activities offered at your destination.	Do your research to optimize your access to exercise equipment or locations. Walk as much as possible.	Try and get up early enough to complete your exercise before you meet for the day.	You will likely be tapering. How will you avoid fatigue but stay active enough for operations?
SLEEP	Aim for 8 hours per night, but be less strict about bedtimes. Wake up without an alarm.	Follow your sleep/wake routine as if you were at home. Be mindful of the time-zone change, if any.	Oftentimes, the least opportunities for sleep. Do the best you can to get adequate sleep before your trip.	Optimize sleep. Stick to a consistent sleep/wake cycle. Get adequate rest when you can before you leave.

Figure 4–4. Different types of travel

NECESSITIES ON THE ROAD

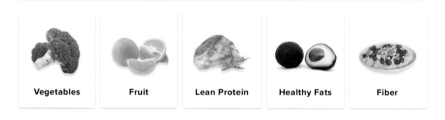

| Vegetables | Fruit | Lean Protein | Healthy Fats | Fiber |

Figure 4–5. Necessities on the road

Avoid "feel bad" foods—the foods that you crave (or that smell good as you walk through the airport or rest stop) but make you feel sick and tired after you eat them. When traveling, it is essential to avoid foods that deplete your energy and deflate your mood (fig. 4–6).

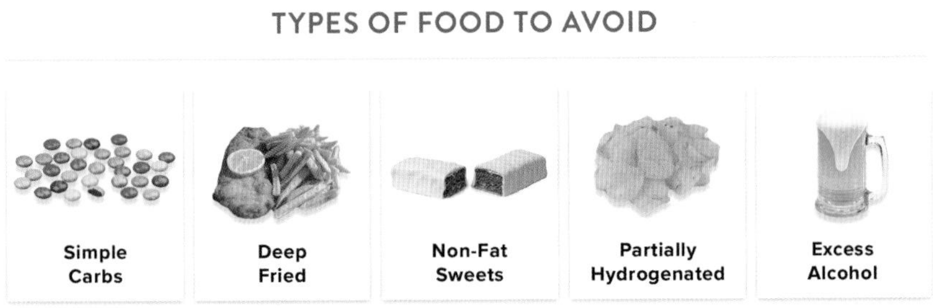

TYPES OF FOOD TO AVOID

| Simple Carbs | Deep Fried | Non-Fat Sweets | Partially Hydrogenated | Excess Alcohol |

Figure 4–6. Types of foods to avoid

Tips and Tricks

Lodging

- Book a hotel that will help you stick to your nutrition plan.
  - Book a hotel with a kitchen or a microwave and refrigerator. If it is unclear on the website whether the rooms have them, call to ask.
  - If a hotel does not have a refrigerator in the room, you can sometimes request one for a small fee. Many hotels have microwaves in the guest common area or the executive lounges.
  - Purchase disposable plastic steam bags. They are good for cooking salmon and vegetables in the microwave.
- Book a hotel that provides a free breakfast each day. Because of the increased emphasis on good nutrition, most buffet-style breakfasts include ingredients for a nutrient-dense meal.
  - *Choose:* hard-boiled eggs, made-to-order omelets, fruit salad, Greek yogurt, oatmeal.
  - *Avoid:* dried fruits, waffles, pastries. They have little nutritional value and many calories, mostly from sugar.
  - *Stock up!* You can store hard-boiled eggs, small boxes of cereal, and whole fruit for later in the day. If you eat a big breakfast, take a little and make it your lunch.
- Scope out restaurants or grocery stores around your destination and then book lodging based on how easily you can access good nutrition and exercise options.

Packing

- Pack plenty of snacks.
  - Sometimes you may get stuck with only the food on your back to support you—have you ever sat on a delayed plane for 2 hours before a 3-hour flight? Pack protein bars and healthy snacks in your bag to prepare. Otherwise, you may get stuck filling up on airline snacks with little nutritional value.
- Pack your supplements.
  - One of the first things in your carry-on bag should be your essential supplements. They are difficult to find on the road and may be more expensive if you need to rely on an airport-based store.
  - If you are a frequent traveler, it might be wise to invest in doubles. Keep a supply in your suitcase and a supply at your house. (This is also a good tip for exercise gear; keep an older pair of running shoes in your suitcase so that you will never be without a pair on the road.)
- When driving to your destination:
  - Pack foods in an inexpensive Styrofoam cooler and bring with you. The cooler is less bulky, inexpensive, and easily replaced at any grocery store.
  - You can load foods into the hotel fridge upon arrival.
  - Restock and refreeze with ice from the hotel ice machine.
  - If you do not have a refrigerator or are staying in a hostel or B&B that does not have one, use the cooler and the ice machine to store food.
- Portable nutrition:
  - Perishable foods that are easy to take on road trips:
    - Raw vegetables
    - Hard-boiled eggs
    - Precooked sweet potatoes
    - Frozen protein shakes
    - Meats (shrimp, chicken, beef that is precut)
    - Single-serving packs of guacamole
    - Slices of raw-milk cheeses, string cheese, or prepackaged cheese
    - Hard fruits (apples, pears, oranges)
  - Nonperishable foods that are easy to take on flights, trains, boats, or road trips:
    - Protein supplements (bars, powder)
    - Jerky/beef sticks
    - Raw nuts and seeds
    - Individual packets of almond butter or coconut butter
    - Individual packets of coconut oil or hemp seeds
    - Wild-caught canned salmon or fresh-water sardines
    - Fruits (apples, bananas, avocados, oranges)

- Pack nutrition that travels well:
  - Canned chicken, canned tuna, canned salmon, tuna pouches, cut veggies, packaged oatmeal, nuts, protein powder, peanut/almond butter, sugar snap peas, and some fruits (oranges, apples, pears).
  - Purchase yogurt and cottage cheese on arrival and keep in fridge.
  - If you know that you cannot refrain from eating an entire box of bars or bag of trail mix, *do not bring them with you.*
- In-flight nutrition:
  - Dry foods and protein bars.
  - Bring a bottle with you so that you can fill it and maintain hydration, or once you are through security at the airport, purchase a large bottle of water for your flight
  - Limit consumption of alcohol on long flights to one or two drinks.
  - Caffeine is OK to drink, but be sure to drink water too and maintain hydration.
  - Fruit juices served in flight are packed with sugars, so stick to tomato juice or water.

Restaurants and eating out

- Research:
  - Find tools and resources to help you keep track of what you eat and the amount of nutrition in each item. Information on foods from fast-food restaurants as well as from popular restaurant chains is available online.
  - Look at the menu online before you get there. Making a decision beforehand can help you skip indulgences and choose the meal with optimal nutrient density.
- Master the buffet:
  - Take a lap before deciding which foods you will have. If you examine all the options and then select your favorites, you will not arrive at the end of the buffet line with an overflowing plate of low-nutrition foods.
  - A good strategy might be to pile most of your plate with vegetables and lean proteins and then go back to add the indulgences. There will be less room for error.
- In the airport or during long layovers:
  - Ideally, eat at a restaurant. Food will be fresh and you can have it made to order.
  - If you do not have time, choose a premade salad with protein (no dressing) or a made-to-order sandwich.
  - Premade sandwiches contain high-fat dressing and bread with little nutritional value.
  - Newsstands carry protein bars and healthy snacks such as fruit and natural meal-replacement bars. (But read the labels and serving sizes.)

- No time for a meal in the terminal? Many flights offer snack packs. Choose one with high-protein snacks. Read labels and avoid foods with low nutritional value.
- Frequent work travel:
  - No matter how conscientious you are, restaurant meals will add extra calories to your diet. If you travel frequently, locate whole food/natural grocery stores in the area. You can easily get a healthy meal from the buffet or build your own salad with little to no extra sauces and dressings. This may be your best option when on the road to eat clean since you will control what is on your plate.
  - Go to the grocer's website and look up store locations so that you can prepare in advance.
- Suggested foods for nutritious eating in restaurants:
  - Omelets
  - Greek yogurt
  - Egg-white breakfast sandwiches
  - Salads with protein (no dressing—try salsa, mustard, cocktail sauce, or lemon juice)
  - *Grilled* meats and seafood (shrimp, chicken, grass-fed beef)
  - *Pan-seared* seafood
  - Vegetable-based dishes (stir-fry, raw platters)
  - "Naked" sandwich, burger, or fish tacos (skip bun and creamy dressing)

EXERCISE ON THE ROAD

The Necessities

When it comes to exercise, many of the necessities revolve around having a plan, being prepared, and knowing your space and time constraints:

- Pack exercise clothing and athletic shoes; do not leave them out of your suitcase because you think you might not have time. Even if you only put on sneakers to walk around the airport when stuck on a long layover or flight delay, you are doing more than if you did not have comfortable shoes.
- Know your surroundings. Sometimes travel derails us because we have a perfect plan in mind of how we will exercise while on the road, but then we arrive and the hotel gym is closed or the hotel is located on a busy interstate. Plan in advance so that you have a realistic idea of your resources (and how you can pack more resourcefully—see below).
- Carve out time. Make physical activity a priority while on the road, even if it is only 20 minutes in the morning before your day starts. The extra energy provided

by a 20-minute walk or a high-intensity hotel-room workout will make a large difference in your health while traveling. You will make wiser food choices and feel better about yourself. Set that alarm a few minutes earlier and make a commitment to yourself that each day you will do *something*. It is much easier to get back into your groove when you get home if you stay somewhat mobile on the road. Remember, an object in motion remains in motion.

- Dress and pack for success. You do not need to take up precious suitcase space with multiple exercise clothes. Bring lightweight things that dry quickly. You can wash them in the hotel sink and hang to dry. Use the laundry bag in the hotel to transport your dirty or wet clothes back home.

- Pack equipment you can use on the go. Minibands, resistance bands, and jump ropes are all portable options you can use anywhere (fig. 4–7).

RESISTANCE BAND WORKOUT

Resistance bands are a great way to maximize your workout while on the road. They are light weight and flexible, and make for a great resistance training option.

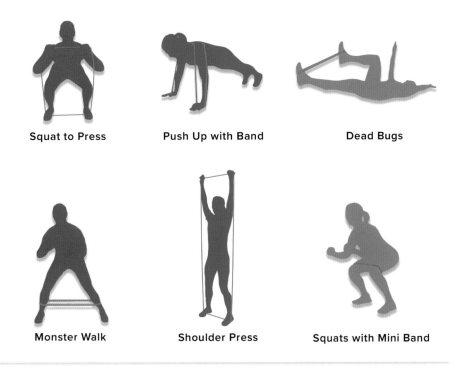

Squat to Press Push Up with Band Dead Bugs

Monster Walk Shoulder Press Squats with Mini Band

Figure 4–7. Resistance band workout

Tips and Tricks

Monitoring

- If you do not already have one, purchase a step counter so that you can keep track of your steps. See if you can come within 75% of your normal step count when you are at home. Seeing your steps increase as you walk through airports, hotels, conference centers, and so on will continue to motivate you.

Lodging

- Book a hotel with a fitness center. Keep in mind that most fitness centers will have one or two treadmills, an elliptical, and maybe a bike. For resistance exercises, it is tough to find weights that are heavier than 50 lbs.
  - Lift anyway. Increase your repetitions and try new exercises.
  - Be prepared to share cardio exercise equipment during peak exercise times (before 8:00 a.m. and after 5:00 p.m.). Try to do 10–15 minutes on different machinery to add variety.
- If you are a runner, ask the front desk for a map of running routes. In major cities and resorts, this is a guaranteed perk.
- Look at a map—are there any parks or bike trails nearby? You can not only get your exercise in, but also have some of the best work-travel experiences from finding a beautiful trail in the mountains or along a river.
- If you are in a congested area, find a shopping center with a large parking lot. Try interval runs or laps in the parking lot.
- If you cannot go outside or use the treadmill in the hotel gym, see below for some alternative exercises and workouts.
- Caution: many hotels will advertise a pool, but many of those pools are too small or shallow for swimming laps. Do not rely on this being your only option. However, it is a good option for a no-impact workout if you choose to swim, tread water, or perform exercises in the water.

Gym membership

- Gyms are everywhere. If you are a frequent traveler, it is worthwhile to find a gym chain that you can access from multiple locations when you are on the road.
- If you are staying at a hotel for a week, you may be able to get a trial membership to a local gym for a small fee. Look for short-term membership or class deals (a great option for those who like indoor-cycling classes, yoga, etc.).

Long-haul flights or international travel

- Use your time in terminals to get extra steps in. You will feel much better after long flights if you stay active between them.
- To avoid deep-vein issues (or swollen feet, a problem in many athletes with low heart rates) purchase compression socks or stockings (15–20 mmHg) to wear on flights. Also, while en route, move your legs as much as you can. Some exercises are ankle rolls, foot flexion, toe stretches, and seated calf-raises.
- If you have time when you arrive at your destination, resist the urge to nap, and instead go for a walk. The sunlight and exercise will help you readjust to the time change. Plus, it is a great way to scope out a new city.
- If you have a long layover, find a local gym or a hotel with a gym for use (do this before you leave). Take the airport shuttle or a cab to the hotel or gym. Pack a change of clothes in your carry-on. You will get the bonus of a shower midtrip after your workout. It is a fantastic refresher, especially if your day started at 3:00 a.m.

Options for exercise

- Walk whenever you can: park your car further from the terminal, avoid the moving walkway and escalators, pace on the plane, walk the terminals, or find a gym or yoga room while on layovers.
- Online before you leave, check local maps and use mobile apps that show running and cycling routes in the areas where you plan to travel. Type your destination into the search field to see routes mapped by locals.
  - If you are a biker, locate a bike shop or outfitter and inquire about renting a bike while in town. You can usually bring your own pedals and shoes.
  - Visit a local running specialty store. Ask about the best local routes. Some running specialty stores offer free group runs.
  - Find a sight-seeing jogging or biking tour. City running or biking tours are a great way to see lots of tourist attractions, meet other runners, and work out at the same time.

Workouts

- Simple: On a short trip with limited time to exercise, make yourself do three or four main exercises per day (fig. 4–8). Keep track of your progress every day on a notepad or digitally. This holds you accountable and motivates you to do more than you planned.
  - Example: 50 push-ups, 1-minute run in place, 50 sit-ups, 50 burpees.
  - Challenge: Increase each exercise by 5–10 reps daily.

WORKOUT ON THE ROAD

On a short trip with limited time to workout, make yourself do 3-4 main exercises per day. Keep track of your progress on a notepad or app.

CHALLENGE = INCREASE 5-10 REPS/SECONDS EACH DAY

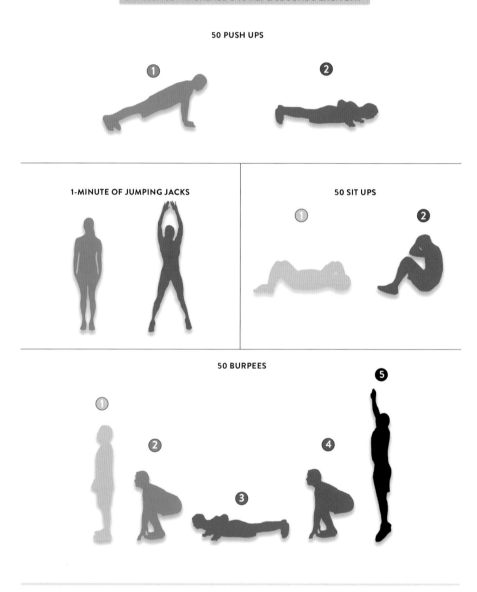

50 PUSH UPS

1-MINUTE OF JUMPING JACKS

50 SIT UPS

50 BURPEES

Figure 4–8. Workout on the road

- More challenging: Turn your hotel room into a circuit (fig. 4–9). You do not need equipment and you will not have to share a small fitness room with other hotel guests.
  - Try to complete it every morning.
  - Increase repetitions by five each day.
  - Forgetting your workout clothes is no excuse to skip exercise.

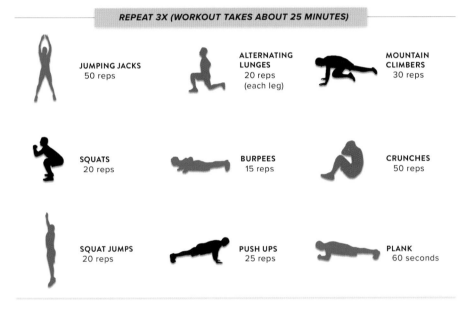

NO NONSENSE CIRCUIT

Turn your hotel room into a circuit. You do not need equipment and you will not have to share a small fitness room with other hotel guests.

1) Try to complete every morning
2) Increase reps by 5 each day
Bonus) Forgetting your workout clothes is no excuse to skip exercising

REPEAT 3X (WORKOUT TAKES ABOUT 25 MINUTES)

JUMPING JACKS
50 reps

ALTERNATING LUNGES
20 reps
(each leg)

MOUNTAIN CLIMBERS
30 reps

SQUATS
20 reps

BURPEES
15 reps

CRUNCHES
50 reps

SQUAT JUMPS
20 reps

PUSH UPS
25 reps

PLANK
60 seconds

Figure 4–9. No-nonsense circuit

- Vacation or long trip challenge: Choose a variety of exercises that incorporate body-weight resistance and cardio intervals.
  - Chart your progress daily.
  - Challenge yourself by increasing the complexity of exercises.
    - Example: Regular push-ups to handstand push-ups.
  - Use local venues to add variety to your workouts.
    - Example: Playground bars for pull-ups, stadiums for stair runs.

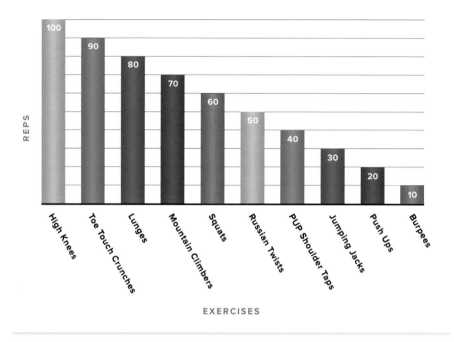

COUNTDOWN WORKOUT

REPS / EXERCISES

High Knees — 100, Toe Touch Crunches — 90, Lunges — 80, Mountain Climbers — 70, Squats — 60, Russian Twists — 50, PUP Shoulder Taps — 40, Jumping Jacks — 30, Push Ups — 20, Burpees — 10

Figure 4–10. Countdown workout

SLEEP ON THE ROAD

The Necessities

All aspects of what you do are impaired when you do not get enough sleep. You will feel irritable and short tempered and will not perform well, from socializing to athletic events.

A few hours of lost sleep combined with travel significantly reduces performance according to a recent study.[1] Travelers perceived themselves as performing at a much higher level than they actually did (a 20% drop).

- Travelers actually performed best during midday, not early morning
- Of those who rated their performance highly, half fell asleep unintentionally on the trip.
- Travelers who exercised during their trip *performed 61% better* than those who did not.
- Study participants registered a total sleep loss of almost 8 hours by the time they returned home, the equivalent of one full night's sleep.

Tips and Tricks

Prepare

- Take the time to prepare for your trip. If you can, take a day off to get things in order before you leave. If you cannot take the time off, try preparing for your trip at least a week earlier than usual.

Manage

- *Jet lag:* Your internal clock prefers to have a longer day rather than a shorter one. For this reason, it is generally harder to adjust to the time change when you are traveling east as opposed to west. Anticipate that you will feel jet lagged and schedule your activities accordingly. Also make an effort to get as much sleep as possible to reduce the effect of jet lag.
- *Naps:* Short bouts of sleep during the day can boost performance.
- *Caffeine:* Use caffeine wisely. Caffeinated beverages will enhance your performance and mood when used strategically. Keep in mind that you may need 100–200 milligrams of caffeine (the equivalent of a 12-ounce cup of coffee or several soft drinks) to get desired results. It takes the stimulant 15–30 minutes to take effect, and it lasts 3–4 hours. Try not to ingest caffeine close to bedtime (3–4 hours) since it will disrupt your sleep. While you may be able to fall asleep, you will not sleep as deep as necessary to feel refreshed.
- *Battle the first-night effect:* If possible, book lodging in areas with familiar noise levels. The National Sleep Foundation recommends using earplugs and eye masks to drown out noise and unwanted light. It is wise to use these on the plane if you are flying overnight.

Recipe for sleep success: Pre-trip

- *Plan ahead:* Pack, finish preparations, confirm flight and hotel information, and secure your boarding pass. Last-minute tasks will delay your pre-trip bedtime and increase stress.
- *Be sleep ready:* Get a sleep kit ready to go and leave it in your toiletry bag. Earplugs and eye covers are extremely helpful on the plane and in the hotel.
- Exercise and eat right the day before your trip
- Be well rested before you start your trip.

Recipe for sleep success: In flight

- *Get comfortable:* Bring your own pillow, earplugs, eye mask, or anything else you may like on the plane. Take off your shoes or loosen the laces to promote optimal circulation.
- *Seating:* A window seat offers you a headrest, and you will not be disturbed by fellow passengers wanting to get out.
- *Nap carefully:* On longer flights, consider waiting until the latter portion of the flight to nap so that you wake feeling refreshed when the flight lands. Napping more than 30–45 minutes can put you in a deep sleep, making you feel more tired when you wake.

Recipe for sleep success: At your destination

- When booking a hotel, ask for a room away from the bar, restaurant, or elevator.
- Check the alarm clock in the room to make sure the alarm is set appropriately.
- Unplug or block any sources of light that are distracting (microwave, nightlight in bathroom, clock illumination). Towels work well under the door.
- Ask for a wake-up call so you do not become preoccupied about missing your alarm.
- Most hotel rooms have light-blocking curtains and controllable thermostats. Be sure that the lighting (as dark as possible) and temperature (66°F–68°F) are ideal for sleeping.

Recipe for sleep success: Bonus tips

- *Time is important on short trips across time zones:* if possible, plan meetings or events using your home time since your body will not have enough time to adjust.
- *Sunshine is critical:* Let as much light into the room as possible when awake and stay active.
- *Give in:* If you are wiped out, take a short nap (10–20 minutes).
- *Reduce caffeine:* Caffeine may stay in your body for up to 14 hours.
- *Alcohol in moderation:* While alcohol may help you fall asleep, as your body clears it from your system, it can cause symptoms that disrupt sleep (e.g., nightmares, sweats, headaches).
- *Exercise:* Exercise can help you sleep. The timing and intensity of exercise plays a key role in its effects on sleep. If you are the type of person who gets energized or becomes more alert after exercise, it may be best to exercise in the morning.
- *Meal planning:* Do not go to bed hungry, but avoid heavy meals before bedtime. Allow at least 3 hours between your final meal and going to sleep.

STRESS MANAGEMENT ON THE ROAD

Managing stress on the road is like the CliffsNotes version of managing stress when you have a steady routine at home; it may just take a little bit more planning and effort to get it done every day. Here are four key components of stress management on the road (they may sound familiar to what you have already read in the main sections of this book):

Control what you can: You have very little control over your fate when you are traveling. Unpredictability could come from airline delays, dealing with mass transportation, crowds, or the potential setback of lost luggage. Reacting to every obstacle or unpredictable setback is not realistic or necessary. If you react to everything that goes wrong or does not go as planned, you will have a consistently elevated blood pressure and heart rate. Instead of reacting, practice mindfulness. Let these moments be a learning experience. Instead, control what you can and deal with everything else as it comes. The things you can control are your attitude and your ability to be kind to anyone who is helping you troubleshoot. Control what you can.

Sweat when you can: We have discussed this in depth throughout the book, but it is always good to remember that exercise releases endorphins that reduce your stress response. Plan to do something that makes you feel relaxed (versus uncomfortable). For example, go for a walk, relax in the hotel pool, take a short hike, or walk around the local shops wherever you are visiting. Travel days can be long, and getting moving when you can will make a big difference in how you feel, physically and mentally.

Find your drive: We talked about finding your drive or visualizing your inner resource earlier in the book—imagining the place where you feel most at peace. When you travel, you can bring things with you that make you feel more comfortable, whether that means wearing comfortable clothes, listening to your favorite music, or bringing food that makes you feel healthy. Having things around you that you appreciate or that remind you of things you love will make you feel more relaxed and at peace. This is the travel version of finding your drive.

Eat well: The importance of proper nutrition has been talked about at length, and is equally important on the road as when you are at home. Foods that are high in omega-3s and B vitamins will help your body manage stress (cortisol levels). Some examples are tuna sandwiches, bananas, fish, dairy, and eggs. And remember the fundamentals of quality, quantity, and timing.

Tips and Tricks

- Be kind. Greet people—from the front-desk clerk to the server at the restaurant. Have a conversation about the area. The combination of pleasantness and interest will put you in a friendly light in that person's mind. They will likely go out of their way to make your travel experience better. Even if they do not, the body reacts to pleasant interactions such as these in a beneficial way.
- It is the body's natural tendency to go into fight-or-flight mode when stressed. Cortisol and adrenaline are produced and both can wreak havoc on our appetites (food cravings), sleep, skin health, and overall physiology. The best ways to manage cortisol and adrenaline are to exercise (even lightly) and enjoy fresh air.
  - Many travelers have long meetings and are stuck indoors with artificial lighting and harsh air-conditioning. Try to incorporate even short walks in the parking lot or outdoors to give your body some exposure to the natural elements.
  - Jet lag is the direct result of chemical imbalances. The body produces less serotonin. Serotonin is important for regulating sleep patterns, appetite, and mood. Be aware of these signals that your body and mind are receiving, and do your best to ignore food cravings or the urge to wallow in a cranky stage. Force yourself to do something (even just listening to music loudly) that will brighten your mood.
- Packing:
  - Packing is stressful! You need to anticipate everything you will need for the next couple of days (or weeks). Make a list of everything you will need—a few days before your trip. You will be able to add things as the date comes closer and pick up things you do not have, rather than having to rush for it at the last minute.
  - Double up. If you are a frequent traveler, it helps to purchase doubles of things such as toiletries and running shoes (or retire an old pair a bit early). Keep your bag halfway packed at all times with your toiletries and running shoes so that you do not forget these essentials.
- Not getting sick:
  - Being cooped up on planes, trains, and automobiles when you are working against a tough sleep, exercise, and nutrition schedule is a surefire recipe to getting sick.
  - Getting plenty of rest and staying hydrated will help you ward off many bugs that come your way. Bring antibacterial wipes and wipe down surfaces that you will be touching (tray tables, phone in hotel room, remote control). Wash your hands at every opportunity you get.

- The inevitable crying child on a long flight:
  - ○ This is stressful for everyone—the kid, the parents, and the travelers. Noise canceling headphones are your best bet to cope when the child cannot be consoled.

SUMMARY

Travel *will not* derail you if you plan properly.

- EAT: You know how to obtain healthy, high-quality foods while on the road.
  - ○ Choose what type of nutrition plan to stick to.
  - ○ Plan ahead to minimize distractions.
  - ○ Stay hydrated throughout your trip.
- SWEAT: Whether in an unfamiliar place or a hotel room, you have the tools to stay active.
  - ○ Decide how much you plan to exercise.
  - ○ Plan how you will make this happen while traveling (when and where).
- THRIVE: Try to sleep at least 6 hours per night.
  - ○ Eliminate things that will keep you awake, and follow good sleep hygiene.
- Practice stress management
  - ○ Be aware of the havoc that travel will induce on chemical signaling in your body.
  - ○ Be more mindful of your behaviors and how you can modify them to minimize stress reactions.

CONCLUSION

By now, you have read about the science behind nutrition, conditioning, and mental performance and how each one plays a role in your work as a tactical athlete. Something we alluded to throughout every chapter is that each pillar is one small part of the whole system. In order to maximize performance, you need to improve each. Without proper nutrition, you will not have the energy you need to train and build strength; and without the physical preparation, you will lack the confidence and skill sets you need to be mentally ready for every call.

While each chapter targets a different component of performance, there are common themes that run through each section. First, whether you are improving your diet, increasing your fitness level, or honing your mental skills, focus on what you can do to make reasonable, incremental improvements. Second, as a tactical athlete you must gear all parts of your training toward job-specific performance and not general fitness. Finally, everything comes back to balance—whether it's planning your meals to ensure you maintain blood sugar stabilization, building a conditioning plan that pairs adequate stress with sufficient recovery, or using mental performance techniques to calm your nerves. Our bodies have evolved to handle stress and return to homeostasis, but as a tactical athlete, you need the resources and skills to face adversity and adapt to extreme levels of job-related mental and physical stress.

Starting with nutrition, by focusing on eating high-quality foods in the proper quantity at the right time throughout the day, you will be fueled to face any challenge. By stabilizing your blood sugar through healthy eating habits, you are less likely to experience spikes and crashes that come with energy imbalances. A balanced diet focused on quality, quantity, and timing will ensure that you are energized and ready to answer any call.

With the proper fuel, you are able to maximize the work you do in your physical training. As a tactical athlete, you have no off-season to focus on preparation and no single event to work toward. Instead, every day could be game day and you must train for performance so that your strength is there when you need it most. This requires a systematic review of your individual and job-related needs and a program focused on building and maintaining energy and strength systems over time. Creating periodized training plans allows you to balance physical conditioning with proper recovery so that you minimize the risk of overtraining and potential for injury, while getting stronger so you are ready when you need to be.

Physical fitness and proper nutrition must be paired with a focus on mental performance. Tactical athletes must understand and recognize the mental stressors that accompany the job. Having this awareness and knowing how to tap into stress-management skills like breathing, mindfulness, and relaxation is key to resetting and building resilience after experiencing any type of stressor.

The final component that impacts every part of performance is sleep. Without enough sleep, our diets suffer, our minds lack clarity, and our bodies lack the ability to fully recover from the daily demands placed on us. Sleep brings our minds and bodies back into balance and provides us a fresh start each day. Sleep is a natural reset button that we must hit in order to maximize performance.

While there are volumes of information and science behind each pillar of the O2X EAT SWEAT THRIVE methodology, what we have provided in this book are the tools to build a strong foundation of mental and physical readiness. Our goal throughout this has not been to simply give you a play-by-play or cookie-cutter formula of exactly what to eat, how to work out, and what to think. Instead, we hope you have learned not just what and how to do it, but also why you need to focus on all pillars of performance as principles to help guide your decisions. This will help keep you accountable in the long run so that the small changes you make become long-term, sustainable lifestyle improvements.

Now that you have the science-backed education and the tools you need to implement incremental changes in your daily life, you are ready to maximize your performance and *finish your career as strong as you started!*

Remember: You have no offseason. What are you waiting for?

NOTES

Chapter 1: EAT

1. Cermak NM, van Loon LJ. The use of carbohydrates during exercise as an ergogenic aid. *Sports Med.* 2013 Nov;43(11):1139–55.

2. Effect of low- and high-glycemic-index meals on metabolism and performance during high-intensity, intermittent exercise. *Int J Sport Nutr Exerc Metab.* 2010 Dec;20(6):447–56.

3. Engin A. Eat and death: Chronic over-eating. *Adv Exp Med Biol.* 2017;960:53–80.

4. Hall KD. Computational model of in vivo human energy metabolism during semistarvation and refeeding. *Am J Physiol Endocrinol Metab.* 2006 Jul;291(1):E23–37. https://www.mayoclinic.org/healthy-lifestyle/nutrition-and-healthy-eating/multimedia/functions-of-water-in-the-body/img-20005799

5. Shirreffs SM, Sawka MN. Fluid and electrolyte needs for training, competition, and recovery. *J Sports Sci.* 2011;29 Suppl 1:S39–46.

6. Edmonds, C. J. Water, hydration status and cognitive performance. *Nutrition and Mental Performance.* 2012:193–211. doi:10.1007/978-1-137-00689-9_11

7. Irwin C, Leveritt M, Shum D, Desbrow B. The effects of dehydration, moderate alcohol consumption, and rehydration on cognitive functions. *Alcohol.* 2013 May;47(3):203–13.

8. Alcohol metabolism. *Clin Liver Dis.* 2012; 16(4):667–85

9. Brosnan JT. Interogran amino acid transport and its regulation. *The Journal of Nutrition.* 2002 June 1;133(6):2068S–2072S.

10. Voet D, Voet JG. (2004) *Biochemistry vol 1,* 3rd Ed. Wiley: Hoboken, NJ. https://publications.nigms.nih.gov/insidelifescience/fats_do.html

11. Bier DM, Brosnan JT, Flatt JP, et al. Report of the IDECG Working Group on lower and upper limits of carbohydrate and fat intake. *Eur J Clin Nutr.* 1999;53(suppl):S177–78.

12. Shirreffs SM, Sawka MN. Fluid and electrolyte needs for training, competition, and recovery. *J Sports Sci.* 2011;29 Suppl 1:S39–46. https://www.ncbi.nlm.nih.gov/pmc/articles/PMC4153275/

13. *Guideline: Sugars intake for adults and children.* Geneva: World Health Organization; 2015.

14. American Diabetes Association. "Statistics about diabetes." 12 Apr 2017. http://www.diabetes.org/diabetes-basics/statistics/

15. Levin RJ. Digestion and absorption of carbohydrates—from molecules and membranes to humans. *Am J Clin Nutr.* 1994;59:690S–698S.

16. Sacks FM, Bray GA, Carey VJ, et al. Comparison of weight-loss diets with different compositions of fat, protein, and carbohydrates. *N Engl J Med.* 2009 Feb 26;360(9):859–73.

17. Leonard WR, Snodgrass JJ, Robertson ML. Evolutionary perspectives on fat ingestion and metabolism in humans. In JP Montmayeur, J le Coutre (Eds.), *Fat detection: Taste, texture, and post ingestive effects.* Boca Raton (FL): CRC Press/Taylor & Francis; 2010. Chapter 1. Available from: https://www.ncbi.nlm.nih.gov/books/NBK53561/

18. Mozaffarian D, Katan, MB, Ascherio A, Stampfer MJ, Willett WC. Trans fatty acids and cardiovascular disease. N Engl J Med. 2006;354(15):1601–13.

19. Di Pasquale MG. The essentials of essential fatty acids. *J Diet Suppl.* 2009;6(2):143–61.

20. Dhaka V, Gulia N, Ahlawat KS, Khatkar BS. Trans fats-sources, health risks and alternative approach—A review. *J Food Sci Technol.* 2011;48(5):534–41.

21. Weylandt KH, Serini S, Chen YQ, et al. Omega-3 polyunsaturated fatty acids: The way forward in times of mixed evidence. *Biomed Res Int.* 2015;2015:143109.

22. Castelli WP, Garrison RJ, Wilson PWF, Abbott RD, Kalousdian S, Kannel WB. Incidence of coronary heart disease and lipoprotein cholesterol levels. The Framingham Study. *JAMA.* 1986;256(20):2835–38.

23. Shenkin A. The key role of micronutrients. *Clin Nutr.* 2006 Feb;25(1):1–13.

24. McRae MP. Health benefits of dietary whole grains: An umbrella review of meta-analyses. *J Chiropr Med.* 2017 Mar;16(1):10–18.

25. Ganesan K, Habboush Y, Sultan S. Intermittent fasting: The choice for a healthier lifestyle. *Cureus.* 2018 Jul 9;10(7).

26. An Increase in the omega-6/omega-3 fatty acid ratio increases the risk for obesity. *Nutrients.* 2016;8(3):128.

27. Ivy, JL. Muscle glycogen synthesis before and after exercise. *Sports Med.* 1991 Jan;11(1):6–19.

28. Kerksick CM, Arent S, Schoenfeld BJ, et al. International society of sports nutrition position stand: nutrient timing. *J Int Soc Sports Nutr.* 2017;14:33.

29. Witard OC, Wardle SL, Macnaughton LS, Hodgson AB, Tipton KD. Protein considerations for optimising skeletal muscle mass in healthy young and older adults. *Nutrients.* 2016;8(4):181. doi:10.3390/nu8040181.

30. Kerksick CM, Arent S, Schoenfeld BJ, et al. International society of sports nutrition position stand: nutrient timing. *J Int Soc Sports Nutr.* 2017;14:33.

31. Kerksick CM, Wilborn CD, Roberts MD, et al. ISSN exercise & sports nutrition review update: Research & recommendations. *J Int Soc Sports Nutr.* 2018;15(1):38.

32. Tucker J, Fischer T, Upjohn L, Mazzera D, Kumar M. Unapproved pharmaceutical ingredients included in dietary supplements associated with US Food and Drug Administration warnings. *JAMA Network Open.* 2018;1(6):e183337.

33. Spriet LL. Exercise and sport performance with low doses of caffeine. *Sports Med (Auckland, NZ).* 2014;44(Suppl 2):175–84. doi:10.1007/s40279-014-0257-8

34. Goldstein ER, Ziegenfuss T, Kalman D, et al. International Society of Sports Nutrition position stand: Caffeine and performance. *J Int Soc Sports Nutr.* 2010 Jan 27;7(1):5.

35. Kerksick CM, Arent S, Schoenfeld BJ, et al. International Society of Sports Nutrition position stand: Nutrient timing. *J Int Soc Sports Nutr.* 2017 Aug 29;14:33.

36. http://www.who.int/news-room/fact-sheets/detail/diabetes

37. Gonzalez de Mejia E, Ramirez-Mares MV. Impact of caffeine and coffee on our health. *Trends Endocrinol Metab.* 2014 Oct;25(10):489–92.

Chapter 2: SWEAT

1. *Mosby's Medical Dictionary*, 9th ed. (St. Louis, MO: Mosby Elsevier, 2013).

2. Haff G and Triplett NT, *Essentials of Strength Training and Conditioning*, 4th ed. (Champaign, IL: Human Kinetics, 2016), 562.

3. Haff and Triplett, *Essentials of Strength Training*.

4. Vorup J, Tybirk J, Gunnarsson TP, Ravnholt T, Dalsgaard S, and Bangsbo J, "Effect of Speed, Endurance, and Strength Training on Performance, Running Economy and Muscular Adaptations in Endurance-Trained Runners," *European Journal of Applied Physiology* 116, no. 7 (July 2016): 1331–41.

5. Silverman GM, *Your Miraculous Back* (Oakland, CA: New Harbinger, 2006).

6. Haff and Triplett, *Essentials of Strength Training*.

7. Nindl BC, Williams TJ, Deuster PA, Butler NL, and Jones BH, "Strategies for Optimizing Military Physical Readiness and Preventing Musculoskeletal Injuries in the 21st Century," *U.S. Army Medical Department Journal* (October–December 2013): 5–23.

8. Parker KN and Ragsdale JM, "Effects of Distress and Eustress on Changes in Fatigue from Waking to Working," *Applied Psychology: Health and Well-Being* 7, no. 3 (November 2015): 293–315.

9. Figure 2.10 adapted from Angie Herbers, "Stress for Success Part 1," *ThinkAdvisor*, July 24, 2012, http://www.thinkadvisor.com/2012/07/24/stress-for-success-pt-1-how-to-handle-the-stress-o.

10. Chris Sherwood, "The Effect of Exercise on Homeostasis," *Livestrong*, September 11, 2017, http://www.livestrong.com/article/480961-the-effect-of-exercise-on-homeostasis/.

11. We want to point out that although Selye's GAS findings have long been applied as a basis of conditioning and resistance training, researchers have recently questioned whether there may be a more appropriate basis. Buckner SL et al., "The General Adaptation Syndrome: Potential Misapplications to Resistance Exercise," *Journal of Science in Medicine and Sport* 20, no. 11 (November 2017): 1015–17. This recent question challenges the application of Selye's finding, but it does not negate the fact that adaptation is a fundamental concept within, and a requirement for, strength and conditioning gains.

12. Søgaard K and Sjøgaard G, "Physical Activity as Cause and Cure of Muscular Pain: Evidence of Underlying Mechanisms," *Exercise and Sport Sciences Reviews* 45, no. 3 (July 2017): 136–45.

13. Hyldahl RD and Hubal MJ, "Lengthening our Perspective: Morphological, Cellular, and Molecular Responses to Eccentric Exercise," *Muscle & Nerve* 49, no. 2 (February 2014): 155–70.

14. Vieira A, Siqueira AF, Ferreira-Junior JB, do Carmo J, Durigan JL, Blazevich A, and Bottaro M, "The Effect of Water Temperature during Cold-Water Immersion on Recovery from Exercise-Induced Muscle Damage," *International Journal of Sports Medicine* 37, no. 12 (November 2016): 937–43.

15. Marqués-Jiménez D, Calleja-González J, Arratibel I, Delextrat A, and Terrados N, "Are Compression Garments Effective for the Recovery of Exercise-Induced Muscle Damage? A Systematic Review with Meta-analysis," *Physiology & Behavior* 153 (January 2016): 133–48.

16. Pearcey GE, Bradbury-Squires DJ, Kawamoto JE, Drinkwater EJ, Behm DG, and Button DC, "Foam Rolling for Delayed-Onset Muscle Soreness and Recovery of Dynamic Performance Measures," *Journal of Athletic Training* 50, no. 1 (January 2015): 5–13.

17. Issurin, VB "New Horizons for the Methodology and Physiology of Training Periodization," *Sports Medicine* 40, no. 3 (March 2010): 189–206. https://doi.org/10.2165/11319770-000000000-00000.

18. Haff and Triplett, *Essentials of Strength Training*, 584–604.

19. This whole concept and the associated chart: 2012 NSCA, Adapted from Landers J, "Maximum Based On Reps," *NSCA Journal* 6, no. 6 (1984): 60–61.

20. Fournier-Farley C, Lamontagne M, Gendron P, and Gagnon DH, "Determinants of Return to Play After the Nonoperative Management of Hamstring Injuries in Athletes: A Systematic Review," *American Journal of Sports Medicine* 44, no. 8 (August 2016): 2166–72.

21. Périard JD, Travers GJ, Racinais S, and Sawka MN, "Cardiovascular Adaptations Supporting Human Exercise-Heat Acclimation," *Autonomic Neuroscience* 196 (2016): 52–62.

22. National Institute of Arthritis and Musculoskeletal and Skin Diseases, *What Are Sports Injuries?* Fast Facts series (Bethesda, MD: National Institute of Health, 2014).

23. *Mosby's Medical Dictionary*, 9th ed. (St. Louis, MO: Mosby Elsevier, 2013).

24. Peerdeman KJ, van Laarhoven AI, Peters ML, and Evers AW, "An Integrative Review of the Influence of Expectancies on Pain," *Frontiers in Psychology*, no. 7 (August 2016): 1270. https://www.ncbi.nlm.nih.gov/pmc/articles/PMC4993782/

25. Chinn L and Hertel J, "Rehabilitation of Ankle and Foot Injuries," *Clinical Sports Medicine* 29, no. 1 (2010): 157–67.

26. Wardle SL and Greeves JP. "Mitigating the Risk of Musculoskeletal Injury: A Systematic Review of the Most Effective Injury Prevention Strategies for Military Personnel," *Journal of Science and Medicine in Sport* 20, suppl. 4 (November 2017): S3–S10

27. Ditmyer MM, Topp R, and Pifer M, "Prehabilitation in Preparation for Orthopaedic Surgery," *Orthopedic Nursing* 21, no. 5 (2002): 43–51; Levett DZ and Grocott MP, "Cardiopulmonary Exercise Testing, Prehabilitation, and Enhanced Recovery After Surgery (ERAS)," *Canadian Journal of Anaesthesia* 62, no. 2 (2015): 131–42.

28. Simic L, Sarabon N, and Markovic G, "Does Pre-exercise Static Stretching Inhibit Maximal Muscular Performance? A Meta-analytical Review," *Scandinavian Journal of Medicine and Science in Sports* 23, no. 2 (2013): 131–48.

29. Postolopoulos N, Metsios GS, Flouris AD, Koutedakis Y, and Wyon MA, "The Relevance of Stretch Intensity and Position: A Systematic Review," *Frontiers in Psychology* 18, no. 6 (August 2015): 1128.

30. Wardle and Greeves, "Mitigating the Risk of Musculoskeletal Injury."

31. Page P, "Current Concepts in Muscle Stretching for Exercise and Rehabilitation," *International Journal of Sports Physical Therapy* 7, no. 1 (2012): 109–19.

32. Haff and Triplett, *Essentials of Strength Training*.

33. Haff and Triplett.

34. Ditmyer, Topp, and Pifer, "Prehabilitation in Preparation for Orthopaedic Surgery."

35. Haff and Triplett, *Essentials of Strength Training*, 93.

36. Haff and Triplett, *Essentials of Strength Training*, 562.

Chapter 3: THRIVE

1. Cohen, S., & Janicki-Deverts, D. (2012). Who's Stressed? Distributions of Psychological Stress in the United States in Probability Samples from 1983, 2006, and 2009. *Journal of Applied Social Psychology*, 42(6): 1320–34.

2. M. Csikszentmihaly, *Flow: The Psychology of Optimal Experience* (New York: Harper and Row, 1990). Jackson, S. A., Thomas, P. R., Marsh, H. W., & Smethurst, C. J. (2001). Relationships between Flow, Self-Concept, Psychological Skills, and Performance. *Journal of Applied Sport Psychology*, 13, 129–153

3. Kamata, A., Tenenbaum, G., & Hanin, Y. L. (2002). Individual Zone of Optimal Functioning (IZOF): A Probabilistic Estimation. *Journal of Sport & Exercise Psychology*, 24, 189–208.

4. American Psychological Association. (2018). Listening to the Warning Signs of Stress. Retrieved October 23, 2018, from American Psychological Association: https://www.apa.org/helpcenter/stress-signs.aspx.

5. McCorry, L. K. (2007). Physiology of the Autonomic Nervous System. *American Journal of Pharmaceutical Education*, 71 (4), 78.

6. McCorry, L. K. (2007). Physiology of the Autonomic Nervous System.

7. Young, H. A., & Benton, D. (2018). Heart-Rate Variability: A Biomarker to Study the Influence of Nutrition on Physiological and Psychological Health? *Behavioral Pharmacology*, 29 (2), 140–151.

8. Young, H. A. & Benton, D. (2018). Heart-rate Variability.

9. Thayer, Yamamoto, & Brosschot, 2009

10. Reardon, M., & Malik, M. (1996). Changes in Heart Rate Variability with Age. *Pacing Clin Electrophysiol.*, 11 (Pt 2), 1863–66.

11. Jon Kabat-Zinn, *Wherever You Go, There You Are* (New York: Hachette Books, 2005), 4.

12. J. Darwin & A. Melling, *Mindfulness and Situation Awareness* (United Kingdom: Sheffield Hallam University, 2011). N. Karelaia & J. Reb, Improving Decision Making through Mindfulness. In *Mindfulness in Organizations: Foundations, research, and applications* (Singapore: Research Collection Lee Kong Chian School of Business, 2015), 163–89.

13. Fraher, A. L., Branicki, L. J., & Grint, K. (2017). Mindfulness in Action: Discovering How U.S. Navy SEALs Build Capacity for Mindfulness in High-Reliability Organizations (HROs). *Academy of Management Discoveries*, 3 (3), 239–61.

14. Bernardi, L. Sleight, P., Bandinelli, G., Cencetti, S., Fattorini, L., Wdowczyc-Szulc, J., & Lagi, A. (2001). Effect of Rosary Prayer and Yoga Mantras on Autonomic Cardiovascular Rhythms: Comparative Study. *BMJ*, 323 (7327), 1446–49.

15. Gilbert, C. (2005). Better Chemistry through Breathing: The Story of Carbon Dioxide and How It Can Go Wrong. *Biofeedback*, 33 (3), 100–104.

16. Jean Marie Williams, *Applied Sport Psychology: Personal Growth to Peak Performance* (New York: McGraw-Hill, 2010).

17. Williams, *Applied Sport Psychology*.

18. Williams, *Applied Sport Psychology*.

19. Sian Beilock, *Choke* (London: Constable, 2010).

20. Grant, A. M., & Gino F. (2010). A Little Thanks Goes a Long Way: Explaining Why Gratitude Expressions Motivate Prosocial Behavior. *Journal of Personality and Social Psychology*, 98 (6), 946–55.

21. "PTSD Statistics," PTSD United, accessed March 29, 2017, http://www.ptsdunited. org/ptsd-statistics-2/.

22. "PTSD Statistics," PTSD United.

23. "Symptoms of PTSD," US Department of Veterans Affairs, last modified August 13, 2015, https://www.ptsd.va.gov/public/PTSD-overview/basics/symptoms_ of_ptsd.asp.

24. Carol S. Dweck, *Mindset* (London: Robinson, 2006).

25. Dweck, *Mindset*.

26. Niemiec, C. P., & Ryan, R. M. (2009). Autonomy, Competence, and Relatedness in the Classroom: Applying Self-Determination Theory to Educational Practice. *Theory and Research in Education*, 7 (2), 133–44.

27. Niemiec & Ryan. (2009). Autonomy, Competence, and Relatedness in the Classroom.

28. Niemiec & Ryan.

29. Shahin, A., & Mahbod, M. A. (2007). Prioritization of Key Performance Indicators: An Integration of Analytical Hierarchy Process and Goal Setting. *International Journal of Productivity and Performance Management*, 56 (3), 226–240.

30. Ahmed, M., Arora, S., Russ, S., Darzi, A., Vincent, C., & Sevdalis, N. (2013). Operation Debrief: A SHARP Improvement in Performance Feedback in the Operating Room. *Annals of Surgery* , 258 (6), 958–63.

31. Luyster, F. S., Strollo, P. J., Zee, P. C., & Walsh, J. K. (2012). Sleep: A Health Imperative. *Sleep*, 35 (6), 727–34. Milewski, M., Skaggs, D., Bishop, G., Pace, J., Ibrahim, D., Wren, T., et al. (2014). Chronic Lack of Sleep is Associated with Increased Sports Injuries in Adolescent Athletes. *Journal of Pedriatric Orthopedics*, 34 (2), 129–33.

32. Hirshkowitz, M., Whiton, K., Albert, S., Alessi, C., Bruni, O., DonCarlos, L., et al. (2015). National Sleep Foundation's Updated Sleep Duration Recommendations: Final Report. *Sleep Health: Journal of the National Sleep Foundation*, 1 (4), 233–43.

33. Barger et al., Harvard Work Hours, Health and Safety Group (2015).

34. Drummond et al. (2005). The Neural Basis of the Psychomotor Vigilance Task. *Sleep,* 9 (28), 1059–68.

35. Van Dongen, H., Maislin, G., Mullington, J. M., & Dinges, D. F. (2003). The Cumulative Cost of Additional Wakefulness: Dose-Response Effects on Neurobehavioral Functions and Sleep Physiology from Chronic Sleep Restriction and Total Sleep Deprivation. *Sleep*, 2 (26), 117–26.

36. Åkerstedt, T., & Wright, K. P. (2009). Sleep Loss and Fatigue in Shift Work and Shift Work Disorder. *Sleep Medicine Clinics*, 2 (4), 257–71.

37. Luyster, F. S., Strollo, P. J., Zee, P. C., & Walsh, J. K. (2012). Sleep: A Health Imperative. *Sleep*, 35 (6), 727–34.

38. Luyster et al. (2012). Sleep: A Health Imperative.

39. Luyster et al.

40. Luyster et al.

41. Luyster et al.

42. Luyster et al.

43. West, K. E., Jablonski, M. R., Warfield, B., Cecil, K. S., James, M., Ayers, M. A., et al. (2011). Blue Light from Light-Emitting Diodes Elicits a Dose-Dependent Suppression of Melatonin in Humans. *Journal of Applied Physiology*, 110, 619–26. Gringras, P., Middleton, B., Skene, D. J., & Revell, V. L. (2015). Bigger, Brighter, Bluer-Better? Current Light-Emitting Devices—Adverse Sleep Properties and Preventative Strategies. *Frontiers in Public Health*, 3, 233.

44. Phillips, B. A., & Danner, F. J. (1995). Cigarette Smoking and Sleep Disturbance. *Archives of Internal Medicine*, 155 (7), 734–37.

45. Fullagar, H. H., Skorski, S., Duffield, R., Hammes, D., Coutts, A., & Meyer, T. (2015). Sleep and Athletic Performance: The Effects of Sleep Loss on Exercise Performance, and Physiological and Cognitive Responses to Exercise. *Sports Medicine*, 45 (2), 161–86.

46. US Olympic Committee. *Jet Lag Countermeasures and Travel Strategies* (Colorado Springs: Government Printing Office, July 2002).

47. Choy, M., & Salbu, R. L. (2011). Jet Lag: Current and Potential Therapies. *Pharmacy and Therapeutics*, 36 (4), 221–24, 231.

48. Driskell, J., Copper, C,. & Moran, A. (1994). Does Mentral Practice Enhance Performance? *Journal of Applied Psychology*, 79, 481.

49. Kabat-Zinn, *Wherever You Go, There You Are*, 4

50. *The Road to Resilience* (Washington, DC: American Psychological Association, 2014), retrieved from http://www.apa.org/helpcenter/road-resilience.aspx.

Chapter 4: HP on the Road

1. Michael J. Breus, P. (n.d.). *Better Sleep Tips for Business Trips.* Retrieved October 2018, from WebMD: https://www.webmd.com/sleep-disorders/features/better-sleep-tips-business-trips#1

INDEX